Healthy Heart, Healthy Brain

THE Proven Personalized Path TO Protect Your Memory, Prevent Heart Attacks AND Strokes, AND Avoid Chronic Illness

Bradley Bale, MD
AND
Amy Doneen, DNP

WITH Lisa Collier Cool

Little, Brown Spark
New York Boston London

Also by Bradley Bale, MD, and Amy Doneen, DNP
with Lisa Collier Cool

Beat the Heart Attack Gene

———————

Little, Brown Spark
Hachette Book Group
1290 Avenue of the Americas, New York, NY 10104
littlebrownspark.com

First Edition: March 2022

Little Brown Spark is an imprint of Little, Brown and Company, a division of
Hachette Book Group, Inc. The Little, Brown Spark name and logo are
trademarks of Hachette Book Group, Inc.

The publisher is not responsible for websites (or their content) that are not
owned by the publisher.

The Hachette Speakers Bureau provides a wide range of authors for speaking
events. To find out more, go to hachettespeakersbureau.com or call
(866) 376-6591.

Library of Congress Control Number: 2021948127

Printing 1, 2022

ISBN 978-0-316-70555-4

LSC-C

Book illustrations by Moss Freedman

Printed in the United States of America

To my wife, Pam, whose love has nurtured me for more than fifty years. She nudged me down the path of preventative care with unwavering support. To my daughter, Brittany, who evolved into my sage colleague and nurse. To my sons, Forrest and Jacob, for their steadfast belief in my healthcare goals.

To our beloved grandchildren, Olivia, Adeline, James, Elliott, Shelby, Peter, Ethan, Marlie, and Cora, may the information in this book enhance your well-being. To my siblings, Shelby, Daryl, Richard, and Phillip, who have regaled in my pioneering spirit.

I also dedicate this book in loving memory of my parents, Joy and Garnett Bale, my sister Barbara, my parents-in-law, June and Peter Barile, and my childhood housekeeper, Mabel Neal. They all encouraged me to follow my dreams and believed in my ability to achieve them. Their spirits continue to infuse my passion for improving the health of others.

—Bradley Bale, MD

In loving memory of my beloved father, Wally "Butch" Hubbard. During the writing of this book, it has been heartbreaking to witness the devastating effects of dementia claim the life of my strong and loving father. My wish is that this book will prevent other families from suffering this catastrophic illness. To my husband, Daren, your love and support have allowed me to follow my passion for my life's work in this field of medicine and prevention. This journey would not be possible without you by my side. To our children, you have shaped my life and taught me so many lessons. Sydney: You teach me to keep a steadfast focus on my goals. Devin: You inspire me to grab hold of all life has to offer. Sophie: You motivate me to follow my heart. To each of you I say, "Follow your dreams as you have supported me to follow mine. I love you all."

—Amy Doneen, DNP

To my husband and best friend, John: Your love, encouragement, wit, and sage advice has nurtured me throughout our life together and during the writing of this book. To our daughters, Alison, Georgia, and Rosalie: I rejoice in your many successes and accomplishments and am proud to be your mom. To our beautiful and brilliant granddaughters, Carson and Alice: you lift my heart and spirit. In loving memory of my father, Oscar Collier, my first agent, editor, and mentor: I shall not look upon your like again. You were gone too soon.

—Lisa Collier Cool

Table of Contents

Part One: The Breakthrough

Part Two: Why Plaque Attacks and What to Do About It

TABLE OF CONTENTS

The Breakthrough

Introduction:
Our Story and Why
Yours Can Be Different

Before we present the revolutionary science behind arteriology—and how this pioneering new medical specialty bridges a dangerous gap in our healthcare system that puts unsuspecting patients in peril—allow us to share a few of the personal experiences that fuel our passion for saving lives, hearts, and brains. One of coauthor Bradley ("Brad") Bale's earliest childhood memories is watching his father—a famous physician—trying, futilely, to save the life of Brad's paternal grandmother after she suffered a massive heart attack at sixty-eight. Just five years old at the time, he will never forget seeing her face in the casket, the smell of the flowers, and the tears in his father's eyes.

As a teenager, Brad mourned the passing of his maternal grandfather, Sidney, from a massive stroke at sixty-five, shortly after Sidney and his wife, Elizabeth, had moved to Beverly Hills, California, in anticipation of a comfortable retirement. Soon afterward, Elizabeth—Brad's maternal grandmother—developed such severe dementia that she was no longer able to manage on her own. She spent her final years living with Brad and his family, in such a state of bewilderment that she no longer recognized them. Decades later, he also witnessed the slow death of his mother from heart failure triggered by a heart attack. In 1997, Brad faced the possibility of losing yet another family member when his eldest brother, Shelby, suffered a near-fatal heart attack at sixty.

Around the same time, Brad, then a family physician, met coauthor Amy Doneen, a doctor of nursing practice (DNP). Together, they began combing the medical literature, searching for anything that might help Brad's brother avoid another heart attack. Intensifying the urgency of this quest was a frightening statistic that still holds true today: About one in four heart attacks and strokes are repeat events, according to the Centers for Disease Control and Prevention (CDC).[1] Additionally, Amy was then conducting a study to identify the most effective ways to detect arterial disease at the earliest, most treatable stages, a topic we'll discuss more fully in part one of this book.[2]

A driving factor behind Amy's study was her own frightening family history: She's lost three of her relatives to heart attacks, including her grandpa Jack, a kind, handsome man who never lost his sense of humor, even as he spent the last years of his life battling Alzheimer's disease (AD), the most common form of dementia. Compounding Amy's intense sorrow at watching AD gradually rob her grandfather of his sharp memory and charming personality was seeing the devastating effect of his illness on her father, Wally "Butch" Hubbard, who spent most of his life in dread of losing his memory. Amy was extremely close to her father and prayed that he'd be spared this disease, which sometimes runs in families. At the time, however, there was no proven way to prevent it. Wally, however, did take an important step to protect his heart and brain health: he quit smoking.

Four years ago, Wally, a retired county planning director, began showing the first signs of Alzheimer's disease at seventy-five. He was a gentle giant, who stood six feet, five inches and weighed 300 pounds, but was remarkably light on his feet and an amazing dancer. He was also devoted to his eight grandchildren and regaled them with tales of his experiences as an Army captain and tank commander, stationed in Germany during the Vietnam War. As his disease progressed, he struggled to recall details of these stories and was no longer able to play cards and chess with his grandkids. Watching Wally disappear into a fog of forgetfulness was heartbreaking for Amy and her entire family, especially her brother, Brian, and Wally's wife Jan. As Wally's dementia rapidly worsened, they experienced the truth of an Alzheimer's caregiver's poignant observation about this scenario: "Knowing the day is coming when your loved one won't know you is the most horrible feeling of all."

Ironically, during Wally's battle with Alzheimer's disease, landmark studies were published in leading scientific journals reporting that with certain specific strategies that will be described in part two of this book, dementia may be preventable. Soon after that, the first guidelines for the prevention of Alzheimer's and other forms of memory loss were published. That knowledge came too late for Wally, who died peacefully at seventy-nine—the same age his father did—as his family was by his side, holding his hands one last time. Amy and her family miss him terribly, but know in their hearts that he's dancing and sending them hugs from above.

Brad and Amy's goal in pioneering the new medical specialty of arteriology is to help patients everywhere have a different story: one in which they can live well, without fear of a heart attack, stroke, dementia, or other chronic diseases. Shelby, Brad's brother, who was one of the first patients treated with our evidence-based approach to prevention—called the BaleDoneen Method—recently celebrated his eighty-fifth birthday. A retired historian who has served as the chief editor of the National Archives, he remains mentally sharp and heart attack free. He feels that the insights gained from our comprehensive prevention-and-treatment plan—coupled with the ongoing care he receives from his cardiologist—have helped him avoid his mother's and grandparents' tragic fates. "Getting the right treatment has added decades to my life," he says, "and that has been a gift and blessing I'd never expected to receive, given my family history."

CHAPTER 1

A Plan That Is Guaranteed to Prevent Heart Attacks and Strokes

"Superior doctors prevent the disease. Mediocre doctors treat the disease before it is evident. Inferior doctors treat the full-blown disease."

— Huang Dee Nai-Chang, from the first known Chinese medical text, c. 2600 BCE

New cars, washing machines, and even toasters come with a warranty. Who would purchase one otherwise? We think that healthcare providers should also guarantee that their care is safe and effective. Since 2008, we have offered all our patients a written guarantee stating that if they experience a heart attack or stroke while under our care, we will refund 100 percent of all fees paid during that year.

To date, we have only had to give three refunds, despite treating hundreds of high-risk patients. These include men and women who have survived previous heart attacks or strokes while under the care of different medical providers. Other patients have major risk factors for suffering these events, such as smoking (past or present), high blood pressure, and obesity, including some patients who weigh as much as four hundred pounds. The three patients who received refunds all chose to continue their treatment with us.

In 2019, we began offering an even more powerful promise of cardiovascular wellness, which is the focus of this book: our new AHA (Arterial Health Assurance) for Life plan, described in depth in chapter two. Drawing on more than twenty years of clinical experience and our landmark research on arterial health and disease reversal, this six-step plan is designed for people who are worried that a heart attack, stroke, dementia, or other devastating complications of cardiovascular disease (CVD) could loom in their future. Rooted in a groundbreaking new medical specialty that we pioneered—called arteriology—as well as the latest peer-reviewed science, our AHA for Life plan provides a proven, easy-to-implement method to protect and enhance your heart and brain health, while also optimizing the wellness of the more than sixty thousand miles of blood vessels that nourish every organ, muscle, and tissue in your body.

We have also observed that patients treated with our holistic approach to arterial wellness have a significantly lower risk for new onset diabetes and chronic diseases of aging, such as AD, Parkinson's disease, vascular dementia, chronic kidney disease, erectile dysfunction, peripheral artery disease, cancer, heart failure, vision loss, high blood pressure, fatty liver disease, and atrial fibrillation. Practiced by healthcare providers all over the world, the BaleDoneen Method has helped thousands of men and women of all ages lead active, healthy, and pleasurable lives, free from the fear of a heart attack, stroke, or dementia.

How Standard Care Can Fail Patients

When we opened the Heart Attack & Stroke Prevention Center in 2001, it was the first facility of its kind in the United States. Our initial goal was to bridge a deadly gap in our healthcare system: When we looked for experts in preventing heart attacks and strokes, we couldn't find any, even though more than 1.6 million Americans suffer heart attacks and strokes each year—and of that number, 775,000 die.[1,2] Recently, rates of these events have gone up among younger adults (those under fifty-five) for reasons that we will discuss in the next chapter, along with the action steps you need to take—today—to avoid them.

Initially, we thought that preventing these life-threatening events was the job of cardiologists. However, in their training and clinical practices, these specialists have traditionally focused on treating patients who are in the later stages of arterial disease. That's because patients are rarely referred to these specialists until they have already developed symptoms of CVD. This condition typically progresses silently over many years. The failure to detect and treat this quiet disease explains why the first sign of a problem is frequently a heart attack, stroke, or cardiac arrest. This results in specialists, such as cardiologists, being so overwhelmed with managing these emergencies that they do not have time to prevent them.

Dr. Pierre Leimgruber, a former interventional cardiologist, told us that, "During the years that I was treating people who had advanced coronary artery disease [CAD], there was so much plaque in their arteries that they were either on the brink of having a heart attack or had already had one. I'd often think, 'What if there was a way to successfully intervene ten or even fifteen years earlier, at the earliest stages of this disease? Would it be possible to *prevent* heart attacks and strokes, instead of doing multiple procedures inside the arteries of the same patients as their CAD continues to progress?'" Dr. Leimgruber, who has been a patient of ours, has become such a staunch supporter of our holistic approach to wellness that he has switched his focus from intervention to prevention, using his thirty-two years of clinical cardiology experience to focus on CVD prevention with the precision-medicine approach of the BaleDoneen Method.

He recently joined our practice as a specialist in heart attack and stroke prevention.

The new medical specialty of arteriology is our answer to Dr. Leimgruber's question. It's designed to transcend the traditional medical silos that result in incomplete, fragmented care for people with blood vessel disorders. For example, patients who suffer strokes are typically managed by neurologists, while those who have heart attacks are treated by cardiologists — even though almost all these events stem from the same cause: Plaque that has been growing silently inside an artery wall becomes so inflamed that it ruptures explosively, like a volcano spewing molten lava. In an attempt to heal the breach, the blood vessel forms a clot. If the clot travels to the brain and blocks one of its arteries, the result is a stroke. If the clot obstructs a coronary artery, a heart attack can occur.

Because arterial disease can literally affect the body from head to toe — causing everything from excruciating leg or chest pain to heart failure, vision problems, erectile dysfunction, chronic kidney disease, non-alcoholic fatty liver disease, digestive disorders, and cognitive impairment — we often see patients who are under the care of multiple specialists, yet continue to experience a relentless progression of their disease. In the next chapter, you will meet a fifty-four-year-old patient named Neal who kept getting sicker despite treatment by numerous specialists, all of whom were doing their utmost to help with the part of the body that was their specialty.

Unlike cardiology, which only focuses on the heart and its major arteries, arteriology encompasses the total care of patients with diseased arteries, since our blood vessels nourish every organ and tissue in our bodies. The primary goal is to prevent arterial inflammation — the fire that sparks most chronic diseases — and empower you to fight back *before* these conditions become manifest. We look at each patient as a unique individual and treat the entire person — not just their cardiovascular disease. Arteriology incorporates the work of many specialists, including family medicine providers (such as nurse practitioners and physician assistants), functional and integrative medicine doctors, sleep specialists, psychologists, nutritionists, cardiologists, neurologists, urologists, geneticists, dental providers, and others who incorporate personalized medicine and genetically guided treatment into their areas of practice.

We use a team approach in which medical and dental providers work together to optimize their patients' oral-systemic wellness. Large studies have shown that one of the simplest—and most effective—keys to a longer, healthier life is to combine regular dental checkups with excellent self-care. Chapter ten includes a detailed, step-by-step guide to optimizing oral wellness, which in turn can help you avoid heart attacks and strokes. Maintaining gum health also reduces risk for many dangerous diseases and conditions, including type 2 diabetes, rheumatoid arthritis, pregnancy complications, digestive disorders, erectile dysfunction, and certain forms of cancer.[3]

Very recently, scientists have identified poor oral health as a potentially modifiable risk factor for Alzheimer's disease and other forms of dementia.[4] Drawing on landmark research published in *The Lancet* by twenty-eight of the world's leading experts in the prevention of Alzheimer's disease and dementia—as well as the first guidelines for risk reduction from the World Health Organization and other, even newer science—we have created an evidence-based three-step plan to protect your memory, which is described in chapter twelve.[5]

Rapid Reversal of Arterial Disease

A recent peer-reviewed study by researchers from the Johns Hopkins Ciccarone Center for the Prevention of Cardiovascular Disease found that the BaleDoneen Method rapidly shrinks and stabilizes arterial plaque in the first year of treatment, helping people avoid heart attacks and strokes. It was also proven that our method eradicated lipid-rich arterial plaque (the most dangerous kind) in 100 percent of cases. Our genetically guided approach also significantly reduced blood pressure, LDL ("bad") cholesterol, and triglycerides in the study participants, while raising their levels of HDL, the "good" cholesterol that helps protect heart health. These trends continued in the second year of treatment and beyond. Published in *Archives of Medical Science,* the study included 328 patients of the Heart Attack & Stroke Prevention Center, who were tracked for five years.[6]

An earlier peer-reviewed study of 572 patients treated with the BaleDoneen Method, published in 2014 in *Journal of Cardiovascular Nursing,* reported dramatic reductions in plaque deposits, fasting blood sugar, LDL cholesterol, blood pressure, and inflammation over an eight-year period.[7] As an added bonus, our method also helps prevent type 2 diabetes—a condition that affects about 30 million Americans, one-third of whom are undiagnosed, greatly escalating their cardiovascular danger—and reduces risk for many other conditions linked to arterial disease, including Alzheimer's and dementia.

These published results explain the success of our original intention: to prevent symptomatic heart attacks and strokes. The findings also help explain an even more exciting revelation that was unintentional. It is now widely recognized that the majority of heart attacks and strokes are silent.[8] Although these events don't cause any obvious symptoms when they occur, they cause hidden damage to tiny arteries (microvessels) that over time can lead to many diseases of aging. Our method extinguishes the chronic inflammation that contributes to these conditions, thus helping to prevent many of the devastating disorders that result in people outliving their health. New research reveals that most people live the final thirteen years of their life in an unhealthy state.[9] Perhaps the greatest benefit of the BaleDoneen

Method is helping our patients achieve a health span that matches their life span.

Throughout this book, you will find the scientific evidence to support each test and treatment we recommend, so you can show it to your healthcare provider and ask for optimal, personalized care. We'll share the stories of several of our patients, including their challenges and the strategies they used to address them. Our goal is to empower you to take charge of your medical destiny by identifying your true risks and what's *really* causing them. You'll also find a guide to the best treatments, including how to lift your lifestyle to the next level, in part three of this book to help you overcome and avoid cardiovascular dangers.

If you are one of the more than 12 million Americans who have had home genetic tests to check for health threats in your DNA, we will also show you how to decode genetic information you may already have and use it to guide the right lifestyle to protect you from those risks, including the diet and exercise plan based on your DNA presented in chapter thirteen. As you will discover, our comprehensive, precision-medicine prevention plan uses inexpensive, noninvasive tests, as well as information that may already be in your medical chart, to answer important questions about your cardiovascular health. Learning the answers—and acting on them—could save your life.

Action Step: Assess Your Heart Attack, Stroke, and Dementia Risk

More than 108 million Americans—nearly half of the adult population—have one or more major risk factors for cardiovascular disease.[10] To find out if you could be at risk for CVD and its devastating conditions, we suggest that you take a few minutes to answer the following questions, which are similar to those we ask our patients during their initial evaluation. The answers will help you identify potential threats to your cardiovascular health and areas you need to work on to prevent a heart attack, stroke, or dementia.

How old are you?

Male younger than 55 years old **1 point**
Female younger than 65 years old **1 point**
Male at least 55 years old **4 points**
Female at least 65 years old **4 points**

Do you have a family history of heart attack, stroke, Alzheimer's disease, or dementia?

No **0 points**
Yes **4 points**

What is your waist circumference, as measured by wrapping a tape measure all the way around your body, level with your belly button? **(Note: Do NOT use your pants size, which often provides an inaccurate waist measurement.)**

If you're a woman: Less than 35 inches **0 points**
If you're male: Less than 40 inches **0 points**
If you're a woman: 35 inches or more **4 points**
If you're a man: 40 inches or more **4 points**

What's your weight range according to BMI? (Check your BMI at https://www.nhlbi.nih.gov/health/educational/lose_wt/BMI /bmicalc.htm?)

Underweight **2 points**
Average **1 point**
Overweight **3 points**
Obese **4 points**

What is your resting pulse?

Less than 60 beats per minute **0 points**
Less than 75 beats per minute **1 point**
More than 75 beats per minute **2 points**
Don't know **2 points**

What is your blood pressure?

Less than 120/80 **0 points**
120/80 to 139/89 **3 points**
140/90 or higher **4 points**
Don't know **4 points**
If taking blood pressure medication, your total count is **3 points.**

What is your total cholesterol level?

Less than 160 mg/dL **0 points**
Less than 200 mg/dL **1 points**
Greater than 200 mg/dL **3 points**
Don't know **3 points**
If taking cholesterol medication, your total count is **2 points.**

What is your HDL (good) cholesterol level?

If you're a woman: Less than 60 mg/dL **0 points**
If you're a man: Less than 50 mg/dL **0 points**

If you're a woman: 60 mg/dL or higher **3 points**
If you're a man: 50 mg/dL or higher **3 points**
Don't know **3 points**

What is your LDL (bad) cholesterol level?

Less than 70 mg/dL **0 points**
70 to 99 mg/dL **1 point**
100 to 130 mg/dL **3 points**
More than 130 mg/dL **4 points**
Don't know **4 points**

Which of the following best describes your triglyceride level?

Less than 100 mg/dL **0 points**
101 to 150 mg/dL **1 point**
More than 150 mg/dL **3 points**
Don't know **3 points**

Do you have diabetes or high blood sugar?

No **0 points**
Yes, I'm prediabetic **3 points**
Yes, I'm diabetic **4 points**
I haven't had my blood sugar tested **4 points**

Do you have bleeding gums? (Check all answers that apply.)

No **0 points**
Yes **2 points**

Which of the following best describes your sleep patterns?

I sleep soundly 6–8 hours a night **0 points**
I sleep restlessly for 6–8 hours a night **2 points**
I sleep less than 6 hours or more than 9 **3 points**

Do you snore?

No **0 points**
Yes, occasionally **1 point**
Yes, frequently and loudly **3 points**
Yes, and I have sleep apnea **4 points**

Do you have rheumatoid arthritis or any other inflammatory disease such as psoriasis or lupus?

No **0 points**
Yes **4 points**

What is your vitamin D level?

At least 50 ng/ml **0 points**
30 to 49 ng/ml **1 point**
Less than 30 ng/ml **3 points**
I do not know my vitamin D level **3 points**

Do you have a history of migraines?

No **0 points**
Yes, with no migraine aura **2 points**
Yes, with a migraine aura **3 points**

How would you characterize your ability to cope with stress?

I'm usually pretty laid back **0 points**
I have healthy ways to cope with stress **1 point**
Sometimes people say that I seem stressed **2 points**
I feel stressed and anxious most of the time **4 points**

Do you spend 11 or more hours a day sitting?

No **0 points**
Yes **4 points**

How much exercise do you get?

At least 30 minutes, 5 to 7 days per week **0 points**
At least 30 minutes, 2 to 4 times per week **1 point**
30 minutes, once a week or less **2 points**
I do not exercise **4 points**

Do you use nicotine in any manner? This would include chewing, cigarettes, cigars, e-cigarettes, nicotine gum, and vaping if nicotine is in the product.

No **0 points**
Yes, but have quit for at least 5 years **1 point**
Yes, but quit less than 5 years ago **2 points**
No, but I am exposed to secondhand nicotine regularly **3 points**
Yes **4 points**

Do you drink regular or diet soft drinks?

Never **0 points**
Rarely drink soft drinks (diet or regular) **1 point**
Once a week (diet or regular) **2 points**
More than once a week **3 points**

Do you watch the amount of carbohydrates in your diet?

I limit my simple carbohydrate intake **0 points**
I know to balance my carbs/proteins **1 point**
I never watch my carbohydrates **2 points**
The majority of my diet consists of carbs **4 points**

(Women only): Did you experience high blood pressure, preeclampsia, or gestational diabetes during pregnancy?

No **0 points**
Yes **4 points**

(Men only): Do you have erectile dysfunction?

No **0 points**
Yes **4 points**

What Your Score Means

2 to 4 points: Congratulations! You're taking excellent care of yourself. Reading this book will help you maintain—and enhance—your cardiovascular health so you will continue to live well.

5 to 10 points: Although you have relatively few cardiovascular risks, you'll benefit from learning how to optimize your heart and brain health with the easy action steps in this book.

11 to 20 points: You have definite risks for arterial disease. This book will alert you to what you should be doing *right now* to counteract these health threats. We also recommend that you follow the six-step prevention plan in chapter two.

21 to 39 points: You're at moderately high risk for cardiovascular disease. In part one of this book, you'll learn how to identify—and overcome—hidden medical problems that may be putting your heart health in jeopardy, including the surprising little-known heart attack, stroke, and dementia red flags that we discuss in chapter three.

40 points or higher: You're at high risk for cardiovascular disease. To prevent a heart attack or stroke, and reduce your risk for dementia, we recommend getting a comprehensive cardiovascular evaluation that includes the tests discussed in part two of this book. In part three, you'll also learn which therapies and lifestyle changes are most likely to help you ward off cardiovascular events and memory impairment.

Read the next chapter to learn something that shocks our patients: Most cardiologists consider themselves "ill-equipped" to handle the complex needs of today's heart patients, who fit a totally different profile than those specialists were taught to recognize in medical school, according to a startling report we'll discuss in the next chapter. You'll also find a simple six-step prevention and treatment plan to help you get optimal cardiovascular care from just about any medical provider, once you know what to ask for. And we will also reveal how heart attacks, strokes, and other devastating complications of arterial disease are potentially preventable with the right personalized approach. And that is a promise that we can confidently back in writing, with the guarantee of arterial wellness that we give to our patients regardless of their risk factors, family history, genes, weight, or a history of previous cardiovascular events.

CHAPTER 2
Arterial Health Assurance (AHA) for Life Program

"A tree's beauty lies in its branches, but its strength lies in its roots."

— Matshona Dhliwayo, author of
Lalibela's Wise Man

When we meet new patients, we always start their first visit by asking, "What are your goals for optimal health?" Some patients say they want to live to be one hundred—or beyond—while remaining mentally sharp and able to live independently. Others want to climb a mountain, run a marathon, or remain physically active and engaged in their favorite sports as they age. Patients frequently tell us that maintaining mobility, having lots of energy, and enjoying life to the fullest for as long as possible with minimal need for medications is very important to them. In other words, they want to have a "health span" that matches their life span.

The health ambitions of one of our patients, Neal, were much more modest: "I'd like to go for a walk and not hurt," the information technology (IT) professional from Spokane, Washington, told us during his initial visit two years ago. Then fifty-two, he was unable to walk more than twenty-five steps before excruciating leg pain from peripheral artery disease (PAD) forced him to stop. About 6.5 million Americans ages forty and older are affected by PAD: narrowing of arteries that transport blood from the heart to other parts of the body.[1] Most commonly, this condition reduces blood flow to the legs and feet, leading to muscle cramps during certain activities, such as walking or climbing stairs, that goes away after a few minutes of rest. Symptoms can also include numbness and weakness in the legs, sores that are slow to heal (or don't heal at all), skin discoloration, and erectile dysfunction. If untreated, PAD can raise risk for heart attacks, strokes, gangrene, and lower limb amputations.

The leading cause of PAD is atherosclerosis (buildup of cholesterol plaque inside the artery walls). This cardiovascular villain, which can affect arteries and smaller blood vessels throughout the body, has more aliases than a career criminal. If it affects the arteries that supply the heart, it's called coronary artery disease (CAD), heart disease, or coronary heart disease. If it affects the brain's blood supply, it's known as cerebrovascular disease or carotid atherosclerosis, and if it affects the smaller vessels, such as the arterioles and capillaries, it's called microvascular disease (MVD), ischemic microvascular disease, or small-vessel disease. The disease that affects the peripheral arteries also has several names, including PAD, peripheral vascular disease, and peripheral obliterative arteriopathy.

Neal was referred to us by his cardiologists because he had all these disorders. After saving his life at least six times through rapid treatment of blockages in his coronary arteries with stents, these doctors told us that they'd run out of treatment options. They asked if we had anything in our toolkit that could help a middle-aged man whose disease kept progressing despite being under the care of numerous specialists, including a neurologist to help him avoid having a stroke; a gastroenterologist to manage chronic GI issues stemming from insufficient blood flow to his gut; a vascular surgeon to treat his PAD; an endocrinologist to deal with his diabetes; a nephrologist to help with his kidney problems; and even a podiatrist to address his unrelenting foot pain.

Even though these doctors were doing their utmost to help with the part of his body that was their specialty, Neal kept getting even sicker. During the initial consultation at our clinic, he described a decade-long medical ordeal that began when he'd needed emergency quadruple coronary bypass surgery at forty-two to treat severely clogged arteries that were putting him at high risk for a heart attack. "It was the worst thing I'd ever gone through," he told us. "They split me open like a clam and after the operation, I was in so much pain I had to go on short-term disability. I told my wife I'd rather die than go through that again." Over the next ten years, he underwent an additional sixteen stenting procedures to reopen clogged arteries all over his body, including those in his heart, legs, kidneys, and gut. Shortly before he was referred to us, one of his doctors said that his only hope of staying alive was a transplant. "A transplant of what?" Neal asked. "My legs? My kidneys? My gut? My heart? My brain? My entire arterial system?"

During our initial visit with Neal, his wife, Ann, was crying so hard that she was unable to speak. Later she told us that she felt as if she was watching her husband of twenty-five years—and the father of their three teenaged children—die before her very eyes from a disease our healthcare system seemed powerless to prevent or even to treat successfully. "Many times, when we see a doctor, it's a ten-minute appointment to discuss what to do about the latest problem—not what we can do to stop his underlying disease from getting even worse," she told us. "I worry all the time about losing Neal—my best friend and the love of my life."

With tears streaming down her face, she added, "I've lain awake so many nights worrying, and if I can't hear him breathing, I put my hand on his back to make sure he's still alive." She feared it might be too late for us to help Neal. However, we assured her that we've successfully treated many patients who were even sicker than he was, including two of the patients you'll meet later in this book: Joe, who was in such poor cardiovascular health when he plugged into our method that he'd been told he needed a heart transplant; and Camille, who told us that after suffering a near-fatal heart attack at forty, she was so terrified she'd have another one that she dreaded going to sleep at night, fearing she wouldn't wake up in the morning.

Arteriology: A Revolutionary New Paradigm in Prevention

What does our AHA for Life plan offer to patients like Neal, Camille, and Joe? Our heart attack, stroke, and dementia prevention method, which we have taught to thousands of health-care providers from all over the world in our American Academy of Family Physicians–accredited training program, is scientifically designed to address the increasingly medically complex needs of men and women with arterial disease, as well as those of people who are at high risk for developing it. As *The Wall Street Journal* recently reported, "Today's heart-disease victim is vastly different from the classic patient doctors and the public were trained to recognize a half-century ago: a smoker, usually male, whose LDL, or 'bad,' cholesterol numbers were 'sky high.' Now, the patients are younger, more obese, much less likely to be smokers and include more women."[2] Many of them, like Neal, had no idea that they were at risk until they'd already suffered heart attacks or strokes, or required emergent procedures to prevent these calamities, such as bypass surgery to route blood around blockages or stents to restore blood flow to clogged arteries.

As recent studies have demonstrated, younger adults, particularly women, often miss out on potentially lifesaving heart health screenings and care, prompting a July 2019 editorial in the *Journal of the American College of Cardiology* to call upon the medical community to "wake up" and "recognize that preventive interventions are occurring too late."[3] To help save the lives of younger, high-risk patients with less advanced disease that is more amenable to prevention, the editorial called upon researchers and medical providers to develop "precision medicine strategies based on genetics, imaging, and other risk factors [so] the next era in cardiovascular disease prevention can begin." That is exactly what arteriology already offers. We use simple, inexpensive, and widely available laboratory tests to detect arterial disease at the earliest, most easily treatable stages. The tests we recommend in this book are available through almost all healthcare providers, once you know what to ask for.

We've been called "disease detectives" because our comprehensive evaluation checks for a wide range of root causes that can lead to arterial disease if they go undiagnosed and untreated. For patients who already have CVD, one of the keys to the success of our evidence-based treatment plan is identifying and treating all the underlying causes of the patient's disease, drawing on the latest scientific research, such as the results of randomized clinical trials published in peer-reviewed medical journals. We also empower our patients with action steps and genetically guided lifestyle changes they can make on their own. In Neal's case, we quickly zeroed in on some previously undiagnosed—and highly treatable—root causes of his CVD that will be discussed later in this chapter. By the end of his first visit, recalls his wife, "We left with something no other doctor had given us: hope."

Rising Rates of Arterial Disease in Younger Adults

Heart specialists are seeing more patients like Neal than ever before: younger adults (those under fifty-five) with a combination of CVD and metabolic disorders, such as diabetes, obesity, insulin resistance (the root cause of about 70 percent of heart attacks, nearly all cases of type 2 diabetes, and many other chronic diseases), or metabolic syndrome: a dangerous cluster of heart attack, stroke, and diabetes risk factors that we'll discuss in more depth in chapter nine. All these conditions have reached epidemic levels in the U.S., collectively affecting about 115 million Americans.[4] Although all these maladies greatly increase a patient's risk for developing arterial disease, they often go undiagnosed and untreated until the person has already suffered a heart attack or stroke. "Nearly all cardiology practices are poorly suited" to manage the care of patients with CVD and metabolic disease (a condition typically managed by endocrinologists), scientists from the Johns Hopkins Ciccarone Center for the Prevention of Cardiovascular Disease recently reported in *American Journal of Medicine*.[5]

The report's authors, cardiologists Robert Eckel, MD, and Michael Blaha, MD, called for a new medical specialty that they've named "cardiometabolic medicine." It would combine internal medicine, cardiology, and endocrinology to improve the care of patients who have CVD and metabolic maladies. Currently, Drs. Eckel and Blaha report that patients with CVD and metabolic disorders are "shunted back and forth among cardiologist, endocrinologist, and primary care physicians — with uncertain 'ownership' of different aspects of the patient's care." In other words, the situation is like a football team without a quarterback to call the plays.

Neal's case highlights the pitfalls of this chaotic care. At thirty-seven, the young dad, who was then carrying 275 pounds on his five-feet-ten-inch frame — putting him in the obese category — was diagnosed with type 2 diabetes, a disease that has been shown in numerous studies to greatly increase risk for cardiovascular events. In fact, a person with diabetes is at as high a risk for a heart attack as a nondiabetic person the same age who has already had one! Yet none of the healthcare providers who were treating him for this blood sugar disease ever warned him of his vascular peril, he reports. Nor was he put on any medications to reduce his heart attack and stroke risk, such as low-dose aspirin, statin therapy, or the other preventive treatments discussed in chapter fourteen.

Incredibly, given the obvious risks posed by Neal's obesity and diabetes, none of his medical providers ever suggested that he be screened for CVD. Had Neal gotten this screening shortly after his diabetes diagnosis—using the testing discussed in this chapter—his doctors almost certainly would have discovered that he had potentially lethal plaque growing in his arteries years before his disease became severe enough to require emergency quadruple bypass surgery.

While we applaud Drs. Blaha and Eckel's advocacy for improved care for people with cardiometabolic disease, which could help many patients like Neal avoid falling through the cracks in standard care, we believe that today's patients need a more holistic approach to arterial wellness. Arteriology is the only medical specialty whose primary goal is to prevent CVD and its many life-threatening conditions. The need for this revolutionary new paradigm has never been greater. CVD now affects 121.5 million Americans—nearly one in two U.S. adults.[6] Not only does it remain the leading killer of American men and women, but heart attacks, strokes, and other cardiovascular events are on the rise among younger adults, despite major advances in prevention and treatment that we will discuss in parts two and three of this book.

Indeed, middle-aged Americans are more likely to die from CVD now than they were in 2011, the CDC recently reported.[7] The key culprit is rising rates of lifestyle-related diseases, particularly obesity and diabetes, which affect many of our patients. Nationally, about 42 percent of Americans twenty or older are obese and another 32 percent are overweight.[8] Indeed, obesity is now considered to be the new smoking. These factors are a key reason why an optimal lifestyle is one of the cornerstones of our evidence-based prevention plan. Unlike standard care, which typically uses a one-size-fits-all approach to arterial disease prevention and treatment based on the average results from large studies, we regard each patient as a unique individual who requires highly personalized therapies to achieve optimal health.

Arteriology embraces the core concepts of precision medicine, which has been defined as "an emerging approach to disease treatment and prevention that takes into account individual variability in genes, environment, and lifestyle for each person."[9] The goal is to pinpoint the specific disease prevention and treatment strategies that will work best for each individual patient. To that end, the National Institutes of Health (NIH) and other groups recently launched a long-term research program called the Precision Medicine Initiative, which seeks to bring this genetically guided approach to all areas of healthcare

What's the difference?

on a large scale. While this may sound like the medicine of the future, personalized care has been a central component of the BaleDoneen Method since its inception in 2001.

A Proven Six-Step Prevention Plan

Our AHA for Life plan has six dynamic elements, each of which is an essential component to taking charge of your arterial health. Following our plan could save your life. The first letters of these foundational elements—Education, Disease, Fire, Root causes, Optimal care, and Genetics—form the acronym EDFROG, which is easy to remember if you think of our method as a frog named Ed. We picture Ed as a health hero who uses leading-edge science as his superpower to outwit and defeat the world's most dangerous—and wily—villain: cardiovascular disease. To high-light key points about our method in presentations to our patients

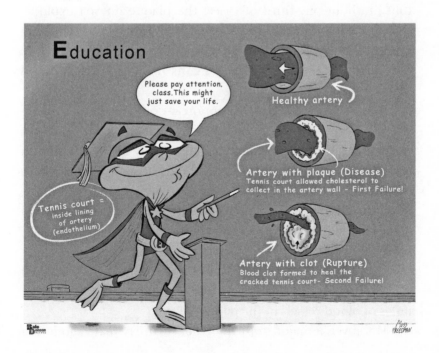

and healthcare providers, we have commissioned an artist, Moss Freedman, to create simple cartoons that you will see throughout this book.

1. Education: What Doctors Don't Tell Patients about Heart Attacks and Strokes

Knowledge is power! Our patients learn how heart attacks and strokes happen, something we call event reality. A common misconception is that arterial disease is a plumbing problem, like grease clogging a kitchen sink, causing an artery to become so obstructed that flow of blood stops, resulting in a heart attack or stroke. However, studies have shown that most of these events occur when plaque inside the artery becomes inflamed and ruptures explosively, like a volcano, leading to the formation of a clot that blocks the flow of blood to the heart or brain.[10] This is called plaque explosion or plaque rupture. It is now recognized that in about one-third of cases, the plaque doesn't explode. Instead, the inner lining of the artery sitting above the plaque erodes, like a sinkhole in the ground. A clot forms to close the breach, while the plaque remains in place. This is called plaque erosion.[11]

Another common misconception—even among many medical providers—is the outdated belief that there is nothing to worry about unless major arteries that supply the heart or brain are at least 70 percent blocked. If that occurs, the patient is often rushed off for invasive procedures, such as Neal's emergency quadruple bypass, to reroute blood around the obstructed areas, or the placement of stents to prop open blocked arteries. However, as he and many other patients have discovered, these costly and potentially risky procedures do not cure CVD because they only treat a few inches of the more than sixty thousand miles of blood vessels in the patient's body.

Moreover, a major study done nearly thirty years ago found

that 86 percent of heart attacks occur in patients whose coronary arteries are less than 70 percent blocked, and 68 percent happen when the major arteries supplying the heart are less than 50 percent obstructed. A number of other studies have similar findings.[12] That's right, most heart attacks do not strike in severely blocked arteries—the ones that interventional cardiologists target for treatment with stents and bypasses! Yet even today, many heart specialists still believe in the "70 percent rule" and describe areas with less than 50 percent blockage as "mild" heart disease. Actually, just as it's impossible to be "a little bit pregnant," there is no such thing as "mild heart disease." If there is plaque in your arteries, it's imperative that it be detected and treated to help you avoid a heart attack or ischemic stroke.

Ischemic strokes are sometimes called brain attacks, because they are like a heart attack that occurs in the brain. About 90 percent of strokes are ischemic, meaning that they are caused by clots. Most of these events happen the same way that heart attacks do: Fatty deposits in arteries that supply the brain become inflamed, leading to plaque rupture or erosion and the formation of a clot that obstructs blood flow. Ischemic strokes can also occur when a clot that forms elsewhere in the body (often in the heart or its large blood vessels) travels to the brain. One of the major culprits in this scenario is atrial fibrillation (AF), a type of irregular heartbeat that can cause blood to pool in the heart's upper chambers (atria) and form clots.

Some strokes only last a few minutes: This is called a transient ischemic attack (TIA) or mini-stroke. TIAs happen when blood supply to part of the brain is briefly blocked and can cause the same symptoms as a full-blown stroke. These include sudden numbness or weakness in the face, arm, or leg—especially on one side of the body—confusion, difficulty speaking or understanding speech, vision problems, and dizziness. Because these symptoms disappear quickly—and are rarely painful—people who have TIAs often delay getting care or don't seek it at all. The key takeaway is that TIAs should be viewed as "warning strokes," and require immediate medical attention, because having one greatly increases risk for having a subsequent full-blown stroke if the patient's arterial disease goes untreated.

It is now recognized that the vast majority of heart attacks and strokes are "silent," causing minimal or no symptoms. Although these events often go undiagnosed and untreated, a silent heart attack can be just as damaging as one that causes such classic symptoms as crushing chest pain, heavy sweating, dizziness, nausea, sudden shortness of breath, and stabbing pain in the arm, neck, or jaw. Several recent studies highlight the dangers of silent heart attacks, including increased risk for strokes, repeat heart attacks, heart failure, and even sudden cardiac death.[13] Also known as silent myocardial infarction (SMI), these events triple a person's risk for dying from CVD.

About 8 to 11 million Americans experience silent strokes each year—more than ten times the number that suffer symptomatic strokes annually (nearly 800,000)—reported a recent scientific statement from the American Heart Association and American Stroke Association (ASA).[14] Indeed, when doctors perform brain scans to evaluate patients for such problems as dizziness, cognitive impairment, or chronic headaches, it's become increasingly common for them to also make an unexpected discovery: areas of scarred brain tissue from previously unrecognized silent strokes that show up as white spots on the scan, the scientific statement reports. Its authors recommend that such patients be treated, since having a silent stroke raises risk for symptomatic strokes, as well as cognitive decline and dementia.

Also known as silent cerebral infarction (SCI), silent strokes are usually caused by clots that block flow to part of the brain, depriving it of oxygenated blood. The result is small areas of dead brain tissue called infarcts. Although the affected part of the brain may be too small to trigger any immediate, dramatic symptoms, over time brain damage can accumulate and start to affect memory and other brain functions, particularly if the person has a series of silent strokes. That is an extremely common scenario, since the person's underlying arterial disease may go unrecognized and untreated.

How can patients find out if they've had a silent event? We use a simple blood test called high-sensitivity troponin T (hsTnT) to check for signs of heart injury in our patients with arterial disease. This biomarker test measures levels of troponin, a type of protein found in heart muscle. Normally, there are very small or undetectable amounts of troponin in the blood, but after a silent or symptomatic heart attack, levels rise because this protein is released by stressed or dying heart muscle cells. The greater the damage to the heart, the higher blood levels of troponin are. Studies have also linked elevated blood levels of hsTnT to future risk for heart attacks, strokes, heart failure, pulmonary embolism, and death from cardiovascular causes, with people with the highest levels of this biomarker being in double the danger for these events than those with the lowest levels.[15]

In fact, hsTnT levels are such a strong predictor of cardiovascular peril that several studies have concluded that it should be used to screen seemingly healthy people to identify high-risk patients and those with silent arterial disease, so they can be treated to help them avoid silent or symptomatic cardiovascular events.[16] Based on this evidence, we recommend this widely available test for all patients with arterial disease, both for insight into whether silent events have already occurred and to evaluate risk for having these or other cardiovascular events in the future. The wonderful news, however, is that both silent and symptomatic cardiovascular events are preventable with the optimal care advised by our AHA for Life plan. Understanding how these calamities occur—and the action steps necessary to avoid them—helps patients make choices that lead to arterial wellness.

2. Disease

Early detection and treatment of arterial plaque is a key element of our evidence-based approach to prevention. To show our patients—and the healthcare providers who attend our continuing medical education programs—what a stealthy predator CVD is, we show them a simple cartoon. It portrays a city square in which a cat is crouched down in a gutter, below street level, licking its chops as it prepares to pounce on an unsuspecting pigeon. The cat symbolizes plaque deposits and the gutter is the arterial lining where plaque lurks. If the cat leaps out of the

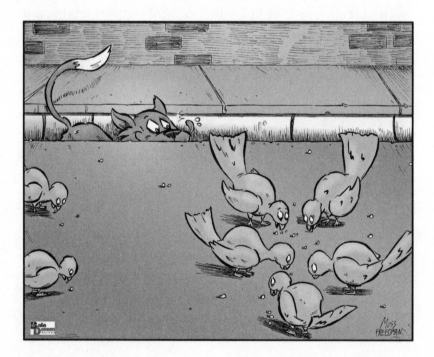

gutter (a plaque rupture), the result can be a heart attack or stroke.

Tragically, many people don't find out that they have diseased arteries until it's too late. About 50 percent of men—and nearly 70 percent of women—who die suddenly from coronary artery disease had no previous symptoms.[17] That's why one of the primary goals of our method is to detect and treat arterial disease *before* it gets severe enough to trigger a heart attack or stroke. Unlike standard care, which considers patients to be "innocent" of CVD unless they have certain risk factors, the BaleDoneen Method considers all patients to be "guilty" of harboring silent, potentially lethal plaque in their arteries unless they are proven innocent through laboratory and imaging tests that directly check for arterial disease.

The key to finding the cat in the gutter before it does irreversible or fatal harm is looking for it in the right place: inside the arterial wall, not the lumen (the open corridor through which blood flows). As we've discussed above, in the vast majority of cases—up to 99 percent, according to some studies— plaque does not obstruct blood flow, so indirect tests that only evaluate blood flow, such as the treadmill test in which people exercise on a treadmill at increasing speeds while hooked up to heart monitors, can miss many cases of arterial disease. In chapter seven, we will take a closer look at the best imaging tests to check for plaque—and also tell you which tests to avoid.

Surprisingly, an ultrasound examination of your neck's largest arteries is one of the best—and safest—ways to check for plaque. Abnormalities that can be detected by this FDA-approved test, known as carotid intima-media thickness (cIMT), are strongly linked to greatly increased risk for heart attacks, strokes, and dementia.[18] This painless fifteen-minute test also provides an estimate of your "arterial age," as compared to your chronological age. Having arteries that are more than eight years "older" than you are is a sign that you're at risk for developing CVD, while finding plaque means that you already have it. Another noninvasive imaging test, coronary artery calcium score (CACS), which will also be discussed in chapter seven, checks for hidden disease in the major vessels that supply your heart.

We recommend screening that includes vascular imaging for everyone over forty and for younger people with any of the red flags discussed in chapter three or with a family history of CVD or diabetes. It's also important for younger adults without these factors to be screened for heart attack and stroke risk. About 20 percent of heart attacks occur in men and women under forty—including men and women in their twenties and early thirties—a recent study reported.[19] Another study reported that rates of stroke have soared by 36 percent among eighteen-to-thirty-five-year-olds and by 43 percent among the forty-five-to-fifty-four age group, compared to the rates in 2003.[20]

It's also important to know the right age to begin screening for risk factors that can lead to arterial disease if they go undetected and untreated. For example, the American Heart Association recommends that everyone should start screening for high blood pressure and high cholesterol at twenty. Parents should also be aware that current medical guidelines call for children nine to seventeen to be checked for high cholesterol, a disorder that can run in families. As we were writing this chapter, a new study reported that cholesterol levels during adolescence are a very important predictor of later risk for developing CVD, highlighting the potentially lifesaving benefits of very early detection and treatment of this major cardiovascular risk factor.

How does the accuracy of our method stack up against that of standard care? We conducted a study of 576 of our patients to compare the two approaches to patient screening and presented the results at the 2009 International Society of Atherosclerosis annual meeting in Barcelona, Spain. When we evaluated the patients with the BaleDoneen Method, using cIMT, CACS, and other tests, we found that 408 of them were at significant risk for heart attacks and strokes, either because they had atherosclerosis or were diabetic, which elevates risk as much as having had a prior heart attack. Analyzing their risk factors—the approach advised in current cardiology guidelines that we'll discuss in depth in the next two chapters—would have missed 86 percent of the at-risk group.

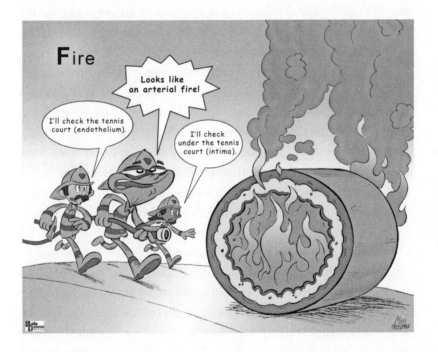

3. Fire in the arteries

Most of the time, inflammation is a potential lifesaver: It's the immune system's defense against viral or bacterial invaders. We've all experienced the typical signs of acute inflammation: swelling, redness, and warmth around a wound. But in some people, particularly those who are overweight, sedentary, eat a poor diet, or smoke, this fiery process becomes chronic. That's when inflammation harms instead of heals, by causing the body to attack normal cells as if they were foreign invaders.

Chronic inflammation has a variety of harmful effects on the lining of the arteries (the endothelium), all of which make it easier for cholesterol to penetrate the arterial wall and form fatty streaks that ultimately turn into plaque. Think of plaque, once formed, as kindling. Inflammation is what lights the match, which can lead to plaque rupture and the formation of a blood clot. If the clot blocks an artery that supplies the heart, the result can be a heart attack. If the clot obstructs one of the brain's arteries, the result can be a stroke.

To help our patients avoid these events, we use treatments designed to cool and heal arteries, including lifestyle changes that will be discussed in part three. In some cases, medication may also be necessary. Statin drugs, for example, are not just cholesterol-busters. Recent studies suggest that they also have anti-inflammatory properties and can reduce rates of heart attacks, strokes, and death from cardiovascular causes in people who have normal levels of cholesterol, but elevated levels of inflammation.[21]

In 2012, two landmark studies published in *The Lancet* were the first to show that chronic inflammation causes CVD. This fiery process is also at the root of many other debilitating or life-threatening conditions, including diabetes and cancer. In fact, it is more dangerous to your arteries than having high cholesterol! In 2017, a clinical trial called CANTOS (Canakinumab Anti-Inflammatory Thrombosis Outcome Study) generated worldwide headlines by reporting that treating patients with therapies to reduce inflammation—without lowering cholesterol—significantly reduced risk for cardiovascular events and cancer.[22] An even newer landmark study by the world's top experts on Alzheimer's disease and other forms of dementia, published in *The Lancet*, was the first to report that these memory-robbing brain disorders may be preventable with strategies that include reducing brain inflammation.

We use a "fire panel" of inexpensive blood and urine tests to check for inflammation. One of the best tests for inflammation is a urine dipstick test that costs just pennies, is covered by virtually all insurance plans, and provides potentially lifesaving information about arterial wall health. These inexpensive biomarker tests, which have been a cornerstone of our method for more than a decade, provide an early warning of danger, so we can quickly initiate therapies—including lifestyle changes—to extinguish the fire smoldering in a patient's arteries. In chapter eight, we will discuss these tests—and the potentially lifesaving information they provide—in more depth, along with easy, natural ways to "fireproof" your arteries, without medication.

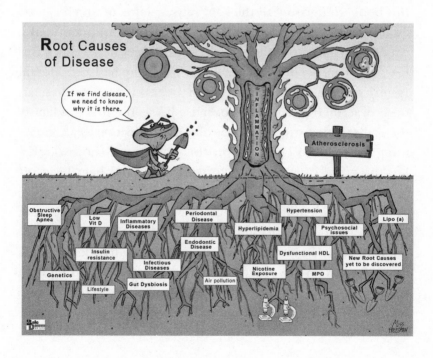

4. Root causes

To put out fire inside the arteries, it's essential to find out what's causing it. For someone who has already had a heart attack or stroke, identifying the root cause is essential to prevent another event. Our method checks for a wide range of root causes that will be discussed more fully in part two, including insulin resistance, metabolic syndrome, high blood pressure (the leading risk factor for stroke), sleep disorders, and a dangerous cholesterol most doctors don't check, even though it has been proven to cause heart attacks!

Very often, arterial disease—as well as heart attacks and strokes—can have multiple causes, including smoking, inflammatory disorders (such as rheumatoid arthritis and psoriasis), autoimmune diseases, obesity, and genetic factors. Frequently it takes medical detective work, using the tests recommended in this book, to uncover all the root causes, some of which can be quite surprising. For example, in Neal's case, we identified a common culprit that most medical providers don't check for: Like the majority of Americans over thirty, he had periodontal (gum) disease. One of our recent peer-reviewed studies has been described as landmark because it was the first to identify the bacteria that trigger this chronic oral infection as a contributing cause of CVD.[23] Later in this book, we'll show you why healthy gums can add years to your life—and help head off heart attacks, strokes, and dementia.

We also identified another previously undiagnosed root cause of Neal's disease. Similar to about 42 percent of the U.S. population, he was deficient in vitamin D.[24] This disorder has been implicated in a wide range of chronic diseases, including high blood pressure, CAD, PAD, diabetes, rheumatoid arthritis, multiple sclerosis, heart failure, and cancers of the prostate, breast, ovaries, and colon. One large study found that men with low levels of vitamin D had double the heart attack risk of those with normal levels, and an analysis that pooled the results of eighteen studies reported that vitamin D deficiency significantly raised the risk for both CAD and early death.[25] Although vitamin D deficiency can be diagnosed with a simple blood test, none of Neal's medical providers had checked him for this extremely—and potentially dangerous—disorder, which can be easily treated by taking a vitamin D supplement.

Identifying the root causes of the patient's disease can also lead to additional treatments to improve outcomes. For example, in Neal's case, our comprehensive evaluation solved the mystery of why his blood pressure remained persistently high even though his doctors had prescribed medications to lower it. Like about 22 million other Americans, he had obstructive sleep apnea (OSA), a disorder marked by brief, repeated episodes in which the person stops breathing during sleep. Characterized by such symptoms as loud snoring, daytime drowsiness, and a dry mouth or sore throat upon awakening, OSA frequently goes undiagnosed. If untreated, this sleep disorder doubles the risk for heart attack, stroke, high blood pressure, heart failure, atrial fibrillation, diabetes, and other cardiovascular problems. Recent studies, however, have shown that treatment of OSA eliminates this excess risk and helps improve blood pressure control.[26] Neal's case bears this out: After he started using a CPAP (continuous positive airway pressure) machine to keep his airways open at night, his blood pressure improved dramatically.

5. Optimal goals

Just as a top-quality construction company may exceed the building code to make homes and offices even stronger and safer from fires, earthquakes, and other catastrophes, in some cases, our AHA for Life plan sets higher standards for treatment and prevention than those set by standard medical care. We recommend working with your healthcare provider to set optimal, individualized goals to modify each of your risk factors. This approach, rather than one-size-fits-all goals set by the standard of care and based on average results from large studies, leads to superior outcomes and more effective heart attack and stroke prevention.

For example, most medical providers will prescribe medication for patients whose blood pressure is 140/90 or higher, while patients with readings between 120/80 and 139/89—a range that used to be known as prehypertension—are often told that their pressure is "a little high but nothing to worry about." However, many large studies have shown that having blood pressure in this range doubles the danger of death from cardiovascular causes and triples heart attack risk, if it goes untreated. Elevated blood pressure is also a leading risk factor for three devastating conditions: strokes, chronic kidney disease, and dementia. Therefore, we recommend that patients whose blood pressure is even slightly above normal (which is a level below 120/80) be evaluated to see if they need treatment. We also believe in setting individual—not aggressive—treatment goals. Certain patients, including those with type 2 diabetes, can be harmed if their blood pressure is reduced to a level below 120/80. In chapter fifteen, we will take a fuller look at blood pressure, including the new numbers to know under recently updated medical guidelines, and how to set optimal goals for both your lifestyle and medical management of conditions that elevate your risk for heart attacks, strokes, and other chronic conditions. We'll also share some inspiring secrets of how to achieve and maintain lifelong wellness, even if you carry high-risk genes. In the appendix, you'll find a detailed chart of all the optimal goals for arterial disease prevention and treatment recommended in this book.

6. Genetics

Basing care on each person's unique genetic makeup is the ultimate in precision medicine. The BaleDoneen Method has used genetic testing for more than a decade both to identify patients with inherited risk for heart attacks and strokes and to guide the best personalized treatments of those risks. For example, like about 50 percent of Americans, Neal is a carrier of the 9P21 gene, which is often called "the heart attack gene," because it is an independent predictor of risk for these events, even when such factors as family history, high blood pressure, diabetes, obesity, and elevated levels of the inflammatory marker C-reactive protein are taken into account. A recent study, however, found that when carriers of the 9P21 and other high-risk genes stay physically fit, they can reduce their risk for CVD by up to 50 percent, highlighting the amazing power of an optimal lifestyle to keep your heart healthy, no matter what is written in your DNA.

Like about 25 percent of Americans, Neal is also a carrier of another high-risk gene called Apo E4. This genotype not only dramatically raises risk for CVD, but it also puts people who carry it at up to twenty times higher risk for developing Alzheimer's disease. In chapter eleven, we will look at these and other high-risk genes more closely and also discuss the best genetically guided strategies people who carry them can use to protect themselves, including a diet and exercise plan based on your Apo E genotype. Using another genetic test that will also be discussed in chapter eleven, we discovered that Neal has a genotype that does best on a gluten-free diet.

Following a genetically guided diet and exercise plan has helped Neal lose weight, and his fitness has improved significantly. Now fifty-four, he reports that after two years of treatment with our method, "I'm not one hundred percent cured, but I feel better than I have in years and can walk further every day. Now that my root causes—and not just my symptoms—are being treated, all my lab results are trending in the right direction and my blood pressure and diabetes are finally under control. Learning that the same genes that put me at risk for having a massive heart attack can also help me avoid one has been such an epiphany. My wife and I are planning to have our children genetically tested so they can follow the right lifestyle now and avoid the disease that nearly killed me when I was forty-two. The doctors who did my quadruple bypass said that if I hadn't had that operation, I would have dropped dead from a massive 'widow-maker' heart attack."

Action Step: Compile Your Family Medical History

Did you know that your family medical history can provide insights into everything from your life expectancy to your risk for heart attacks, strokes, high blood pressure, diabetes, obesity, dementia, and even dental problems? Finding out which disorders run in your family—and sharing this information with your medical provider—could save your life. For example, your provider might recommend lifestyle changes to reduce your risk for these conditions, order screening or diagnostic tests that might not otherwise be considered, or advise more frequent checkups to look for early signs of these diseases.

What's more, working together with your relatives to develop a shared family medical history could help them stay healthy, too. Family get-togethers—whether in person or on a Zoom call—are an ideal time to kick off this project. New online resources make compiling your family's health data easier than ever before. Here's how to compile a family medical history and gain a priceless gift: knowledge that will help you and your loved ones live well. Ideally, your family medical history should include three or more generations. Gather data about your grandparents, parents, siblings, aunts, uncles, first cousins, nieces, nephews, children, and grandchildren. Also include your own health history. For each family member, record as much of the following data as possible:

Date of birth
Sex
Ethnicity
Medical conditions, including the age at which they occurred
Dental disorders, such as gum disease, oral infections, and
    tooth loss

Pregnancy complications, such as gestational diabetes, preeclampsia (high blood pressure and protein in the
urine), miscarriages, and stillbirths
Mental health conditions
Red flags for heart attack, stroke, and dementia, such as
those listed in chapter three
Lifestyle, including smoking, substance abuse, and diet and
exercise habits
For deceased relatives, list the age at death and the cause

If anyone in your extended family was affected by CVD, try
to determine the earliest age at which it manifested. For example, if one of your grandparents died from arterial disease at
eighty-five, it is important for your medical provider to know if it
triggered a heart attack or stroke at fifty-five, since that might
put you at increased risk for developing CVD at a younger than
usual age.

CHAPTER 3

The New Red Flags for Heart Attack, Stroke, and Dementia Risk

"Ignoring the signs is a good way to end up at the wrong destination."

— CAREFREE CONTESSA, "THE SITUATIONSHIP CHRONICLES"

Two of our patients, J.P. and Camille, were always very diligent about getting annual physicals, and both turned to their family doctors when they developed troubling symptoms. J.P. scheduled a checkup after noticing that it was hard for him to keep up with friends when backcountry skiing, even though he was usually one of the better skiers. He was also bothered by sluggishness, anxiety, fatigue, and sleep disturbances, all of which were unlike anything he'd experienced. Camille was concerned about an episode of shortness of breath. In fact, she became so winded while climbing the stairs to her provider's office to discuss this problem that she passed out—and fell down a flight of stairs.

Although all these symptoms can be warning signs of heart disease—or even an impending heart attack, especially in women—both patients were assured that there was no cause for concern. As J.P. recalls, "The doctor said, 'You're forty-two, you have two kids and three auto dealerships—you're under a lot of pressure.' He also said that my levels of good cholesterol were really low and my blood pressure was a bit high at 130/90, but nothing to worry about. After prescribing blood pressure and anti-anxiety medication, he told me that I was as healthy as a horse. I left feeling that the only problem was that I was a bit stressed out."

After Camille literally collapsed on her doctor's doorstep, she was diagnosed with a panic attack. Like J.P., she was handed a prescription for tranquilizers and was also put on an antidepressant. Her shortness of breath went away and during a subsequent annual physical, the then forty-year-old financial services analyst received good news. "After checking my cholesterol and blood pressure, the doctor plugged the numbers into a software program and said that my risk for having a heart attack in the next ten years was less than one percent." The doctor also advised Camille that her cholesterol was a bit high and asked if she wanted a statin, which she declined. Why risk drug side effects when she'd just been assured that her heart was healthy— and almost certain to stay that way?

You may have guessed where these stories are headed. Five months later, Camille had a massive heart attack at work. Attributing her extreme dizziness, nausea, shortness of breath, and chest pain to a panic attack, she waited six hours before seeking medical help. "By the time I got to the ER, I was in so much pain that I could hardly stand and my left arm felt icy cold," she recalls. "The ER doctor said that if I'd waited any longer, I would have died, because there was no blood flow to the right side of my heart. I was terrified and my former husband almost fainted," adds Camille.

On the Fourth of July—one month after the checkup in which J.P. was pronounced to be as healthy as a horse—he developed chest pain while mountain biking with a friend. In the ER, tests showed that he'd had the most dangerous type of heart attack. Known as "the widow maker" because of its high fatality rate, it occurs when the left anterior descending coronary artery becomes completely blocked, depriving the heart of one of its major sources of oxygenated blood. In J.P.'s case, several smaller coronary arteries were also partially obstructed. He was wheeled into the catheterization lab, where cardiologists hooked him up to monitors and threaded a tiny balloon-tipped tube through an artery in his groin up to his heart. Then the balloon was inflated to reopen the blocked artery, which was treated with a stent, a tiny scaffold-like device that props the vessel open to restore blood flow.

After the procedure, a cardiologist prescribed several medications and told the young dad to come back for a checkup in six months. Then the heart specialist offered some advice. "First he said that I needed to exercise. I told him that I already did, twice a day," recalls J.P., an avid backcountry skier, mountain biker, and weightlifter whose fitness routine also includes resistance training, planking, and high-intensity workouts on his elliptical machine. "Then he said I should stop smoking. I told him that I didn't smoke. I left the hospital very confused about why I'd ended up there—and what else I could do to avoid another heart attack when I already ate a healthy diet and worked out seven days a week."

Balloon angioplasty and stenting also saved Camille's life. "After three days in the cardiac ICU, I was sent home with a handful of pills and advice to remember my symptoms and call nine-one-one if they happened again. That's when I realized that the doctors were already preparing me for my next heart attack, instead of telling me how to prevent it," says the young mom. "When I got home, I was so terrified that I'd have another heart attack that I couldn't sleep at night, fearing that I wouldn't wake up in the morning."

Medical Neglect, Misjudgments, and Misdiagnosis Put Young Lives in Danger

What happened to Camille and J.P. is more common than you might think. All too often, young adults aren't identified as being at high risk until they've already suffered heart attacks or strokes. In a recent study of young heart attack survivors, ages eighteen to fifty-five, almost all of them had at least one of the following five modifiable—and highly treatable—cardiovascular risk factors: high blood pressure, smoking, obesity, diabetes, and high cholesterol.[1] About two-thirds of the patients had three or more of these factors.

Yet only half of these young men and women knew they were at risk prior to their life-threatening events—and even fewer had ever discussed their heart risks and how to reduce them with their medical providers. That's an extremely dangerous form of medical neglect, given that numerous studies have shown that having even one of these five risk factors greatly magnifies the threat of having a heart attack or stroke at a young age—and the more risk factors a patient has, the greater the danger. A recent study found that people in their thirties or forties with at least two of these factors are at *ten times higher risk for stroke than those with none.*[2] Another study found that young adults with elevated blood pressure or abnormal levels of LDL or HDL were *at up to thirty times higher risk for having heart attacks or dying from cardiovascular causes after forty than those with normal levels.*[3]

Often called "a silent killer," high blood pressure is one of the most dangerous cardiovascular risk factors, particularly if it goes undetected and untreated. Nearly half of U.S. adults—108 million people—have hypertension (blood pressure of 130/80 or above) and only one in four of them have their condition under control. If you struggle with hard-to-control blood pressure, later in this chapter we'll tell you about a common red flag that can reveal an often-undiagnosed, but highly treatable root cause of this disorder. We'll also alert you to other red flags that signal increased risk for CVD, dementia, and other chronic conditions and what to do if you have any of these warning signs or traditional cardiovascular risk factors.

Women were particularly likely to be left in the dark about their cardiovascular danger and to miss out on potentially life-saving tests, treatments, and even counseling about how to protect their heart and brain health, such as making lifestyle changes, as compared to young men the same age with identical risk factors. For example, along with high cholesterol, Camille had another extremely obvious cardiovascular red flag that her doctor had apparently overlooked: her weight, which had climbed since she had given birth to her son eight years earlier. At the time of her heart attack, she was carrying 246 pounds on her five-foot-four-inch frame, putting her in the obese category. In addition, she was so busy with her demanding office job that she

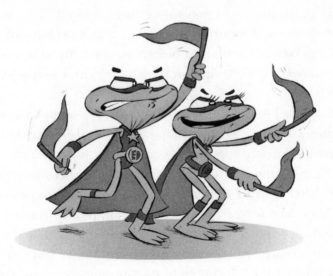

had little time to exercise. Some studies suggest that obesity is just as dangerous to heart health as smoking is, particularly when it's coupled with a sedentary lifestyle.

Lifeguards put up red flags to warn beachgoers of hidden danger lurking in the water, such as a powerful undertow or sharks hunting for prey near the shoreline. Similarly, we educate our patients about cardiovascular warning signs for a very important reason: In many cases, a heart attack or stroke is the first symptom of arterial disease. Sixty-four percent of women—and about 50 percent of men—who die suddenly from these events were previously unaware that they had CVD and had no prior symptoms.[4]

Even when young patients do develop early warning signs of an impending heart attack, they are frequently misdiagnosed. For example, a 2020 study of young heart attack survivors reported that about 30 percent of the women and 22 percent of the men had consulted their providers about similar symptoms prior to their heart attacks. Of this group, 53 percent of the women and 37 percent of the men reported that their doctors didn't think their symptoms were heart related.[5] It's common for early signs of an impending heart attack, which can occur days, weeks, or even months before the event, to be brushed off as anxiety, particularly in women of all ages and young adults of both sexes.[6]

Because J.P. and Camille had both received a psychological diagnosis before their heart attacks, both misinterpreted their symptoms when these events occurred, a mistake that nearly cost Camille her life. Cardiologists say that there is a "golden hour" after a heart attack when treatments are most likely to save lives. As one heart specialist we know puts it, "Time is muscle and muscle is life. Every minute you wait after that golden hour, the more heart muscle will die. And once you lose it, it's not coming back." Fortunately, despite Camille's long delay in seeking care, she avoided permanent heart damage and ultimately made a full recovery.

J.P. shudders to think about what might have happened if he'd been mountain biking alone. "Fifteen minutes into the ride, I was struggling to keep up. My friend looked back and saw that I was holding the handlebars with one hand and massaging my chest with the other. I figured that I'd overdone it with weightlifting the day before and wanted to power through the pain." His friend, however, insisted that they turn back. "When we walked into the house, a curtain came down. The last thing I remember before passing out was the proverbial feeling of an elephant sitting on my chest," adds the young dad. "If I'd been on my own, I probably would have dropped dead on that mountain trail, because I had no idea that I was at risk for a heart attack."

What's Wrong with This Picture?

Camille and J.P. received standard medical checkups. She was correctly diagnosed with high cholesterol and he was accurately diagnosed with high blood pressure, and both patients were offered appropriate medications for these conditions. However, Camille unknowingly turned down a potentially lifesaving treatment that would have helped prevent her heart attack—statin therapy—and J.P. rarely took his blood pressure pills before his event, believing that the medication was unnecessary. That's because both patients were lulled into a false sense of security by their seemingly low risk for cardiovascular events.

Why wasn't their cardiovascular peril recognized before they landed in the cardiac ICU, fighting for their lives? In Dr. Jerome Groopman's book *How Doctors Think,* he describes several common "cognitive traps" that cause medical providers to deliver poor care or seriously harm patients. These errors in thinking are also the underlying reason for 80 percent of medical misdiagnoses, he reports. One of the more common cognitive traps stems from overreliance on one-size-fits-all medical algorithms and decision trees. These tools are intended to help busy doctors who are juggling a heavy patient load provide fast, efficient diagnoses and prescribe evidence-based treatment through standardizing their approach to patient care.

However, these tools can also lead well-intentioned physicians to make critical and even dangerous misjudgments. For example, current medical guidelines advise providers to check patients' cholesterol and blood pressure numbers and plug them into a cardiovascular risk calculator, along with the person's age, gender, and smoking status. The algorithm then crunches the data and provides an estimate of the patient's ten-year risk for heart attacks and strokes. That's how Camille's doctor arrived at the conclusion that her risk for these events was less than 1 percent. However, as we'll explain more fully in the next chapter, these widely used risk score calculators can be dangerously unreliable, especially for women and younger patients. For example, when we plugged J.P.'s pre–heart attack numbers into the latest guideline-recommended version of this tool, we were (mis)informed that his likelihood of having a heart attack in the next decade was only 1.4 percent!

It's also common for doctors to be overly influenced by their first impressions of the patient. For example, J.P. is physically fit with rosy cheeks and looks much younger than his chronological age, all of which convey powerful associations with vigor and good health. As a result, his doctor may have considered him much too young and healthy to be a candidate for a heart attack, despite his abnormal blood pressure. Similarly, Camille's doctor may have been influenced by the long-held myth that heart disease is mainly a threat to old men—not forty-year-old women.

An Often-Overlooked Cardiovascular Risk

Another common cognitive trap that physicians fall into is failing to consider that the patient may have more than one disorder. For example, there were glaring red flags that Camille was at high risk for type 2 diabetes: One of her grandparents had this disorder, which often runs in families. In addition, she was obese and between juggling the demands of her hectic office job and childcare, the young mom rarely had time to exercise. Being overweight, particularly when coupled with a sedentary lifestyle, is the leading risk factor for type 2 diabetes. Indeed, a recent study reported that obese women have a *twenty-eight times higher* risk for developing the blood sugar disease than women of normal weight.[7]

Given these red flags, Camille's doctor should have screened her for diabetes with the two-hour oral glucose tolerance test (OGTT) we recommend in chapter nine. Ranked as the gold standard in accuracy by the American Diabetes Association and the BaleDoneen Method, this inexpensive test is covered by many insurance plans. If Camille had received this test, it would have revealed that she had insulin resistance (IR), the root cause of most heart attacks, nearly all cases of type 2 diabetes, and many chronic illnesses.

Very often, patients don't discover that they have IR or full-blown diabetes until they've already suffered a heart attack or stroke. Yet with early detection and lifestyle changes, including losing as few as seven to ten pounds, IR can often be reversed, as we'll discuss more fully in chapter nine. Although IR and diabetes are most common in people who are sedentary and overweight—especially around the belly—these disorders can also occur in physically fit people with flat bellies.

We recommend that everyone with known arterial disease

get the OGTT, regardless of their weight or BMI. Here's why: If you have atherosclerosis, there is a 70 percent risk that you also have IR or diabetes. J.P. is a case in point. Despite his highly athletic lifestyle, the auto dealer was rather overweight at five-ten and 221 pounds. One of the culprits was dining out frequently (a red flag for cardiovascular risk that we'll discuss later in this chapter).

The Strongest Predictor of Heart Attack, Stroke, Diabetes, and Dementia Risk

J.P. and Camille also had another glaring red flag for cardiovascular risk: Both have close relatives who needed open-heart and other surgeries to treat severely blocked blood vessels. In Camille's case, she told us, "On my dad's side of the family, all the men passed away from heart disease before forty." J.P.'s father has had many mini-strokes and one full-blown stroke that left him with impaired speech, memory, and motor skills. Family history is one of the strongest predictors of cardiovascular risk, with many studies reporting that having a parent or sibling with heart disease doubles or even triples risk for developing it. Moreover, having second-degree relatives (such as a grandparent, aunt, uncle, or half-sibling) with heart disease, stroke, or diabetes also dramatically escalates heart risk.[8]

If you have a family history of heart disease, diabetes, dementia, or other chronic conditions, make sure your medical provider is aware of it and screens you for arterial disease, using the tests advised in part two. Genetic testing revealed that both Camille and J.P. are carriers of the 9P21 "heart attack gene" and other high-risk genes. However, as they and many other high-risk patients treated with the BaleDoneen Method have discovered, their DNA doesn't have to be their destiny, since genetic data can also guide the best personalized treatments to prevent it.

For example, Camille did need a statin, but the one that was prescribed after her heart attack wasn't an effective therapy for people with her genotype. And as we'll explain in chapter four, another patient, Casey, had an inherited cholesterol disorder that most American doctors don't check for, even though it's been shown to cause heart attacks and strokes, often at a young age. Yet this dangerous disorder, which affects about one in five Americans, is easily detectable with a twenty-dollar blood test your healthcare provider can order at the same time as the conventional cholesterol test. Once diagnosed, this condition can be treated with medically prescribed dosages of an inexpensive vitamin, niacin (vitamin B3), which should only be taken under the close supervision of your healthcare providers.

Heart Attack, Stroke, and Dementia Red Flags That Even Surprise Doctors

Here's a look at ten common red flags for cardiovascular peril, all of which you can diagnose yourself, without any medical tests. *Even if you don't have any noticeable symptoms of heart disease—and don't consider yourself a candidate for stroke, dementia, or other chronic illnesses—if you have any of these conditions, you need to take action to protect yourself.* Alert your medical provider if you have any of them and ask for the comprehensive EDFROG assessment you read about in chapter two. Early detection and treatment can stop the cat in the gutter in its tracks, allowing you to live well without fear of a heart attack, stroke, or dementia, even if you have many red flags.

Erectile dysfunction

Difficulty in achieving or maintaining an erection firm enough for sex is one of the most common early warning signs of arterial disease in men—and doubles risk for a cardiovascular event in the next three to five years, according to recent studies.[9] One of these studies reported that the increased danger was independent of such traditional risk factors as high cholesterol, smoking, and high blood pressure. "Our results reveal that erectile dysfunction is, in and of itself, a potent predictor of cardiovascular risk," said the study's lead author, Dr. Michael Blaha. For example, Neal began to struggle with impotence at thirty-seven, five years before his CVD became severe enough to require quadruple bypass surgery. Unfortunately, however, the cardiovascular danger posed by his erectile dysfunction (ED) went unrecognized at the time.

Although a variety of conditions can interfere with a man's sexual performance—including stress, sleep disorders, diabetes, alcohol consumption, smoking, anxiety, depression, and the use of certain medications—CVD is the leading culprit. A 2019 analysis pooling the results of studies of more than 150,000 men found that those with ED were 59 percent more likely to have CVD, prompting Harvard-affiliated cardiologist Dr. Ron Blankstein to report, "In many cases, [ED] might be the first warning sign of underlying cardiovascular disease."[10] He compares the penile artery to the proverbial canary in the coal mine. This artery, which delivers oxygenated blood to the penis, has a relatively small diameter, he explains. "It's the smaller blood vessels which show the first signs of disease."

The key message from the latest research is that ED is preventable through risk factor modification. Many of the same conditions that cause arterial disease and microvascular disease also increase risk for ED, including smoking, high cholesterol, obstructive sleep apnea (OSA), low vitamin D, and obesity.

Migraine headaches

Migraine headaches, particularly those preceded by sensory symptoms known as an aura (such as seeing flashing lights or zigzag lines, or a disturbed sense of smell, taste, or touch), are strongly linked to increased risk for stroke, particularly in women. A recent analysis of studies reported that having migraines with aura more than doubles a woman's risk for stroke, and nearly quadruples it if she is under forty-five.[11] In one woman-only study, migraineurs with aura were twice as likely to suffer heart attacks, angina (heart-related chest pain), and fatal CVD, as compared to women without headaches.[12] Migraine head-aches also raise men's risk for stroke, but not as much.

About 30 million Americans, 75 percent of whom are women, suffer from migraines: debilitating, recurrent headaches, which are sometimes accompanied by nausea, sensitivity to light, and weakness. Only about one in five migraine sufferers experience aura, which typically starts about ten to thirty minutes before head pain strikes. Although the link between migraines and strokes isn't fully understood, people who experience aura may be more prone to developing blood clots, which in turn could predispose them to ischemic stroke. Women with migraines shouldn't use birth control pills, which raise risk for blood clots and strokes.

Bleeding gums

If your gums bleed even a little when you brush, floss, or eat abrasive foods (such as apples), that's a warning sign of peri-odontal disease (PD), a chronic oral infection of the gums that affects about 50 percent of Americans over thirty. One of our studies has been called landmark because it was the first to iden-tify oral bacteria from PD as a contributing cause of CVD.[13] If untreated, these bacteria often enter the bloodstream and inflame arterial plaque, leading to blood clots that can cause heart attacks and strokes. Other research has shown that people with gum disease are at 70 percent higher risk for Alzheimer's disease than those with healthy gums, and among those who already have the memory-robbing disorder, cognitive decline progressed six times faster in those with PD.[14]

Oral pathogens have also been linked to an increased threat of many other chronic conditions, including diabetes, rheumatoid arthritis, and even colon cancer.[15] A 2021 study of more than five hundred patients with COVID-19 reported that those with gum disease were 3.5 times more likely to need ICU care, 4.5 times more likely to be put on a ventilator, and nearly nine times more likely to die, compared to those without gum disease.[16] Conversely, as we'll explain in chapter ten, taking excellent care of your teeth and gums can add years to your life and greatly reduce your risk for a wide range of chronic illnesses, including CVD, respiratory infections, dementia, chronic kidney disease, several forms of cancer, high blood pressure, IR, and other devastating conditions, including erectile dysfunction.

Psoriasis and other autoimmune diseases

Psoriasis isn't just skin deep. In severe cases, it puts younger adults at up to 2.5 times higher risk for a fatal heart attack or stroke, compared to people the same age without this skin disorder. People with severe psoriasis may suffer their first CV event by forty.[17] Characterized by itchy, scaly patches, most commonly on the knees, elbows, trunk, and scalp, and, in some cases, swollen joints, this disease affects more than 3 million Americans. It's been linked to increased risk for high cholesterol, high blood pressure, obesity, diabetes, and metabolic syndrome.

Psoriasis is part of a family of more than a hundred autoimmune disorders, all of which work the same way: The body turns on itself because the immune system mistakes healthy cells, tissues, or organs for foreign invaders, unleashing normally protective reactions, such as inflammation, that never end. A recent systematic review of studies that included about 500,000 people found that on average, those with autoimmune disorders are at 20 percent higher risk for CVD and diabetes than those without them. However, the effect on heart risk can vary widely, depending on which autoimmune disorder you have. Of all the conditions the researchers studied, the one with the least cardiovascular impact was Crohn's disease (a bowel disorder), which hiked CVD and diabetes risk by 6 percent over an eleven-year period.[18]

Other research suggests that people with lupus—an autoimmune disorder best known for causing a butterfly-shaped rash across the nose and cheeks—are particularly vulnerable to heart disease. A 2018 study found that young women with this disease *are fifty times more likely to die from a heart attack than young women without lupus.* Researchers believe that immune system cells called neutrophils may be the culprits: A recent study found that in lupus patients, these normally protective cells go rogue, leading to stiff, inflamed, and plaque-filled arteries.[19] This discovery could lead to new therapies to combat these molecular villains.

Dining out frequently

Most of us have heard that eating a Mediterranean-style diet that is high in fruit, veggies, fish, and low-fat dairy products is better for your heart than a Western diet that's high in processed grains, red meat, full-fat dairy, and sweets. Recently a large study identified an even more unhealthy diet that they called the "social-business" eating pattern.[20] About 20 percent of the more than four thousand initially healthy middle-aged adults they studied followed this pattern, which included frequent restaurant meals. Like J.P., people who follow this pattern tend to eat a lot of red meat, premade meals, fried foods, sugary beverages, and excessive amounts of alcohol, all of which takes a toll on heart health. In the study, those with social-business eating habits were 31 percent more likely to have a dangerous buildup of arterial plaque, boosting their risk for heart attacks and strokes—and were also at increased risk for diabetes and high blood pressure—as compared to those who followed the Mediterranean pattern. The study also found that people who dine out frequently consume about 475 more calories a day, explaining why this pattern is also linked to increased risk for obesity. Later in this book we'll tell you how to personalize your diet for optimal arterial wellness.

Snoring or trouble sleeping

Loud snoring or frequently waking up in the night for no apparent reason are both common symptoms of OSA. As you learned in chapter two, this often-undiagnosed sleep disorder is one of the most common root causes of high blood pressure that doesn't respond to prescribed medications, as turned out to be the case with both Neal and J.P. If you fit this scenario, talk to your medical provider about having a sleep study, even if you don't think you snore, since many people with OSA are unaware of their symptoms. Several studies have also shown that having OSA doubles risk for heart attacks, strokes, and other CV events. The good news is that if this sleep disorder is treated, the excess risk can be eliminated. That's why it's important to let your doctor know if you have any symptoms of this condition, whether or not you have high blood pressure.

Gout

J.P.'s medical records also revealed another important clue to his risk for cardiovascular disease and its most common root cause: insulin resistance. Three years before his heart attack, he was diagnosed with gout, an inflammatory form of arthritis that occurs when uric acid builds up in the body, leading to joint pain and swelling, especially in the big toes. Although gout and diabetes are different diseases, people who have one are more likely to get the other. If you have gout even occasionally, we recommend having your blood sugar checked with the OGTT, since discovering and treating this very common condition is a key component of our prevention plan. When we tested J.P. after his heart attack, he turned out to be prediabetic.

Here's why people with gout need evaluation with the Bale-Doneen Method: A recent study found that *people with gout are at nearly 50 percent higher risk for coronary artery disease (CAD) than those without gout.*[21] Having this inflammatory disorder puts people who already have heart disease in significantly greater danger of heart attacks, strokes, and death from CV causes, as compared to heart patients without gout, according to a 2018 study by Duke University researchers.[22] Gout has also been shown to raise women's stroke risk by 34 percent.[23] However, treating gout with anti-inflammatory medications dramatically reduces these risks, leading the authors of a large 2020 study to conclude that gout is a modifiable risk factor for arterial disease.[24]

Working long hours

Not only is clocking long hours on the job stressful, but it can take a toll on your cardiovascular health. In a recent analysis of studies that included more than 600,000 initially healthy men and women, those who worked fifty-five or more hours a week had a 13 percent higher rate of heart attacks and 33 percent higher rate of strokes, compared to those who worked thirty-five to forty hours a week.[25] The participants were tracked for seven to eight years. Working long hours has also been linked to increased likelihood of weight gain, smoking, and excessive drinking.[26]

Asthma

Having persistent asthma symptoms can double your risk for a cardiovascular event, such as a heart attack, stroke, or related complication of arterial disease, a recent study found.[27] Another study found that taking daily medication (such as oral or inhaled corticosteroids) for chronic asthma boosts risk for such events by 60 percent over a ten-year period, as compared to having intermittent asthma that doesn't require controller medications.[28]

What's the link between asthma—a respiratory disease that affects about 25 million Americans—and heart risk? Inflammation plays a key role in both conditions, as do genes. In fact, children are up to five times more likely to develop it if their mother has asthma and up to twice as likely if their father does.[29] In the study of users and non-users of asthma control medications, those with persistent symptoms requiring daily treatment had much higher levels of systemic inflammation than those with intermittent symptoms. The findings align with a large body of research tying other inflammatory conditions, such as rheumatoid arthritis and HIV (human immunodeficiency virus) to an increased threat of heart problems.[30] In chapter eight, we'll take a closer look at chronic inflammation and how to tell if your arteries are on fire.

Divorce

Eight years after Camille's heart attack, she requested an urgent reevaluation of her arterial health. At the time, she was under intense stress because in the span of just six months, she'd lost her home to foreclosure and her husband had left her. During her divorce, she was also caught up in a custody battle over the couple's son and was facing the loss of her job, putting her under enormous financial strain. She was right to be concerned, since studies show that divorce can literally be heartbreaking, especially for women. For example, a 2015 study found that one divorce raises women's heart attack risk by 30 percent—and two divorces doubles their risk! The same study found that men must be divorced at least twice to have any increased heart attack risk.[31]

When we checked Camille's inflammatory markers with the fire panel of tests we discuss in chapter eight, we found an alarming increase. Her arteries were ablaze and we immediately changed her treatment to help her avoid a repeat heart attack. Now fifty-eight, she recently told us that she feels that life has given her a "bonus round" and she's determined to make the most of it. After losing her home, she managed to buy and remodel a new one on a shoestring. She also returned to college to get associate degrees in business and accounting and found a better job, while also raising her son as a single mom.

While she continues to struggle with her weight, she's now down to 189 pounds—a loss of fifty-seven pounds from her heart attack weight—and exercises regularly, allowing her to be fit enough to participate in half marathons. Throughout all these ups and downs, she says, "In every aspect of my life, I did what everybody said couldn't be done. In terms of my health, I am living proof that despite my genetic predisposition to heart disease and diabetes, the AHA for Life plan really does work."

A green flag that makes people smile

Along with a wide range of red flags that warn of cardiovascular danger that may lie ahead, researchers have also found a factor that protects and enhances heart health: optimism. People with an upbeat outlook have a 35 percent *lower* risk for heart attacks, strokes, angina, and death from CV causes, according to a 2019 analysis of studies that included nearly 130,000 men and women who were tracked for about fourteen years.[32] The findings held true even when the researchers considered numerous potential risk factors.

Why does focusing on the positives do the heart good? The 2019 findings suggest that optimistic people may have healthier habits, such as eating a better diet and getting more exercise. Or they may have better coping skills that help them get through tough times without turning to unhealthy behaviors, such as smoking or substance abuse. By contrast, pessimism may erode arterial wellness by making people more predisposed to inflammation, suggested lead study author Dr. Alan Rozanski, a researcher at the Icahn School of Medicine at Mount Sinai in New York City. "Optimism has long been linked to better performance in school and in such jobs as sales, sports, political endeavors, and social relationships, but it's also an important health issue that has not been well studied until now," he said in a news release.

To find out if people were optimistic, many of the studies the team analyzed used "life orientation" tests that asked participants to answer six questions about their future expectations, such as what they expected during uncertain times or how likely they were to anticipate the best possible outcome. Based on such measures, J.P. is now very optimistic. Last year, on July Fourth, he celebrated five years of being heart attack free by going mountain biking on the same path near his vacation home where his near-fatal heart attack occurred.

"Now that I'm on the right medications, as well as a diet based on my DNA, we've seen a significant shrinkage of the plaque in my arteries," says the father of two, who remains an avid mountain biker and backcountry skier. After literally having a peak experience pedaling up the steep mountain path where he'd nearly lost his life five years earlier, J.P. followed his annual tradition of going to an Independence Day picnic with his wife and daughters at their country club. "After that, we watched the fireworks light up the sky over the lake and appreciated how truly blessed we are," he says. "Without this deep dive into my medical situation to find and treat *all* my risk factors, I probably wouldn't be here today."

And while very few people would describe having a near-fatal heart attack as "almost a blessing," Camille does. Why? "I survived it and am stronger now," she told us. She recently celebrated sixteen years of being heart attack and worry free, she adds. "Life gave me a bonus round and I'm determined to make the most of it."

Action Step: Look in the Mirror or at a Selfie

An intriguing 2020 study suggests that in the future, sending a selfie to your medical provider could be an easy, low-cost way to be screened for CAD without a medical exam. This landmark research is the first to show that a deep learning computer algorithm can identify patients with CAD by analyzing four photos of the person's face. In the study, the algorithm was 80 percent accurate when tested on 1,013 Chinese patients who also underwent heart scans. While further large-scale research is needed to see if this tool is equally reliable in ethnically diverse populations, in the study it outperformed conventional methods of predicting heart attack and stroke risk, such as the Framingham Risk Score and other widely used risk calculators that we'll discuss in the next chapter, all of which can be dangerously unreliable, especially for younger adults and women of all ages.

Previous research shows that there's a lot you can learn about your heart and arterial health simply by looking in the mirror. For example, when we teach healthcare providers about cardiovascular red flags in our continuing medical education (CME) course, we show them a photo of coauthor Brad Bale's earlobe, which has a diagonal crease called Frank's sign. People with this tiny wrinkle or fold, which looks like the backslash on your computer, are at more than three times higher risk for CAD than those without it, according to a recent study.[33] Another study concluded that Frank's sign is a better predictor of risk for severe CAD, heart attacks, and peripheral artery disease than such well-known risk factors as smoking, high blood pressure, and high cholesterol.

What's the link between earlobe creases and heart health? More than four decades after these associations were first discovered, scientists still don't know.[34] Nor can they explain why

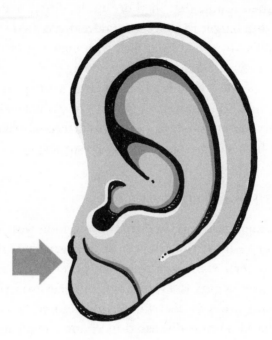

hypertension, metabolic syndrome, and obesity appear to strike people with Frank's sign at higher rates than those without it.[35] Here are some other physical red flags to check for—and what to do if you have any of them.

Male pattern baldness

A 2014 study linked this form of hair loss, which affects the front and top of the scalp, to a 40 percent rise in heart attack risk, as compared to that of men the same age with a full head of hair.[36] And the earlier this pattern of hair loss begins, the stronger its impact on cardiovascular risk, the researchers reported. Although scientists don't yet know the reason for this link, other studies have reported similar findings. For example, a 2017 study of two thousand men found that in those under forty, male pattern baldness was a bigger risk factor for developing CAD than obesity is.[37] That's why even young men with male pattern baldness should get a comprehensive cardiovascular evaluation with the tests recommended in this book. Such a workup would have identified Neal, who started to go bald in his early thirties, as being at very high risk—long before his arterial disease grew so severe that he needed emergency bypass surgery.

Prematurely gray hair or wrinkles

The researchers also reported that young men with heart disease were more likely to have prematurely gray hair than their healthy counterparts, suggesting that accelerated aging may play a role. Going gray at a young age, or excessive wrinkling in sun-protected areas is also linked to elevated heart risk in women. The cIMT test discussed in chapter two can reveal if your arteries are "older" than your chronological age. If so, the personalized lifestyle moves we recommend in chapter thirteen can often reverse accelerated aging and help you look and feel younger—on the inside and outside.

A ring around the colored part of your eye

Primarily found in people with an inherited form of extremely high cholesterol (familial hypercholesterolemia, or FH), this condition creates a deposit of cholesterol and triglycerides in an arc on either the top or bottom of the iris (the colored portion of your eye), inside the cornea.[38] Because people with FH are at extremely high risk for heart attacks and strokes, early detection and treatment can be lifesaving. If untreated, people with FH are twenty times more likely to develop CAD than those without FH—and are up to 50 percent more likely to suffer a fatal or nonfatal heart attack by fifty.[39]

Yellowish, waxy skin growths

Known as xanthoma, these fatty growths can be a sign of high cholesterol. They can be as small as a pinhead or as big as a grape and can occur in many areas, including the corners of your eyes, your hands, and the back of your legs. In one large, long-term study, people who had them were at a 48 percent higher risk for heart attacks.[40] Getting your cholesterol under control may help clear up these growths, as well as helping prevent life-threatening heart disease. In the next chapter, we'll tell you about a dangerous type of cholesterol most American doctors don't check—even though it's been shown to cause heart attacks and strokes! You'll also learn which lipid test can detect this extremely common and often overlooked disorder, which is easily treatable with an inexpensive vitamin.

CHAPTER 4

How Faulty Medical Guidelines Harm "Healthy" Patients

"Illness is a puzzle scattered in pieces. Find a way to make whole all the parts, and you can find wellness."

— TERRI GUILLEMETS,
ANTHROPOLOGIST

Casey is one of the world's strongest men. The businessman from Sherman, Texas, has competed internationally in clean and jerk weightlifting events and has been ranked number one in the U.S. in his age and weight categories and number five in the world. He also holds several masters' titles in his sport—and has the powerful, ripped physique to prove it. When Casey, then forty-five, accompanied his wife, Melinda, to our center last year, he had no intention of becoming our patient. Instead, he was only there to provide emotional support for Melinda, who had turned to us for help after suffering a seemingly inexplicable stroke. (Her story appears in chapter six, including how we solved a medical mystery that had baffled her neurologists, using a simple test that none of them had ordered.)

Before Melinda's initial evaluation at our center, says Casey, "I'd made up my mind that I wasn't going to spend any money on testing for myself, because I wasn't having any medical issues—and had always been told that my blood pressure and cholesterol were completely normal." To keep in peak condition for weightlifting competitions, Casey, a lifelong nonsmoker, ate an optimal diet and worked out intensely every day, including doing back squats with barbells that weigh twice as much as he does. He and his two teenaged sons also enjoyed a wide range of other sports, including wakeboarding, basketball, and golf. Other than breaking his leg in a sledding accident at nineteen and a couple of mild bouts of psoriasis when he was in his thirties, the young dad had always considered himself to be in perfect health.

During Melinda's initial assessment, which included examining her with the carotid intima-media thickness (cIMT) test discussed in chapter two, we asked Casey if he'd like to have his arteries scanned. After learning that this painless, noninvasive ultrasound test is FDA-approved and only takes fifteen minutes, he said, "Sure, why not?" Although the weightlifting champion had expected the scan to show that he was in perfect cardiovascular health, it detected a massive plaque deposit lurking inside his arterial walls. He didn't just have a cat in the gutter—this was a lion lying in wait for its unsuspecting prey!

"I was very shocked—and alarmed—by my cIMT results," says Casey. "I had even worse arterial disease than my wife— and she'd already suffered a stroke!" A pair of 2006 studies suggests that the weightlifting champion was right to be concerned about the health of his most important muscle, his heart, and his most important organ, his brain.[1] Both studies analyzed the accuracy of cIMT as a five-year predictor of risk for major cardiovascular (CV) events. One study reported that men with the amount of plaque we found in Casey's neck arteries were four times more likely to suffer CV events—particularly heart attacks—than other men the same age with normal cIMT

HEALTHY HEART, HEALTHY BRAIN

results. The other study suggests that without treatment, Casey would have had a 75 percent chance of having a stroke at some point in his life.

"I feel very fortunate that I went to that appointment with Melinda, because without that cIMT test, there's no telling what might have happened to me," says Casey, who immediately scheduled a full evaluation at our center. "It's very possible that scan saved my life, because without it, I'd be walking around with a ticking time bomb in my arteries."

A Dangerously Unreliable Screening Tool for Heart Attack and Stroke Risk

Our patients are often shocked to learn that most medical providers still screen patients for arterial disease in the same way they did in the 1990s, when Bill Clinton was president, the macarena was the hottest dance craze, and going online required enduring several minutes of electronic screeches while waiting for your dialup line to connect. In that era, a then-new screening tool called Framingham Risk Score (FRS) was introduced to help providers identify which patients might be at increased risk for heart attacks and strokes, so they could receive preventive care to protect their arterial health.

The FRS uses a risk scoring formula derived from an ongoing study of the residents of Framingham, Massachusetts, that began in 1948. There are several versions of this scoring system, which estimates patients' ten-year risk for having a heart attack or stroke based on their age, gender, cholesterol levels, blood pressure, and smoking status. Despite many studies showing that most initial cardiovascular events do not occur in people deemed at high risk by this formula, it is still recommended in the 2019 ACC/AHA guidelines.[2] As an example of how wildly inaccurate the latest version of the ACC/AHA's risk scoring

74

algorithm can be, we plugged in Casey's numbers from his initial evaluation at our center and were (mis)informed that his risk for having a heart attack or stroke in the next ten years was a mere 2 percent.

When we ran Brad's brother Shelby's numbers from an exam performed ten days before his 1996 heart attack, this tool estimated his ten-year risk for having one at 6.6 percent—even though he was a long-time smoker. He also had other red flags that the FRS failed to take into account, then and even now, including something as obvious as his weight. Although Shelby was carrying 230 pounds on his six-foot frame (putting him in the obese category), had a very sedentary lifestyle, and ate a poor diet, the FRS estimated that his risk for a heart attack or stroke was the same as that of a male triathlete with ideal eating habits who weighed fifty pounds less. Given the false sense of security that Shelby gained from his seemingly low cardiovascular risk, based on his completely normal blood pressure and cholesterol levels, he even continued to smoke—right up to the day when he was rushed to the hospital in the throes of a near-fatal heart attack!

Shelby's family history—and that of Casey—was another huge red flag, since both had many relatives who suffered cardiovascular events. Casey's maternal grandfather died of a stroke at fifty-nine and his maternal grandmother spent her final years battling both carotid artery disease and Alzheimer's. Many studies have shown that family history is one of the best predictors of CVD risk—and the more relatives that are affected, the greater the danger—yet neither FRS nor the ACC/AHA risk calculator take family history into account. However, they should, since Casey's family history should have alerted his medical providers that he was at increased risk, despite his lack of the Framingham factors.[3]

Another risk prediction algorithm, the Reynolds Risk Score (RRS), does take family history into consideration, but in a very limited manner.[4] Introduced in 2007, the RRS uses a formula that includes the traditional Framingham factors, plus two additional factors: if one of the patient's parents experienced a cardiovascular event before sixty (as a measure of genetic risk) and if the patient's level of the inflammatory blood marker high-sensitivity C-reactive protein (CRP) is high.

At best, the RRS, which is not widely used in current medical practice, only offers modest improvement over the FRS and only for certain patients. For example, Casey's grandfather's fatal stroke at fifty-nine didn't count because this tool ignores the solid science showing that it's important to look at a patient's full family history, not just that of their parents. Nor did the young athlete have elevated levels of CRP. As a result, the RRS yielded the same results as the ACC/AHA tool: It predicted that there was only a 2 percent chance that he'd have a heart attack or stroke in the next ten years.

Genetic testing at our center revealed that Casey carried several high-risk genes that were one of the root causes of his extensive arterial disease. Similar to about 50 percent of Americans, he's a carrier of the 9P21 "heart attack" gene. People with two copies of this gene, like Casey, have double the usual risk of developing CVD, often at a relatively young age, and are far more likely to develop severe coronary artery disease affecting multiple blood vessels, both at a young age and over a lifetime. He also carried one copy of the Apo E4 gene, which predicts increased risk for both CVD and Alzheimer's disease.

Moreover, he had a variant of the haptoglobin gene called Hp 2-2 that raises lifetime risk for arterial disease as much as smoking does, and also increases the likelihood of developing autoimmune diseases and cancer.[5] Not only is this gene probably related to Casey's psoriasis—an autoimmune disease that is known to increase heart attack and stroke risk—but, more significant, people with his genotype do best if they follow a gluten-free diet. He also got some genetic good news from our tests: He carries a copy of the heart-protective Apo E2 gene, which may counteract the danger posed by his Apo E4 gene. In chapter eleven, we will take a closer look at these genes and show you how to personalize your diet to optimize your arterial wellness. You will also learn why an inexpensive dietary supplement that is harmful for most people can be potentially lifesaving for people with type 2 diabetes who carry the Hp 2-2 genotype.

The Dangerous Cholesterol Most Doctors Don't Check

Our testing also identified another culprit in Casey's disease, one that astonished him. Because he'd had his cholesterol checked a few years before he visited our center, he assumed that he'd already been screened for all harmful forms of cholesterol that might explain why he had such a large plaque deposit. After all, the test he had, which is widely used in standard care and recommended in current cardiology guidelines, certainly sounds comprehensive. Known as a lipid profile or a coronary risk panel, it measures levels of several blood fats: total cholesterol, high-density lipoprotein (HDL), low-density lipoprotein (LDL), and triglycerides.[6] Because he'd been told that his results were normal, he assumed that his arterial disease wasn't caused by a cholesterol problem.

However, all these assumptions were wrong. A twenty-dollar blood test performed at our center revealed another of the root causes of his arterial disease: He had elevated levels of lipoprotein (a), also known as Lp(a). We call this inherited cholesterol disorder the mass murderer—it triples risk for heart attacks and strokes, often at a relatively young age.[7] Unlike LDL—the infamous "bad" cholesterol—Lp(a) isn't affected by lifestyle, nor can it be effectively treated with cholesterol-lowering statin drugs if it's elevated, according to a 2018 study published in *Circulation*.[8] The researchers report that patients with one copy of the gene responsible for elevated Lp(a) levels are 58 percent more likely to develop coronary heart disease (CHD) while taking a statin for prevention than those without the gene, while risk for CHD is more than doubled in statin users with two copies of the Lp(a) gene!

The study also found that aspirin therapy didn't have much, if any, effect on Lp(a) levels. These findings suggest that the two drugs most commonly prescribed for heart attack and stroke prevention are *not* protecting the 20 percent of patients with this inherited condition, most of whom are undiagnosed and unaware of their peril. In 2010, the European Atherosclerosis Society (EAS) issued a scientific statement calling for routine screening and treatment of elevated Lp(a) levels as "an important priority to reduce cardiovascular risk."[9] Yet more than a decade later, in the U.S., it's *still* not the standard of care to treat—or even measure—this dangerous form of cholesterol that is found at elevated levels in up to one-third of heart attack victims.

At our center, we frequently see patients who have already survived a heart attack or stroke—or even multiple events—who still haven't been checked for a cholesterol villain that has been shown to trigger these calamities! Have *you* ever had your Lp(a) levels checked? Has your medical provider ever told you about this test? If the answer is no, consider this: Being left in the dark about this crucial test nearly cost several of the patients you'll meet in this book, including Casey, their lives.

Also witness what happened to celebrity fitness trainer Bob Harper, famed for his role as the host of the hit TV show *The Biggest Loser*. When he suffered a massive widow-maker heart attack in 2017 at fifty-two that left him in a coma for two days, he and his doctors were completely baffled. Harper was the picture of health—and always passed his annual physicals with flying colors. A year later, he learned that he had perilously high levels of Lp(a), a discovery that inspired him to work to raise awareness of the value of Lp(a) testing. As he recently told *The New York Times*, "Being healthy is not about what you can do in the gym. It's not about what you can do on the outside. It's what's going on in the inside."[10]

Because the Lp(a) test checks for an inherited condition, if your levels are normal, there's no need to be tested more than once because your genes don't change. We recommend that everyone get this inexpensive blood test, which can be performed at the same time as conventional cholesterol testing. If your levels are elevated, the best treatment is niacin (vitamin B3), which should only be taken under medical supervision. The EAS reports that niacin therapy can lower Lp(a) levels by up to 40 percent—a potentially lifesaving benefit. Decreasing Lp(a) was shown to reduce risk for cardiovascular events by about 75 percent in the *Circulation* study discussed earlier, highlighting the value of getting tested and treated if your levels are elevated.

Are You Getting the Best Cholesterol Test to Predict Cardiovascular Risk?

For decades, LDL cholesterol has been vilified as public enemy number one by the medical profession. Yet none of the hundreds of cholesterol studies performed to date has ever shown that LDL causes heart attacks. This unscientific belief has become so ingrained in medical thinking—as well as cardiology guidelines—that it's been termed "the great cholesterol hoax." Indeed, a large body of research suggests that your level of LDL is the *worst* lipoprotein predictor of your heart attack risk.[11]

Instead, the most predictive measurement is apolipoprotein B-100 (ApoB), which can be checked with a twenty-dollar blood test available through almost all medical labs. Widespread use of this test—and the potentially lifesaving information it can provide—could prevent 500,000 heart attacks and strokes over the next ten years, according to a recent paper published in *Journal of the American College of Cardiology*.[12] ApoB testing has also been shown to identify young adults at risk for developing heart disease decades before any traditional risk factors manifest, creating opportunities for very early intervention, using lifestyle changes and possibly medications.

What does the ApoB test measure? Cholesterol, a waxy substance produced by the liver, is ferried through the bloodstream by molecular "submarines" known as lipoproteins. ApoB is a major component of the four lipoprotein particles that are most harmful to the arteries when found at elevated levels: LDL, intermediate density lipoprotein (IDL), very low-density lipoprotein (VLDL), and Lp(a). Since each of these particles contains one ApoB molecule, measurements of ApoB reveal the total burden of dangerous lipoprotein particles circulating in your blood. This test is similar to counting the number of submarines in an enemy attack force to assess how great a threat they pose.

Conversely, the standard cholesterol test only measures the amount of cargo, such as LDL cholesterol, that the fleet of submarines is carrying. Why does this distinction matter? In a recent study called JUPITER, there was *no* correlation between the 11,186 participants' initial blood levels of LDL (as measured by the standard test) and their subsequent rate of heart attacks, strokes, and other cardiovascular (CV) events over the next two to five years, while their baseline numbers for ApoB and triglycerides (TG) strongly predicted future CV risk.[13]

In many cases, ApoB testing can reveal hidden cardiovascular peril that would have been missed, had the patient only been checked with the conventional test. For example, our testing found that Casey had high levels of ApoB, while his LDL was only very mildly elevated. Although each of the four cholesterol bullies that comprise ApoB, including LDL, can contribute to the development of arterial plaque, LDL is arguably the wimp of the gang.

Wondering if you should get the ApoB test instead of the standard test? We recommend that you get both tests—as well as the Lp(a)—because each of them provides valuable information about your heart and metabolic health. For example, having high triglycerides isn't just a heart attack and stroke risk factor. It can also be an early warning sign that you're headed for type 2 diabetes. In a ten-year study of nearly fourteen thousand initially healthy young men, those whose TG levels rose the most during the study period were *twelve times more likely* to develop diabetes than those whose TG levels remained normal.[14]

The study also found that men who started off with high TG but lowered their levels through healthy lifestyle changes had the same diabetes risk as men who never had high TG at all, highlighting the value of early detection and treatment of this lifestyle-linked lipid abnormality. In chapter nine, we'll take a closer look at the triglycerides/diabetes connection, as well as other surprising insights about your overall health and risk for several chronic diseases that you can glean from your standard cholesterol test results. In chapter fourteen, we will discuss a variety of therapies—including dietary changes, supplements, and medications—that help lower ApoB levels. Our patients are also pleasantly surprised to learn that a number of studies have shown that cinnamon can have beneficial effects on levels of several lipids, including LDL, ApoB, and triglycerides, and can also help reduce blood pressure and blood sugar.[15,16,17]

The Perils of Not Treating Plaque

An online version of the ACC/AHA risk scoring tool developed for patients told Casey that his then-risk for developing heart disease or having a stroke were so low that he wasn't a candidate for medications to prevent these conditions, such as low-dose aspirin or statins. Instead, the tool urged him to exercise regularly, eat a heart-healthy diet, maintain a healthy weight, and avoid all forms of nicotine—all of which he was already doing. Similarly, most doctors would have congratulated the weightlifting champion on his excellent lifestyle, assured him that he was at extremely low risk for heart attacks and strokes, and told him to keep up the good work.

What would have happened if we'd followed the ACC/AHA latest screening guidelines and only looked at Casey's risk factors—not his arteries?[18] The landmark 2001 CAFES-CAVE study has revealed the extreme danger of not treating plaque.[19] The researchers recruited ten thousand low-risk, healthy men and women who were thirty-five to sixty-four at the start of the study; all of them were screened for plaque using cIMT and a similar test (femoral IMT) that measures the intima-media thickness of leg arteries. Even if plaque was found, the volunteers did not receive any medical treatment, such as low-dose aspirin or statins. The participants were tracked for ten years, with their rate of cardiovascular events (such as heart attacks and strokes) and deaths correlated with their initial IMT results, with the following findings:

Class I (normal arteries)

The ten-year rate of CV events in this group was 0.1 percent, with no deaths.

Class II (artery wall thickening)

Nearly 9 percent of this group suffered CV events, also with no fatalities.

Class III (plaque deposits that didn't block blood flow)

Nearly 40 percent of this group had heart attacks and strokes, including fatal events.

Class IV (obstructive arterial disease)

More than 81 percent of these people suffered heart attacks or strokes, and of all CV-related deaths among the study participants, the vast majority occurred in this group.

Based on this study, the largest of its kind ever conducted, Casey's true risk for a heart attack or stroke was *nearly twenty times higher than his ACC/AHA risk score had predicted,* if he'd gone untreated, even though he had no symptoms of disease. In other words, without proper treatment, Casey really would have been walking around with a ticking time bomb in his arteries. It could have exploded at any time, quite possibly leading to a fatal cardiovascular event like the one that killed his fifty-nine-year-old grandfather!

Only through vascular screening (testing to check the symptom-free, seemingly healthy patient for arterial diseases) did he learn that he was in potentially life-threatening danger, despite his apparent outward good health and reassuringly low risk score. Yet the latest ACC/AHA guidelines only recommend the use of imaging tests to screen patients in one specific scenario: cases in which healthcare providers are having trouble deciding if a patient's ten-year risk for heart attacks and strokes is high enough to merit a statin prescription to lower it.

What's the Best Way to Be Screened for Heart Attack, Stroke, and Dementia Danger?

Standard care divides patients into two categories. People who have not yet experienced heart attacks or strokes are considered potential candidates for what's now called primary prevention, treatments to reduce their risk for these events, such as lifestyle changes and in certain cases, medication. People who have already suffered one or more heart attacks and strokes are deemed to need what's now called secondary prevention, treatments aimed at helping these patients avoid repeat events, a topic we will discuss more fully in part three of this book.

However, as you've seen in this chapter, dangerously unscientific screening guidelines are putting unsuspecting patients in peril. Millions of men and women miss out on potentially lifesaving interventions, simply because they don't have the specific risk factors that healthcare providers are instructed to check. Therefore, in one of our recent peer-reviewed publications, we have proposed a completely different approach to risk assessment. Instead of looking solely at patients' risk factors, we recommend that healthcare providers also look at the body system they are treating: the patient's arteries.[20] We further propose a three-tiered classification, based on the presence or absence of arterial disease, as follows:

Primary prevention

There is no cat in the gutter and our mission is to keep it feline free through optimal lifestyle and management of all the patient's risk factors and cardiovascular red flags. This also includes making sure the patient is getting the right dental care and following a genetically guided diet and exercise plan. Even if patients in this category have many risk factors, they still don't need medications like low-dose aspirin or statins, because risk factors don't cause heart attacks and strokes—plaque does, if it becomes inflamed and ruptures, leading to the formation of a blood clot. A key part of our primary prevention plan is helping you avoid chronic inflammation, the fire that damages the arterial lining and makes it easier for cholesterol particles to cluster in blood vessel walls.

Secondary prevention

As Casey would put it, people in this category have a ticking time bomb in their arteries, and our mission is to safely defuse it before it explodes. In part three, we'll discuss the best treatments for plaque, including some that will surprise and even delight you. For example, we recommend that our patients eat a daily dose of dark chocolates (in small amounts) as part of their secondary prevention plan. We'll also discuss fun ways to get a cardiovascular workout, including dancing, laughter, yoga, and mindful meditation—natural stress-busters—and why getting sounder, more refreshing sleep does your heart and blood vessels good.

Tertiary prevention

The cat has already leapt out at least once and our mission is to make sure that never happens again. In chapter six, you will meet two women who suffered seemingly inexplicable strokes at relatively young ages, including Casey's wife, Melinda, and we'll explain why it only took us fifteen minutes to solve the medical mystery that had stumped their neurologists. Throughout this book, we will zero in on common root causes of heart attacks and strokes and how to treat or even reverse them. We will also show you why your dental provider can be a potentially lifesaving member of your heart attack, stroke, and dementia prevention team, how to make sure you are getting the right medications at the right dose to halt and reverse your disease, and why the right lifestyle is the ultimate miracle cure.

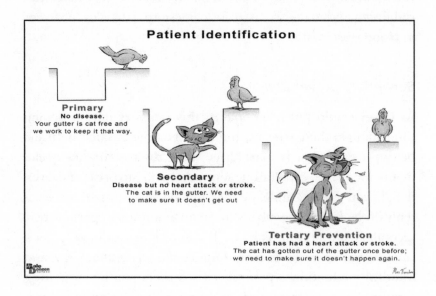

Action Step: Learn How to Be Your Own Medical Detective

Until recently, most medical knowledge, guidelines, treatments, and research on CVD was focused on men, and even today, women's arterial disease remains underdiagnosed and under-treated, leading to worse outcomes and a deadly gender gap in survival after a heart attack. To help women fight back—and save their own lives—the next chapter includes our top ten prevention tips for women. We will also alert you to red flags for heart attack, stroke, and dementia risk that are unique to women and tell you why men need to know about them, too. In fact, one of the risk factors we discuss puts male relatives of women who have it at just as high risk as the women themselves! Think of these factors as clues that a detective would use to uncover a criminal conspiracy—and arrest the perpetrators in time to foil their plot.

Learning how to be a medical detective—and sharing the knowledge you've gained from assessing your red flags with your healthcare provider—is especially important for women. As you'll learn in the next chapter, there are several common myths about women's heart health that many doctors believe. As a result, all too often, women are not identified as being at high risk until they've already had a heart attack or stroke. We'll bust the myths and empower women with the facts they need to advocate for themselves and offer a message of reality and hope: By following our AHA for Life Plan, heart attacks and strokes won't come as a surprise to women. By knowing the warning signs to watch for, you can take action to protect your heart, brain, and arterial wellness. Nor are chronic diseases inevitable as you age. In the next chapter, you'll learn how every woman can achieve a health span to match her life span.

CHAPTER 5

The Truth About Women and Heart Disease

"Women belong in all places where decisions are being made."

— RUTH BADER GINSBURG

It was nearly seven a.m. and Juli was worried that she'd be late to work. The customer service representative was hastily applying makeup when she felt a stabbing pain in her chest. It shot down her right arm, making her fingers grow numb and tingly. Suddenly, she found herself struggling to breathe. "Honey, I need help!" she yelled to her husband, Matt, who was in the next room with their four-year-old daughter, Selah. The pain grew so intense that she collapsed on her bedroom floor, gasping and vomiting.

As Matt drove her to the ER, with Selah in the backseat, Juli tried to figure out what was triggering her terrifying symptoms. Could it be a panic attack, brought on by the stress of rushing around that morning? Then she came up with a scary theory. "I thought, 'There's no way I could be having a heart attack at thirty-seven,' but this is what I thought one would feel like," she recalls. After a long wait in the ER, a doctor dismissed her concerns. "He hooked me up to an EKG, said everything was normal, and told me if it was a heart attack, the pain would be [in] my left arm — not the right," says Juli, who was then asked if she ever felt stressed or anxious. She replied, "Every day, but not like this."

The ER doctor attributed her chest pain, shortness of breath, and vomiting to bacterial pneumonia. After getting IV medication, she felt better and was sent home with a packet of powerful antibiotics. "The nurse said, 'This will get rid of your cough.' I said that I didn't have a cough, but she told me to take the pills and get a checkup afterward," adds Juli. The antibiotic seemed to help and when she had a checkup five days later, the doctor pronounced her lungs to be clear. But that night, when Selah was sitting in her lap, Juli was struck with similar symptoms. This time, however, her back and jaw hurt and she felt nauseated, with a strong feeling of pressure in her chest.

Chalking it up to another bout of pneumonia, she went to bed early, only to wake up repeatedly as the pain steadily intensified. Matt wanted to rush her to the ER, but Juli was worried about the cost under their high-deductible health plan. She insisted on toughing it out until the urgent care center opened at eight a.m. "By the time we got there, I felt like I'd been hit by a truck," says the mom. "When the doctor heard my story, I saw him shaking his head and I could tell that he wasn't buying the pneumonia diagnosis." The physician ordered blood tests, which showed an abnormally high level of cardiac enzymes.

"The doctor said my heart was damaged and wanted to call an ambulance," adds Juli. Again, concerned about costs, and unsure of what the results meant, she asked Matt to drive her to the ER, where the physician had told her that a cardiologist would be standing by to provide immediate care. Instead, she spent two hours in the waiting room, still in excruciating pain, while other patients were treated ahead of her. When she was finally seen, she received another EKG and was assured, an hour later, that the results were normal. "Soon after that, a lot of doctors and nurses came running in, looking frightened, because the blood test results had just come back," reports Juli. "That's when I found out what elevated cardiac enzymes mean: You've had a heart attack."

In fact, as she soon found out, it was her second heart attack: She'd been misdiagnosed during her first visit to the ER five days earlier. The antibiotic that was mistakenly prescribed, azithromycin, is extremely dangerous for someone in the throes of a heart attack. A 2020 study of nearly 3 million people found that those treated with this antibiotic had nearly twice the risk of dying from cardiovascular or other causes in the next five days, as compared with people treated with amoxicillin, an anti-biotic not associated with CV events.[1] Three previous studies have reported increased risk for cardiovascular deaths, serious heart arrythmias, or heart attacks in patients who received azithromycin.[2] While deaths linked to this widely prescribed antibiotic are rare, the highest rates were seen in patients with cardiovascular disease.

As Matt held Juli's hand, ER physicians explained the full significance of elevated cardiac enzymes: Some of the muscle cells in her heart had died from lack of oxygenated blood—and without immediate treatment to reopen the blocked artery, more extensive or fatal damage could occur. Then she was faced with a frightening decision. "The doctors wanted me to sign a consent form for angioplasty, but they explained that I could die if the blockage was knocked loose during the procedure." Dazed from pain and fear, she scrawled her name and was wheeled off to the OR.

The procedure went smoothly and three days later, she was discharged with prescriptions for a beta blocker and a high-dose statin. "When I asked why I needed a statin when I'd been told my cholesterol numbers were 'beautiful, like a teenager's,' the answer I got was, 'This is what we do after a heart attack,'" recalls Juli, who quit taking the statin after developing a side effect (a mild skin rash). "The only advice I got was to schedule a follow-up appointment in two weeks." At that appointment, she adds, "I was seated in the waiting room next to a sixty-year-old man who had smoked for his whole life, and thought, 'What am I doing here? I don't smoke, I go to the gym, and my blood pressure is on the low end of normal.'" What's more, the young mom was at an ideal weight.

During her recovery, recalls Juli, "I was an emotional wreck because nobody could explain why I'd had a heart attack. I felt extremely anxious and lost. I was constantly checking for any symptom that might signal another heart attack. I kept praying for a medical Sherlock Holmes who could figure out what was wrong and fix it. One day, two different people told me that I needed to go to the Heart Attack & Stroke Prevention Center. I took that as a sign from God that I'd find answers there."

A Staggering Rise in Heart Attacks and Chronic Illness in Young Women

What happened to Juli is not as unusual as it may sound. Heart attacks are increasingly common in young women, who account for nearly one-third of all female heart attack patients, compared to about one-fifth twenty years ago, according to a 2019 study.[3] The researchers analyzed medical records of nearly thirty thousand people who were hospitalized for heart attacks between 1995 and 2014. They found that over that time span, rates of heart attacks remained fairly stable among young men and decreased in older adults.

Among women ages thirty-five to fifty-four, however, the rate of heart attack hospitalizations soared from 21 percent at the start of the study to 31 percent at the end—an increase the researchers described as "staggering in the background of the aging general U.S. population." The study also found that young women who were hospitalized for heart attacks were more likely than their male counterparts to have high blood pressure, diabetes, or chronic kidney disease or to have suffered a stroke before their heart attacks and to develop heart failure afterward.[4] Other research shows that rates of dementia are on the rise among older women. Indeed, two-thirds of Americans with Alzheimer's disease are women and U.S. deaths from this memory-robbing disorder have soared by 145 percent between 2000 and 2017.[5]

Another frightening fact: Since 2010, heart disease fatalities have been steadily increasing every year among young women, a nationwide study reported in 2021.[6] "There is a misconception that women are not at risk for heart disease before menopause, yet one-third of their cardiovascular problems occur before 65," lead study author Dr. Erin Michos of Johns Hopkins University School of Medicine stated in a news release. "Young women in the US are becoming less healthy, which is now reversing prior improvements in heart disease deaths," she added. "With worsening epidemics of diabetes and obesity across developed countries, our findings are a warning sign that we need to pay more attention to the health of young women."

Women have unique cardiovascular risks. One of those that we'll discuss in this chapter puts the male relatives of women who have it at equally high risk for cardiovascular events as the women themselves. It's also important for men to know that their family history, including that of their mothers, grandmothers, aunts, sisters, and other female relatives, can provide insights into everything from their risk for heart attacks and strokes, to high blood pressure, diabetes, obesity, dementia, and even dental problems. And married men can play a key role in helping their wives—and themselves—avoid these and other chronic diseases. Traditionally, many women take on the role of being the family's chief medical officer, taking care of everybody's health but their own. However, as you'll learn in this chapter, arterial disease is an equal opportunity assassin that men and women each need help to avoid at every age—not just in their later years.

The Deadly Gender Gap in Women's Cardiovascular Care

Decades of research have documented a wide range of horrifying disparities in women's cardiovascular care, leading to worse outcomes. For example, women are up to three times more likely than men to die after a heart attack, due to unequal treatment, according to a 2018 study published in *Journal of the American Medical Association* (*JAMA*).[7] The researchers found that women are less likely to be given the same diagnostic tests, resulting in women being initially misdiagnosed at a 50 percent higher rate than their male counterparts. An earlier study found that younger women are particularly likely to have their heart attack symptoms mistakenly attributed to other causes, such as anxiety.[8] The researchers found that when women under fifty-five go to the ER in the throes of a heart attack, they are *seven times more likely than men* the same age to be misdiagnosed and sent home untreated.

The *JAMA* study also found that after a heart attack, women often miss out on potentially lifesaving therapies or are undertreated—leaving them in danger of repeat events. For example, women with high blood pressure were less likely than men to receive medications to treat this dangerous disorder at guideline-directed dosages. As a result, the women were more likely to have poorly controlled blood pressure, a condition that is often described as a silent killer, because it's a leading risk factor for heart attack, stroke, dementia, chronic kidney disease, and many other devastating complications.

Similarly, women with high cholesterol are less likely to be treated with lipid-lowering statins, despite their proven efficacy for the prevention of heart attacks, strokes, and other CV events, according to a 2019 study of nearly six thousand patients (43 percent women).[9] Although all the patients in this study met medical criteria for statin therapy because they either had heart disease or were at high risk for developing it, statin therapy was only prescribed for 67 percent of the women, versus nearly 80 percent of the men. What's more, the women in the study, on average, had *higher* cholesterol levels than the men, yet were significantly less likely to receive guideline-recommended statin dosing than their male counterparts. As a result of this medical neglect, the female patients were undertreated—if they received a statin prescription at all—leaving them in cardiovascular peril.

The *JAMA* study found that even after a heart attack, women received statin prescriptions at lower rates than men, despite evidence-based guidelines advising medical providers that these medications can be lifesaving for heart patients of both sexes. The researchers also reported that when female heart attack patients received *all* guideline-directed therapies, the gender gap in survival rates was dramatically reduced. Yet many women miss out on lifesaving care during cardiovascular emergencies, a 2019 editorial in *The Lancet* reported.[10] "U.S. data…showed that women with heart attack symptoms were less likely to receive aspirin, be resuscitated, or be transported to the hospital in ambulances using lights and sirens than were men."

Until recently, most heart-related studies have focused on men, so less is known about which treatments and diagnostic approaches are best suited to women. "The historic failings of cardiology to take a balanced approach to research have led to fundamental flaws in the care for women with heart disease and have cost the lives of many women," the *Lancet* editorial stated.[11] And even today, the editorial's authors note, women "are dramatically under-represented in clinical trials for coronary heart disease and heart failure," in which the treatments of the future are tested for safety and effectiveness. That's alarming since women respond differently to certain drugs than men do. Until women are equally represented in trials of tomorrow's therapies, they will remain at risk for getting new heart medications that may work superbly for men, but could be worthless or even dangerous for women.

In chapter fourteen, we'll tell you about a new genetic test that can help patients of both sexes get the safest, most effective medications at the right dose. For example, like about 40 percent of Americans, Juli has a KIF6 genotype that makes the statin her doctors had prescribed after her second heart attack, Lipitor (atorvastatin), ineffective when taken as a sole therapy.[12] That meant she was getting zero protection against heart attacks, strokes, and other complications of arterial disease. Other research suggests that this medication doesn't work as well in women as in men, and is also less effective for people with insulin resistance. Because many doctors are unaware of these individual differences in statin response, Lipitor is so widely prescribed to patients of both sexes that it's the world's bestselling drug.[13] A key reason for its popularity: In clinical trials that mostly included men, Lipitor was spectacularly successful at saving lives—in male heart patients with a certain KIF6 genetic variant.[14]

Why Do Women's Heart Attacks Come as a Surprise?

All too often, women don't find out that they have a disease in the wall of the artery until it's too late. Sixty-four percent of women who die suddenly from a heart attack were unaware that they had CVD. Why aren't doctors doing a better job of identifying high-risk women *before* they have heart attacks and strokes? One key factor is the long-held myth that heart disease is mainly an "old man's disease." Most women—and many doctors, including cardiologists—mistakenly believe that breast cancer is the leading killer of women, according to a shocking 2017 survey of women and physicians published in the *Journal of the American College of Cardiology*.[15]

In reality, cardiovascular disease is the number one cause of death in women. One in thirty-one women dies from breast cancer each year, while heart disease kills one in three women. That's about one death every minute![16] Although heart disease kills more women annually than all forms of cancer combined, only 39 percent of the physicians surveyed ranked it as a top health concern in women. Nor did most primary care doctors consider themselves well prepared to assess female patients for heart disease, the researchers reported.

It's easy to see how this stunning lack of awareness among primary care physicians endangers women: The doctors that women are most likely to turn to for checkups and health advice aren't finding heart disease in women because they aren't looking for it in female patients! Although most of the women surveyed had a routine physical or wellness exam in the previous year, only 40 percent had received a heart health assessment. The study also found that 71 percent of women had never asked to be checked for CVD. Instead, they assumed that their provider would alert them if there was a problem.

Another disturbing finding: Although the American Heart Association (AHA) and the American College of Cardiology (ACC) have been issuing female-specific guidelines for the prevention of CVD in women since 2011, the study found that very few of the primary care physicians and cardiologists surveyed followed them.[17] For example, these guidelines tell medical providers to check women for both traditional heart disease risk factors and female-specific risks. These factors, which we will discuss in more depth later in this chapter, include early menopause, certain pregnancy complications, recurrent miscarriages, and autoimmune diseases, all of which have been linked to higher risk for developing arterial disease.

However, instead of checking women for female-specific risks, about half of the doctors used risk prediction calculators, most of which are based on studies of men. And despite studies showing that women with even one female-specific risk factor are in significantly greater danger of suffering heart attacks, strokes, or other complications of CVD, the AHA/ACC's latest risk scoring tool, introduced nearly a decade after these groups started telling doctors to factor female-specific risks into women's heart health evaluations, still doesn't include any of these factors.[18]

The survey also found that doctors aren't doing a very good job of checking women for conventional risk factors, either. Although nearly 75 percent of the women polled reported having at least one of these factors—such as smoking, high blood pressure, high cholesterol, or a family history of heart disease—only 16 percent had ever been warned of their cardiovascular peril by their medical provider. As a result, many women have a false sense of security about their heart health. Indeed, 63 percent of the women polled admitted that they sometimes put off going to their medical provider, feeling that they had little need of medical care because they looked and felt healthy.

However, as we have emphasized in earlier chapters, even seemingly healthy, young women with no obvious risk factors can harbor silent, potentially lethal plaque in their arteries. Our advice to women of all ages is to be bold—ask for the screening tests recommended in this book, even if you feel fine. For example, had Juli known about the twenty-dollar cholesterol test discussed in chapter four, and asked her doctor to order it, she would have learned that she had elevated levels of lipoprotein (a), the inherited cholesterol disorder that we call the mass murderer because it triples risk for heart attacks and strokes, often at an early age.

Armed with the knowledge that she was in much greater danger than her "beautiful" levels of LDL (bad) cholesterol suggested, she could have been treated with an inexpensive vitamin (niacin) and the other therapies advised in part three of this book—helping her avoid having to be rushed to the ER twice in the same week in the throes of two heart attacks. Like many of our patients, Juli was shocked to learn that 50 percent of heart attacks and many strokes occur in people who have normal or even optimal LDL.[19]

Ten Heart Attack Warning Signs That Women Often Ignore—and Doctors Often Misdiagnose

Imagine that someone is having a heart attack. What do you think that would look and feel like? Chances are that you pictured an older man clutching his chest in agony and dropping to the floor, feeling as if an elephant was sitting on his chest. This scenario is often described as a classic or typical heart attack, because these symptoms are indeed typical—in men.

In yet another example of the deadly gender bias in cardiology, women's heart attack symptoms are frequently misdiagnosed because they can be very different than the classic male warning signs that physicians are taught to recognize in medical school. Women's symptoms can be much more varied and subtle than those in men and may not involve the chest at all. Although such symptoms are often labeled as atypical, they are extremely common in 51 percent of the population: women. In addition, these lesser-known heart attack symptoms can sometimes occur in men, so both sexes need to know *all* the warning signs to watch for.

Because many women—especially younger women—don't perceive themselves as being at risk for heart problems, they frequently wait much longer than men do before seeking help for potential signs of a heart attack. And when women do go to the hospital, their symptoms often go unrecognized until it's too late, causing them to miss out on lifesaving treatments.

A study of more than 1.1 million heart attack patients found that almost 15 percent of the women died in the hospital after a heart attack, compared to 10 percent of the men, largely due to misdiagnosis and delays in getting care.[20] Younger women with atypical symptoms were at 20 percent higher risk for death after a heart attack than their male counterparts.

Remember how the ER doctor quickly concluded that Juli's pain was unrelated to her heart because it was in the "wrong" arm? The researchers analyzed the frequency with which ten common heart attack symptoms occurred in men and women. They found that almost 62 percent of the women had pain in three or more areas other than the chest, compared to 54 percent of the men. Women also had higher rates of dizziness, shortness of breath, nausea, and stomach pain.[21]

If there is any suspicion a person may be having a heart attack (see the ten warning signs listed below), it is best to be cautious and call 911 immediately, because every second counts. Patients who arrive by ambulance usually get faster care — and treatment can start on the way to the hospital. Tell medical providers that you think it's a heart attack and don't let them brush off the symptoms as anxiety, heartburn, or other noncardiac causes without doing tests. EKGs frequently have normal or inconclusive findings in heart attack patients, particularly in women, so you should insist on having your levels of cardiac enzymes measured, using a blood test called high-sensitivity troponin, which checks for elevated levels of proteins that are released when muscle cells in the heart are damaged, as occurs during a heart attack.[22]

At some hospitals, it can take a couple of hours to get results from high-sensitivity troponin testing. Many large hospitals now have a rapid version of this test, with results available in ten to fifteen minutes. The longer a heart attack goes untreated, the more damage occurs. Be aware of the following symptoms which can occur with a heart attack. If the reason for the symptom is not obvious, consider the possibility of a heart attack and seek medical advice.

Pain in areas of the upper body, including the jaw, neck, back, shoulders, or arms

Fullness, squeezing, or pressure in the chest or a choking sensation that may feel like heartburn

Dizziness or feeling light-headed

Nausea with or without vomiting

Shortness of breath

Abnormally heavy sweating or breaking out in a cold sweat that may feel stress-related

Unusual fatigue, extreme weakness or anxiety, or a sense of impending doom

Rapid, irregular, pounding, or fluttering heartbeats

Sudden confusion

Abdominal pain that may feel like indigestion or severe abdominal pressure that may feel like an elephant is sitting on your stomach

The Women's Disease That Also Endangers Their Male Relatives

Polycystic ovary syndrome (PCOS) is the most common endocrine disorder in women, affecting up to 19 percent of women during their childbearing years. Its name describes the hallmark of this disease: numerous small cysts (fluid-filled sacs) in the ovaries. Although the exact cause of PCOS is unknown, in women who have it, the ovaries produce abnormally high levels of male sex hormones called androgens, which can lead to excessive amount of facial and body hair, male pattern baldness or thinning hair, and weight gain, especially around the belly. Other symptoms include infrequent or irregular periods, infertility, acne or oily skin, and dark skin patches under the breasts, in the armpits, and on the back of the neck.

Women with PCOS are at increased risk for chronic diseases, including diabetes, obesity, high blood pressure, and CVD. The disorder is also strongly associated with insulin resistance, and many women who have it also meet medical criteria for metabolic syndrome, a gang of five cardiovascular bullies that we'll look at more closely in part two. These include high blood pressure, high cholesterol, high triglycerides, and a large waistline—and when they attack in tandem, risk for heart attacks and diabetes soars.[23]

Not only does having PCOS greatly magnify a woman's risk for cardiometabolic disorders, but their first-degree relatives (mothers, fathers, sisters, and brothers) are at a similarly high risk for the same clusters of abnormalities, according to a recent analysis of fourteen earlier studies.[24] Indeed, some researchers have reported that the brothers of women with PCOS are at just as high risk for insulin resistance and metabolic syndrome as the women themselves!

Pregnancy Is a Stress Test for Women's Bodies — Here's Why

A woman's reproductive history can contain important clues to her future risk for heart attacks and strokes. In Juli's case, we detected a previously overlooked red flag for cardiovascular peril: Long before her heart attack, she'd suffered two miscarriages. In a 2015 study of more than sixty thousand women, those who had experienced at least two pregnancy losses were at 75 percent higher risk for heart disease as compared to women with no miscarriages, even when other health factors were taken into account.[25]

Many other studies have identified two other common pregnancy complications, gestational diabetes and preeclampsia, as strongly predictive of a woman's risk for heart disease and other chronic disorders. For example, having gestational diabetes (elevated blood sugar during pregnancy) puts women at eight times higher risk for subsequently developing type 2 diabetes, and doubles their risk for heart attacks, strokes, and other CV events, compared to moms-to-be whose blood sugar remains normal throughout their pregnancy.[26] Preeclampsia—a very dangerous or, in some cases, potentially life-threatening pregnancy complication marked by high blood pressure, protein in the urine, and sudden swelling of the legs, hands, and feet— doubles women's future risk for heart disease and quadruples it for heart failure, according to a recent study of more than 6.4 million women.[27] Researchers have also linked delivering a premature baby or having two or more pregnancies to increased risk for CVD.

What's the link between pregnancy and heart disease? Pregnancy acts as a natural stress test for women's hearts and blood vessels in several ways. To nourish the developing fetus, an expectant mom's blood volume increases by about 50 percent during the first trimester and remains high throughout the pregnancy.[28] This dramatic rise in blood volume forces the heart to pump much harder than usual; the heart rate typically increases by ten to fifteen beats per minute. Like many young women with heart problems, Juli wondered if the stress of pregnancy would be safe for her. We were able to reassure her that like many women with heart disease, she could have a successful pregnancy and recommended that her prenatal care be managed by a high-risk obstetrician, while we would continue her cardiovascular care.

Four years after surviving two heart attacks, Juli and her husband welcomed a son, Soren, to their family, as a little brother to Selah. She was so excited that she texted us from the delivery room, saying, "Wow, we did it! Thanks so much for getting us here!" Later, she brought Soren to our center so we could meet this adorable little fellow with fuzzy red hair that looked like a mini-mohawk. "I'm over the moon with joy," she told us, as we cradled Soren in our arms. "Having Soren seemed even more miraculous than giving birth the first time."

Is Hormone Replacement Therapy Helpful or Harmful to Women's Hearts?

Introduced in the 1960s, hormone replacement therapy (HRT) reached its zenith of popularity in the 1990s, when it was widely prescribed to postmenopausal women for long-term use, both to relieve hot flashes and other vexing menopause symptoms and as a "fountain of youth" that purported to roll back the years, benefiting everything from women's looks, sex life, and bone density to their heart health. Over the past two decades, however, there has been intense scientific controversy about the cardiovascular effects of HRT, fueled by wildly conflicting studies.

In the early 2000s, millions of women were scared away from HRT by frightening media reports about the potential dangers of its most common form: combination therapy, which combines doses of two hormones that regulate women's menstrual cycles— estrogen and progesterone. This type of HRT is the only option for women who have not had a hysterectomy, since the other form of HRT, which only contains estrogen, raises risk for uterine cancer. The addition of progesterone prevents this problem.

In 2002, data from the Women's Health Initiative (WHI), a large, U.S. government–run clinical trial, triggered an avalanche of alarm by reporting large increases in heart attacks, strokes, blood clots, heart disease, and breast cancer in women who received HRT that contained the hormones estrogen and progesterone, compared to women who had received a placebo.[29] At the time, these findings were deemed so scary that the estrogen-and-progesterone arm of the trial was immediately halted for safety reasons, and two years later, the estrogen-only arm was also stopped after increased rates of heart attacks and strokes were reported among participants who took that type of HRT.

Flash forward to 2012, when researchers reanalyzed the WHI data and reported that millions of women were suffering needlessly from menopause symptoms that could have been safely relieved with HRT. Other studies were published around the same time reporting that the use of HRT soon after menopause and in younger women (fifty to fifty-nine) was beneficial to cardiovascular health and *lowered* risk for heart disease.[30] For example, a 2012 study suggested that in women under sixty, HRT may even be *more* beneficial to the heart than statins or low-dose aspirin.

These and other studies with similar findings inspired a theory that's been dubbed "the timing hypothesis." It holds that there is a critical "window of opportunity" after menopause during which HRT helps ward off CVD in recently menopausal women who are under sixty, while not providing the same benefits in older women. Proponents of this hypothesis point out that women enrolled in the WHI were older (average sixty-three) and, on average, had started HRT twelve years after their periods had stopped. The trial, which sought to find out if HRT helped prevent heart disease and other chronic illnesses, even included first-time HRT users as old as seventy-eight.

Even today, more than a decade after this still-popular theory was first proposed, the American Heart Association and the U.S. Preventive Services Task Force continue to recommend *against* taking HRT for the prevention of any chronic illness, including heart disease, in either younger or older postmenopausal women. Understandably, this ongoing controversy has left women confused and concerned when faced with a thorny decision after menopause: Should they take HRT? Up to 80 percent of women experience vexing symptoms during and after the menopausal transition, which can sometimes be severe and persist for years. These include hot flashes, night sweats, mood swings, bladder-control issues (including frequent or urgent urination), trouble concentrating, diminished libido, vaginal dryness, and painful sex.

Loss of estrogen after menopause is also associated with several factors that elevate risk for CVD, including increases in blood pressure, lipid levels, vascular inflammation, reduced glucose tolerance, and changes in body fat distribution, leading to a larger waistline and more belly fat. In addition, postmenopausal women often experience sleep disturbances or insomnia, both of which also magnify the threat of developing arterial disease. A 2020 study found that women who experience early menopause, either naturally or due to a hysterectomy, before forty-one are nearly three times more likely to develop chronic illnesses—including heart disease, stroke, diabetes, high blood pressure, asthma, breast cancer, and osteoporosis (brittle bones that can lead to fractures)—compared to women whose periods stopped when they were fifty or older.[31]

What's the bottom line on HRT, the timing hypothesis, and heart health after menopause? To find out, a 2019 analysis pooled data from thirty-five randomized, controlled clinical trials (the gold standard of scientific research) that included more than forty thousand postmenopausal women.[32] The researchers then compared rates of fatal and nonfatal cardiovascular events in women under sixty with those in women over sixty. They found that both younger and older HRT users were at increased risk for stroke, mini-stroke (transient ischemic attack), and blood clots, compared to women the same age who didn't use HRT, and that risk for these events rose with age among women who take hormones. However, younger HRT users were not at increased risk for fatal or nonfatal heart problems, including heart attacks.

Here's our takeaway: We recommend that the HRT risk/benefit analysis needs to be personalized for each woman, factoring in her age, medical and family history, and health concerns. As one ob/gyn recently put it, "Each patient is like a Rubik's Cube and you have to find the right solution for her. Hormones are neither a panacea nor a weapon of mass destruction." Personalized care is one of the cornerstones of our AHA for Life plan, so we believe in sharing the latest science with women and empowering them to make a truly informed decision about what's right for their bodies. *We recommend that if you do decide to take HRT, after weighing the risks and benefits discussed in this chapter and consulting your medical provider, that treatment should start soon after menopause, at the lowest possible dose for symptom relief, taken for the shortest time possible.*

Also talk to your provider about non-pill options. HRT is now available in a wide range of forms, including sprays, gels, skin patches, vaginal rings, and suppositories. Applying HRT topically reduces the systemic effects by reducing the amount of estrogen in your bloodstream, which may decrease risk for arterial and other side effects. The delivery method should be matched to the symptoms being treated. For example, pills and skin patches can be helpful with a wide range of symptoms, including hot flashes, while low-dose vaginal preparations (inserted in the form of a ring, cream, or suppository) can be an excellent option to relieve vaginal dryness, the most common culprit for painful sex.

For postmenopausal women with vaginal dryness and atrophy (age-related shrinkage), vaginal HRT really can be a fountain of youth. It improves lubrication and, over time, gradually makes vaginal walls become plumper and more elastic as they start to regain some of their youthful folds and creases—all of which heightens sexual pleasure. As one gynecologist we know puts it, "The vagina is one place where women *want* to have wrinkles!"

That said, we also emphasize that menopause is not a disease—it's a natural condition and not all women experience symptoms. If you do, we encourage you to talk to your provider about all the options to manage them, including lifestyle improvements. For example, a study of more than seventeen thousand postmenopausal women found that those who shed at least ten pounds or 10 percent of their body weight over a year were much more likely to end hot flashes and night sweats, compared to a control group of women whose weight was unchanged.[33] And if you smoke, here's some powerful motivation to snuff out the deadly nicotine habit: Female smokers have twice as many hot flashes as nonsmokers and also reach menopause a year earlier than those who don't light up.[34]

Regular exercise can reduce the severity of hot flashes, improve sleep quality, reduce depression and anxiety, and help you avoid weight gain, which is a common problem in postmenopausal women. Middle-aged spread can have serious implications for your health, since it's the leading indicator that you're at risk for insulin resistance, which in turn escalates risk for heart attacks, strokes, dementia, type 2 diabetes, and other chronic diseases. Fortunately, this dangerous disorder is both preventable and highly treatable—if it's caught early. In fact, as you'll learn in chapter nine, in about 70 percent of cases, IR can be reversed without medication by making two simple lifestyle changes. In part two, we'll also look at other common reasons why plaque attacks—and the best ways to fight back against this wily predator. Turn the page to learn our top ten prevention tips for women and why they can save your life and those of the women you care about.

Action Step: Stop Heart Disease in Its Tracks with Our Top Ten Prevention Tips for Women

Get educated.

The more women know about heart disease, the easier it is for them to partner with their healthcare providers and avoid their leading health threat. Every year, heart disease claims the lives of nearly 300,000 U.S. women. That's about one woman every sixty seconds![35] What's more, older women who survive a heart attack are twice as likely to develop dementia and cognitive impairment as those with no history of heart problems.[36] The wonderful news is that this disease is both preventable and highly treatable. Women need to be their own best advocates, demand top-notch personalized care, and make cardiovascular wellness a priority. The advocacy group Go Red for Women reports that more than 670,000 women with a family history of heart disease have saved their own lives by making healthy choices—leading to three hundred fewer deaths a day among women at high genetic risk. Throughout this book, you'll meet men and women who are living proof that once patients are empowered with the knowledge they need to protect and enhance their heart and brain health, they take the action steps that lead to arterial wellness and a health span that matches their life span.

Move more.

Exercise has such powerful mental and physical benefits that it's been called the ultimate wonder drug. To keep your heart healthy, the American Heart Association and the BaleDoneen Method recommend a minimum of 150 minutes of moderate physical activity a week, such as walking, jogging, biking, or swimming.[37] Workouts that target belly fat also have important benefits: A recent study reported that losing just two inches from your waist can significantly reduce blood pressure, cholesterol, and other heart attack risks.[38] Always check with your medical provider before starting a new workout to make sure it's right for you.

Follow a healthy lifestyle.

An optimal lifestyle reduces heart attack and stroke risk by up to 90 percent![39] Take excellent care of your heart by following these simple tips: Shake the sugar habit. A high-sugar diet has been shown to triple the risk for fatal CVD, while a diet that's high in fruit and vegetables has the opposite effect.[40] Maintain a healthy weight: If getting to your ideal weight seems daunting, start with a more modest goal. Shedding as few as seven to ten pounds reduces risk for type 2 diabetes (a major risk factor for heart disease) by up to 70 percent, even if you are already pre-diabetic.[41] Look for ways to tame tension: A large study in fifty-two countries found that psychological factors, including stress, nearly tripled heart attack risk.[42] You'll find tips on easy, fun ways to dial down your stress level in chapter thirteen.

No nicotine.

Every year, exposure to secondhand smoke kills an estimated forty-one thousand Americans, with heart disease accounting for nearly thirty-four thousand of these fatalities and lung cancer the culprit in seven thousand, reports the CDC.[43] Smoking (and other types of nicotine use, such as vaping or chewing tobacco) triples the risk for fatal CVD. What's more, young women who smoke are at more than thirteen times higher risk of heart attack than nonsmokers the same age![44] Even one cigarette daily has been shown to dramatically increase a woman's risk for heart attack, stroke, cancer, or early death.[45] Conversely, quitting smoking at any age reduces risk for numerous serious or fatal diseases, and kicking the habit before forty cuts risk for early death by about 90 percent, as compared to continuing to smoke.[46]

Check blood pressure.

Nearly 50 percent of U.S. adults—108 million people—have high blood pressure (a reading of 130/80 mm Hg—millimeters of mercury—or above) and millions more have elevated blood pressure: systolic blood pressure (the top number) between 120 and 129 and diastolic pressure (the bottom number) below 80.[47] Most of them aren't aware of their condition or don't have it under control. Yet high blood pressure is highly treatable with weight loss, dietary and lifestyle changes, and, in many cases, medications. Even very small reductions can be lifesaving for people with hypertension: A very large 2021 study found that for each five mm Hg drop in blood pressure, a patient's risk for heart attacks, strokes, and other major cardiovascular events in the next four years fell by 10 percent![48] Discuss your numbers with your medical provider. In chapter fifteen, we'll take a closer look at the latest blood pressure guidelines and the best ways to reduce your blood pressure if it's too high.

Have your cholesterol checked at least once a year.

Starting at twenty, have your cholesterol checked annually (or more frequently, if advised by your provider) with both the conventional test and the ApoB test discussed in chapter four. If you haven't had your levels of lipoprotein (a) checked yet, consider this: Being kept in the dark about this twenty-dollar blood test nearly cost Juli her life. Our testing revealed that she had high levels of this dangerous cholesterol, which is now being treated with niacin. Had she been tested and treated sooner, she might have avoided two terrifying trips to the ER in the same week, while in the throes of a heart attack.

Get checked for prediabetes.

It's very common for people to be diagnosed with diabetes or insulin resistance (IR), a disorder also known as prediabetes, shortly after they suffer a heart attack. While these conditions may sound unrelated, IR is the underlying cause of 70 percent of heart attacks and many strokes. It's also one of the root causes of many chronic diseases, including dementia. Our studies and other research have proven that the most accurate screening test for IR and diabetes is the two-hour oral glucose tolerance test (OGTT), which will be discussed more fully in chapter nine, along with the best ways to prevent insulin resistance and diabetes.

Get dental care at least twice a year.

If you haven't seen your dentist lately, here's some powerful motivation to make an appointment: Keeping your gums healthy could help you avoid a heart attack! Conversely, having peri-odontal (gum) disease due to certain high-risk oral bacteria can *cause* cardiovascular disease. In chapter ten, you'll find our easy four-step plan to optimize your oral health, which includes being checked for gum disease and high-risk oral pathogens and a program of home care to disinfect your mouth.

Sleep well.

Regardless of other risk factors, people who don't sleep enough face an increased threat of CVD. In fact, one study of about 200,000 people reported that those who snoozed less than five hours a night were nearly twice as likely to suffer a stroke as people who slept six to eight hours a night.[49] Skimping on slumber has also been linked to higher risk for heart attacks, obesity, cancer, high blood pressure, heart failure, chest pain, irregular heartbeats, and diabetes.[50] The sweet spot for slumber is six to eight hours a night. In part three, you'll find natural ways to get the sound, refreshing sleep you need for optimal heart health, all of which are backed by solid science.

Save a life.

Tell and teach a friend what you learned in this chapter. You could save a life! And please help us spread an important message: The cat in the gutter doesn't attack out of nowhere after women's periods stop. All women are at potential risk, even young, seemingly healthy premenopausal women like Juli. In the next chapter, we'll look at why rates of stroke are skyrocketing in young adults, particularly women. We'll also tell you about a simple, noninvasive test that can reveal if you're at risk in just fifteen minutes and how we used it to solve two medical mysteries that had baffled numerous specialists.

Why Plaque Attacks and What to Do About It

CHAPTER 6

Lifesaving Lessons We've Learned from Looking at More than Ten Thousand Arteries

"All the secrets of the world worth knowing are hiding in plain sight."

— ROBIN SLOAN, *MR. PENUMBRA'S 24-HOUR BOOKSTORE*

Melinda and Nikki don't know each other, but they have a lot in common. They're both slim, physically fit nonsmokers who eat a heart-healthy diet. Both are forty-something moms and get regular medical checkups, and both have consistently been praised for their excellent lifestyle. Melinda, a nutrition counselor and personal trainer from Sherman, Texas, has spent many years teaching yoga, cycling, Pilates, and fitness group and boot camp classes. She and her husband, Casey, are particularly enthusiastic about CrossFit and weightlifting. Not only do they exercise intensely, but the couple used to own a gym where they coached others on their two favorite workouts. Nikki, a second-grade teacher from Spokane, Washington, is so dedicated to fitness that she gets up at four a.m. every day to run several miles before work. Her doctor has frequently told her that, "You are the healthiest patient I've seen all day." Melinda has received many similar compliments from her doctor.

Yet both of these athletic young moms suffered seemingly inexplicable cardiovascular events when they were in their early forties. While watching a football game with her family and friends, Nikki suddenly developed a stabbing pain behind her left eye. "I started seeing double and had to close my eyes, then everything started spinning around," she says. "I got very nauseated and became so dizzy that I couldn't walk in a straight line." The headache intensified and she started vomiting. Assuming that the culprit was a virus or something she'd eaten, she went to bed early, figuring that she'd sleep it off.

The next day, her symptoms grew worse and she landed in the ICU, where tests showed she'd suffered a stroke. "Getting that diagnosis at forty-two was surreal," she adds. "It took a long time to sink in and I kept thinking, *How can this be? I thought I was doing everything right.* And I have no family history of anything like this. The neurologists said, 'We're not sure why this happened, but we're putting you on a statin because that's what we do,' even though my cholesterol was normal. Later, I was told that I didn't need the statin. After I left the hospital, I went from doctor to doctor, trying to get answers and do everything I could to stay alive."

Melinda had a similar ordeal. When she developed nausea and vertigo, she initially chalked it up to Ménière's disease, an inner ear disorder that she'd experienced in the past. Over the next several days, the dizzy spells and spinning sensation intensified—and she had a persistent sense of uneasiness, as if something was terribly wrong. She consulted a doctor, who ordered a brain MRI. "I was shocked and frightened when the scan showed that I'd had a stroke," says the then forty-three-year-old nutritionist and CrossFit coach. "There were never any red flags in my checkups. My blood pressure and cholesterol were always fine and I'm a lifelong fitness advocate and exercise enthusiast.

Maintaining a healthy lifestyle—and training people how to do vigorous, enjoyable workouts and eat an optimal diet—isn't just my job; it's what I love."

Her doctor prescribed a statin, then referred her to a medical center that specialized in neurological disorders. There, she received what the medical community calls the million-dollar workup: an extensive—and extremely expensive—battery of diagnostic tests to look for the cause of her stroke. Although Melinda doesn't know the exact cost of her evaluation, most of which was covered by her health plan, it certainly seemed comprehensive. She underwent MRI, CT, and ultrasound scans of her brain and its arteries, numerous blood tests to check for clotting disorders and other conditions, and even an invasive procedure to examine her heart for blood-flow abnormalities, with none found. Her doctors also hooked her up to a portable monitor that continuously tracked her heart rhythms for a month, with no irregular heartbeats detected.

After weeks of being poked, prodded, and scanned by various specialists, she was told that her healthcare team considered her case a medical mystery. "One of the doctors said that 25 percent of the time, they can't pinpoint what happened," recalls Melinda, who also consulted her family doctor and her gynecologist. "Although it was unsettling that none of these specialists could explain my stroke, they told me they'd checked for everything." Although she never took the statin—believing it to be unnecessary—her symptoms disappeared. "I started feeling great again, so I tried to put the mystery of my stroke on a back burner and go on with my everyday life."

That proved harder than the young nutritionist had expected. "Over the next several months, I started having other health issues, including a flare-up of a hip injury, and worried about every little twinge or symptom," she adds. "Sometimes it was hard to sleep at night and I was feeling more and more stressed. Sometimes my heart would start racing or I'd get flushed. I was having some confusion and brain fog, then I started having the same uneasy feeling I did during the stroke. I didn't know if it was paranoia—or a warning sign that I might be headed for another one—but I knew I urgently needed answers."

A Global Medical Mystery?

Before we share the lifesaving lessons that we've learned from looking at more than ten thousand arteries—and why it only took us fifteen minutes to solve the mystery that baffled all of Nikki and Melinda's doctors—let's take a look at some alarming stroke trends and how most doctors evaluate patients who have suffered these potentially life-threatening events. Strokes rank as one of the most expensive—and devastating—medical conditions. Every forty seconds, someone in the U.S. has a stroke and every four minutes someone dies from one.[1] Of those who survive, only 10 percent make a full recovery and 25 percent recover with minor impairments, according to the American Stroke Association. The rest experience moderate to severe impairments, with about 10 percent of stroke survivors requiring care in a nursing home or other long-term care facility.

Although most people think of strokes as primarily being a threat to the elderly, rates among younger adults, such as Melinda and Nikki, are skyrocketing. A very large 2017 study found that between 1995 and 2012, U.S. hospitalizations for ischemic strokes—the most common type of stroke—nearly doubled for men eighteen to forty-four and rose by more than 53 percent among women in this age group.[2] The study also found that young adults who suffer these events are twice as likely as their healthy counterparts to have three or more of the following stroke risk factors: high blood pressure, diabetes, obesity, tobacco use, and abnormal cholesterol levels.

Since then, the incidence of stroke has continued to climb

among young people, particularly women. A large 2020 study reported that women twenty-five to forty-four had a 30 percent higher rate of stroke than their male peers—even though young women have a much lower rate of traditional cardiovascular risk factors than their male counterparts.[3] Recent studies in Europe have also reported that rates of stroke are rising faster in young women than in men the same age, while the incidence of strokes among older adults of both sexes hasn't changed much in recent years.[4,5]

"It has been a mystery why the number of strokes in young adults has been growing," the 2020 study's lead author, Michelle Hu Leppert, MD, assistant professor of neurology at the University of Colorado School of Medicine in Aurora, told *Medscape Medical News*.[6] "This is a trend seen worldwide." Some neurologists took the findings as a call to conduct even more exhaustive investigations of the causes of strokes in younger adults, who are more likely than older people to suffer cryptogenic (medically unexplained) strokes.

Finding the Hidden Cause of Most Strokes

Many experts argue that devoting more attention and healthcare spending on extensive diagnostic testing—such as Melinda's million-dollar workup—to check for rare causes *after* young people have already suffered strokes could distract medical providers from a lifesaving public health mission: preventing these events from occurring in the first place through wider use of screening tests. (Examinations to check seemingly healthy, symptom-free people for hidden signs of disease.) If you do have symptoms, *diagnostic* tests are used to find out what's triggering them.

The authors of the 2017 study discussed above recommend that cardiovascular screening starts when people are in their teens or twenties. That's because their study found that micro-vascular and large-vessel arterial disease are increasingly common culprits in strokes among younger adults, starting at thirty. Therefore, they advocate that the best way to prevent the tragedy of strokes at an early age is to identify at-risk patients through screening, before their disease becomes severe enough to trigger these events.

In this chapter, we'll share six lifesaving lessons we've learned from looking at scans of more than ten thousand arteries. You'll also get an overview of the many benefits of vascular imaging, which has been a vital part of the BaleDoneen Method for more than two decades. After we started using it in our practice to identify and guide the treatment of at-risk patients, rates of heart attacks, strokes, and new-onset type 2 diabetes in our patients fell to near zero. We also observed that our patients had extremely low risk for developing chronic diseases of aging, including dementia, cancer, erectile dysfunction, heart failure, and chronic kidney disease.

Yet even today, despite decades of evidence from numerous large studies about the potentially lifesaving value of vascular imaging, the latest guidelines for the prevention of CVD still don't advocate its routine use. Think about it. If ER doctors suspected that you had a broken leg, would you want them to analyze your risk factors, or would you want them to order an X-ray? Almost all medical specialties use imaging technology to look at the organ they are treating, yet most cardiovascular care providers still rely on guesswork to decide which patients need treatment. A doctor we know has compared this approach to "throwing medication-tipped darts in the dark and hoping they hit the right patients."

Without the benefits of looking at the patient's arteries, cardiovascular disease has remained the leading killer of Americans. In chapter seven, we will provide an in-depth guide to commonly used vascular imaging tests. However, it's important to realize that there is no one specific test that provides a complete evaluation of your cardiovascular health. That's why this book highlights the best tests—including vascular imaging—to provide a comprehensive, personalized assessment of your overall risk for heart attacks, strokes, and dementia. We also recommend that testing, including vascular imaging, be personalized based on your age, medical history, genetics, and cardiovascular red flags. Here is a look at six lifesaving lessons we have learned from looking at more than ten thousand arteries, and how they can help pilot you to the right destination: optimal arterial health.

Lifesaving Lesson No. 1: To Find Out Which Patients Are in Cardiovascular Danger, You Need to Look at Their Arteries—Not Just Their Risk Factors.

When we met Nikki, it was easy to see why her doctor had considered her to be the healthiest patient he'd seen all day. She looked lean, fit, and strong. In fact, she told us that after her stroke, she'd competed in two half-marathons and had set a personal speed record in one of them. Melinda also said that she was feeling great physically, but continued to struggle with the emotional aftermath of her stroke: She felt stressed, anxious, and frightened nearly every day, not knowing why this potentially life-threatening event had occurred or if another one might be looming in her future.

What happened to Nikki and Melinda isn't as unusual as it might sound. About 80 percent of strokes—and 70 percent of fatal heart attacks—occur in people who have never previously been diagnosed with CVD. Very often, these men and women had no prior symptoms of arterial disease, which typically develops silently. As Nikki and Melinda's cases highlight, these events can occur in young people with none of the traditional Framingham risk factors we discussed in chapter four. Indeed, when we plugged their pre-stroke numbers into the American Heart Association/American College of Cardiology's latest risk scoring tool, it estimated their chances of having a heart attack or stroke in the next ten years at a mere 0.1 percent (the lowest possible risk score). Therefore, neither woman would have been considered a candidate for any type of treatment that could have helped prevent her stroke, such as low-dose aspirin or other medications.

Lifesaving Lesson No. 2: To Find Arterial Disease, You Have to Look in the Right Place.

Although Nikki and Melinda had been told that their various specialists had "checked for everything," both women were convinced that their medical teams had missed something. They were right: We immediately noticed some glaring omissions in their seemingly comprehensive workups when we reviewed their medical records. Both women had been checked for arterial blockages and narrowing in the neck's two largest arteries, the carotids, using an ultrasound test called carotid duplex, which will be discussed more fully in the next chapter. Because no blockages were found, their doctors concluded that they didn't have atherosclerosis, the leading cause of ischemic stroke in men and women of all ages.

Although this test sounds similar to the cIMT test you read about in chapter two—and can be valuable for patients who have had a stroke or transient ischemic attack (TIA, also known as a mini-stroke)—it has a very different purpose. Carotid duplex only evaluates one aspect of blood vessel health: the rate of blood flow through the artery's lumen (the "pipe" through which blood flows). It's similar to the police using a radar gun to see how fast vehicles are traveling on the highway. But just as a radar gun can't alert police to dangerous situations that are *not* blocking traffic—such as a fiery car crash at the side of the road, with injured accident victims screaming for help—carotid duplex can't detect plaque inside the arterial wall, even if it's highly inflamed (the kind that sparks heart attacks and strokes).

Therefore, the lack of blockages in Melinda and Nikki's arteries was *not* proof that they were free of atherosclerosis. What most patients—and many doctors—don't know is that 99 percent of plaque—including areas of highly inflamed plaque—does not block blood flow at all, according to a startling 2004 study by Dr. Steven Nissen of the Cleveland Clinic.[7] These findings suggest that tests that only check for blockages, such as carotid duplex and treadmill stress tests, may miss up to 99 percent of people at risk for heart attacks and strokes. Melinda and Nikki are cases in point. When they were checked with the cIMT test discussed more fully in the next chapter, this fifteen-minute ultrasound scan detected plaque in their neck arteries, solving the mystery of why they'd had strokes.

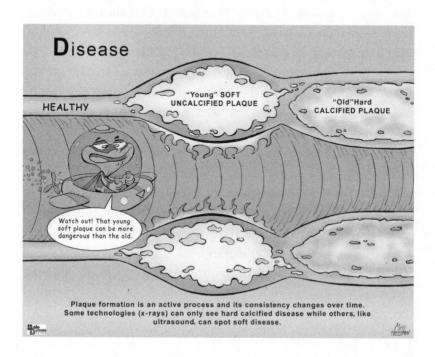

Plaque formation is an active process and its consistency changes over time. Some technologies (x-rays) can only see hard calcified disease while others, like ultrasound, can spot soft disease.

Lifesaving Lesson No. 3: Vascular Imaging Helps Save Lives AND Money.

Unfortunately, insurance plans may not pay for some of the vascular screening tests discussed in this chapter. One of our patients, a nurse, recently told us that her primary care doctor doesn't even tell his patients about these tests because he thinks they wouldn't want to pay for them out of pocket. She is a firm believer in our method and educated her doctor about their value. If you think you are too young—or too healthy—to need vascular screening, which costs about one hundred to two hundred dollars, consider this: Only through vascular imaging did Melinda's husband, Casey, find out that he had a ticking time bomb in his arteries that almost certainly would have caused a stroke or heart attack, if it had gone untreated. Such screening could also have helped Melinda and Nikki avoid potentially life-threatening events, huge medical bills, and the stress of living in daily fear of having yet another seemingly inexplicable stroke.

Rising rates of strokes in young adults are a key factor in the skyrocketing cost of these events, a 2020 study found.[8] The researchers calculated the total annual cost of strokes in the U.S. at $103.5 billion—a number that the American Heart Association has predicted will soar to an astounding $2.2 trillion in 2050, putting a massive strain on the U.S. economy. Currently, younger stroke victims account for the majority of the direct costs (such as medical treatment), even though strokes are more common among older adults. That's because younger adults are more likely to have seemingly inexplicable strokes, leading to exhaustive medical testing to look for the cause, such as Melinda's million-dollar workup.

Along with expensive diagnostic tests and the other short-term costs—such as an ICU stay, which can cost up to $30,000 a day at some U.S. hospitals—younger stroke survivors also face a much heavier long-term financial burden than their older counterparts. There are two reasons for this, the researchers report. First, most stroke victims don't make a full recovery and need ongoing treatment for lingering impairments. As a result, medical bills for someone who has a stroke at a young age will be far higher than those for an elderly stroke survivor, since the older person has a shorter post-stroke life span. Second, people whose stroke occurs at a younger age also have much higher indirect costs, such as missed workdays, lost wages, career setbacks, and/ or unemployment due to illness, as compared to someone over sixty-five, who may already be retired.

When the researchers crunched the numbers, they found that strokes cost younger adults $2.2 billion a year more than they do older adults — even though strokes occur at a higher rate among the elderly. On average, each young stroke survivor incurred $4,317 more in direct and indirect costs annually after their event than a healthy person of the same age.[9] Given the devastating financial and physical toll of strokes — which currently rank as the third leading cause of death in the U.S. and the leading cause of long-term disability — researchers and medical providers are looking for the most cost-effective ways to identify at-risk patients *before* a stroke occurs. We'd argue that compared to the cost of a stroke, the imaging tests we recommend, each of which costs two hundred dollars or less, offer an extremely safe, accurate, and relatively inexpensive screening tool to help save lives, hearts, brains, *and* healthcare dollars.[10]

Lifesaving Lesson No. 4: Even Small Plaques Can Be Potentially Lethal, If Untreated.

As it turned out, Melinda had a much smaller area of plaque than her husband did, yet she had a stroke and he didn't. The reason is simple. Any size "cat" can cause a cardiovascular event. What matters most is how "hot" the cat is. Decades of research have shown that the overwhelming majority of heart attacks and strokes occur in people with nonobstructive plaque.[11] The most frequent culprit is inflammation that causes plaque inside the artery wall to rupture explosively, like a volcano spewing molten lava. Therefore, we had a second mystery to solve: What caused the cat to leap out of the gutter? In Melinda's case, we found an important clue in her medical records: Shortly after her stroke, she had been treated for a severely infected tooth, which required extraction. It's our belief, supported by solid scientific data, that inflammation from the then-undiagnosed infection in her mouth was a major culprit in her stroke.

In a 2019 study of blood clots removed from patients' brains after an ischemic stroke, 84 percent contained DNA from oral bacteria.[12] The researchers—who did a previous study of clots removed from heart attack patients, with similar findings— report that oral bacteria have several harmful effects on the blood vessel lining, making people more susceptible to developing arterial plaque. In those who already have it, these pathogens promote arterial inflammation that can lead to plaque rupture and the formation of a blood clot, which in turn can trigger a heart attack or stroke.

In Nikki's case, we also checked a part of the head that most doctors ignore: her mouth. A dental evaluation revealed that she had previously undiagnosed periodontal (gum) disease. About 50 percent of Americans over thirty have this chronic oral infection, which has also been linked in very recent studies to increased risk for developing memory impairment and loss. Like many of these patients, Nikki, who has a beautiful smile, was unaware that she had high levels of periodontal bacteria circulating in her bloodstream until she had a simple oral-swab DNA test that will be discussed in chapter ten.

Lifesaving Lesson No. 5: Arterial Imaging Helps Patients Get the Right Diagnosis and Potentially Lifesaving Treatment.

During her initial visit to our center, Melinda told us that she'd never taken the statin her doctors had prescribed, believing it to be unnecessary. One of Nikki's doctors had also prescribed a statin after her stroke, then another doctor told her that she didn't need it, leading her to quit this treatment. Actually, both women did need a statin. As we'll explain more fully in chapter fourteen, statin therapy is one of the cornerstones of our evidence-based disease reversal plan for patients who have arterial plaque.

Very large studies have shown that this medication helps prevent heart attacks, strokes, and deaths from cardiovascular causes in people at increased risk for these events—even if they have normal cholesterol levels. What many patients—and some doctors—don't know is that statin therapy has powerful anti-inflammatory effects and reduces risk for blood clots. That's why it's a key component of our disease reversal plan. Therefore, finding out that Melinda and Nikki had atherosclerosis was central to determining the best treatments to prevent repeat events.

Although Melinda thought that she didn't have a cholesterol problem, a twenty-dollar blood test revealed that she had extremely high levels of lipoprotein (a), or Lp(a), the dangerous cholesterol that you read about in chapter four. In fact, she had the highest level of any patient we've ever tested at our center! In a 2019 study, people with the highest levels of Lp(a), which we call the mass murderer, had a 60 percent higher risk for having a stroke in the next ten years than those with the lowest levels.[13] The study included nearly fifty thousand initially healthy men and women.

Although Lp(a) was first discovered in 1963,[14] it wasn't

known to cause heart attacks and strokes until 2009, when three conclusive genetic studies involving hundreds of thousands of patients were published in *Journal of the American Medical Association* and *The New England Journal of Medicine*.[15] Linked to genes on chromosome 6, Lp(a) appears to be a genetic "misfire" that occurred millions of years ago. Only found in humans, Old World monkeys, and hedgehogs, Lp(a) can directly promote arterial disease through contributing to the buildup of cholesterol plaque inside the arterial wall, another 2019 study found. The researchers also reported that people with elevated levels of Lp(a) also have increased arterial wall inflammation, which may also explain why they are at high risk for heart attacks and strokes.[16]

Once plaque has formed, Lp(a) also contributes to heart attack and stroke risk in another way. It has an almost identical molecular makeup as plasminogen, a protein involved in blood clotting. That's hazardous because when a plaque rupture occurs, the body normally sends out two chemical signals. One of them tells the affected blood vessel to form a clot to close the breach, just as your body would form a scab over a cut. Because the body is smart and recognizes that clots circulating in your bloodstream can lead to heart attacks and strokes, it also sends out a second signal to dissolve the clot by breaking down plasminogen.

In people with elevated Lp(a), however, the body mistakenly tries to break down these cholesterol particles—instead of plasminogen—an action that has no effect on blood clots. Therefore, in these patients, the clotting signal wins out over the normally protective anti-clotting signal. To counteract these perils, we prescribed niacin (vitamin B3), which has been shown to be the most effective therapy for this disorder. There's also some evidence that keeping levels of LDL (bad) cholesterol as low as possible helps people with elevated Lp(a) avoid cardiovascular events.

Our testing also revealed that Melinda had elevated levels of another dangerous cholesterol most doctors don't check: ApoB. As you learned in chapter four, this twenty-dollar blood test can identify young adults at risk for heart attacks and strokes decades before *any* conventional risk factors manifest. Had any of her medical providers ordered this simple test, which is available through almost all medical labs, she could have gotten a comprehensive screening with the BaleDoneen Method at a small fraction of the cost of her million-dollar stroke workup. What's more, the lifesaving information provided by this test could have helped Melinda—and thousands of other young stroke victims—avoid developing the leading cause of these events: atherosclerosis.

Lifesaving Lesson No. 6: It's Never Too Late — or Too Soon — to Take Charge of Your Arterial Health.

In 1994, coauthor Brad Bale performed his first arterial scan—on himself. Due to his frightening family history, he'd always strived to take optimal care of his heart. Then forty-six, he was so fit that he'd completed a half Ironman race, climbed Mount Rainier, and then held the world record for one-day vertical feet in heli-skiing. To check for early signs of CVD, he consulted a cardiologist annually, who evaluated his heart health by hooking him up to an EKG (electrocardiogram) machine that monitored his heartbeat while he walked and then ran at increasing speeds on a treadmill. The aim is to see how the heart performs during the stress of exercise.

Brad always passed the stress test and breathed a sigh of relief, believing that he'd managed to dodge the disease that had killed several of his family members. And according to his Framingham Risk Score, his ten-year risk for a heart attack or stroke was only 2 percent. When a local cardiologist, Dr. Jerry Shields, purchased a new vascular imaging technology called electron beam tomography (EBT) in 1994, Brad asked to try it out, assuming the scan would confirm that he was in perfect heart health. Instead, the scan showed that despite his athletic lifestyle, Brad was a heart attack or stroke waiting to happen. In fact, he had such a high level of plaque in his coronary arteries that it was amazing that he hadn't already had one!

Brad often wishes that he'd been able to plug into the Bale-Doneen Method at a younger age, as coauthor Amy Doneen did. When we founded our personalized approach to arterial disease prevention and reversal in 2001, Brad was fifty-two and already had horribly diseased arteries. In fact, when his heart arteries were scanned with another imaging test, coronary artery calcium score (CACS), which will be discussed in more depth in the next chapter, his score of 1,756 was far above the number that has traditionally been considered to represent the highest possible risk for major cardiovascular events (a score of more than 300).

In other words, instead of having a cat in the gutter, Brad's coronary arteries were a lion's den packed with ferocious predators. With Amy as Brad's arteriologist over the last twenty years, her aim has been to stop the progression of his disease. Very often, it's impossible to get rid of the cat—even with optimal treatments—in patients with severely diseased arteries because they may have dozens or even hundreds of plaque deposits throughout their arterial tree. Instead, the goal is to stabilize soft, vulnerable plaque (the most dangerous kind) so it becomes calcified. Think of it as building very strong cages so the cats—or lions—can't leap out.

How effective was Brad's treatment? Compared to people with a score of 0 (indicating no calcified plaque was found), those with a score above 1,000 are at five times higher risk for suffering major cardiovascular events, such as heart attacks, strokes, or the need for emergency procedures to prevent these catastrophes, and have double the ten-year risk for death from any cause.[17] People with high CACS are also at increased risk for dementia, cancer, and other chronic diseases.[18] Compounding Brad's cardiovascular risk, he's a carrier of the 9P21 heart attack gene. Yet decades after Brad's initial diagnosis, he remains heart attack and stroke free, with no chronic diseases of any kind, thanks to the therapies we recommend in part three.

Coauthor Amy Doneen is often asked if she uses the Bale-Doneen Method for her own cardiovascular care. The answer is yes, as she also has genetic risks, including a family history of heart attacks, strokes, type 2 diabetes, and Alzheimer's disease. She also carries the heart attack gene and two other high-risk genes (KIF6 and Hp 2-2) that will be discussed in chapter eleven. With Brad as her arteriologist, she has been applying the BaleDoneen Method to her own care for the past twenty years. When she started being his patient in 2001, she was thirty-one and free of arterial disease. Amy is a passionate athlete and has completed more than twenty marathons, works out every day, and eats a diet based on her DNA. She also sees her dental provider every three months to safeguard her oral health. For the past twenty years, she's had her neck arteries scanned with cIMT annually, with no abnormalities of any kind detected. When she turned fifty, she also had her coronary arteries scanned with CACS, and received a score of 0.

Recognizing that everyone is at risk for CVD—and that risk rises with age—Amy plans to continue being screened for this disease with vascular imaging and the other potentially lifesaving tests recommended in this book. Recently, an inexpensive blood test revealed that she had low levels of vitamin D. Nearly 40 percent of U.S. adults, many of whom are undiagnosed, are deficient in the sunshine vitamin, putting them at increased risk for heart attacks, strokes, heart failure, type 1 and 2 diabetes, high blood pressure, osteoporosis (the brittle-bone disease that leads to fractures), several common, deadly cancers, and a wide range of other maladies.[19] Once diagnosed, low levels of vitamin D are easily treated with a vitamin supplement.

Throughout this book, we'll alert you to simple steps that will help you protect and enhance your arterial health, enabling you to learn the most important lifesaving lesson of all: With the optimal care and lifestyle advised by our AHA for Life Plan, arterial disease is preventable, treatable, and beatable! What's more, taking action now, by getting the inexpensive vascular screening we recommend in the next chapter, can help you avoid landing in the ICU with a seemingly inexplicable stroke, as Melinda and Nikki did.

Action Step: Talk to Your Provider About This Easy — and Often Overlooked — Way to Find Out If You Have Arterial Plaque.

Before seeing new patients, we always carefully review their medical and dental records, including any imaging studies the person may have already had, such as mammograms, medical or dental X-rays, and CT scans. Patients are often surprised to learn that imaging studies performed for other purposes can sometimes reveal the presence of plaque, thus enabling the diagnosis of arterial disease without the need for a vascular scan. For example, research has recently revealed that mammograms, which are widely used to check for early signs of breast cancer, can also detect hidden signs of heart disease.

In a 2016 study, 292 seemingly healthy women received both a mammogram and a CT scan called coronary artery calcium scoring (CACS).[20] As we will explain more fully later in chapter seven, this widely used vascular imaging test checks for calcified plaque in the arteries that feed the heart. In the study, half of the women under sixty had breast artery calcification (BAC), indicating plaque in those arteries, and of this group, 83 percent also had coronary artery calcium, indicating that they had heart disease. The researchers reported that BAC was a very strong predictor of coronary artery disease in symptom-free women — and was more accurate than standard cardiovascular risk factors for the identification of high-risk women. An earlier study, conducted in 2008, reported that women with BAC were more than twice as likely to have suffered a cardiovascular event as those without it.[21]

Similarly, a 2006 study found that routine panoramic X-rays performed by dental providers to evaluate patients' oral health can reveal calcification of the carotid arteries (plaque that contains flecks of calcium).[22] The researchers reported that among men with this dental finding, 26 percent suffered a cardiovascular event within the next 3.5 years. Other studies have found similar links to increased CV risk in people whose arm or leg X-rays, brain imaging, or abdominal scans had detected areas of calcification.[23] The key takeaway is that if calcified plaque is found in *any* of your arteries—not just those that supply the heart and brain—it is a strong indication that you are at potential risk for a heart attack, stroke, or dementia. That means you need the comprehensive BaleDoneen evaluation recommended in this book to identify the root causes and best treatments to reverse your disease.

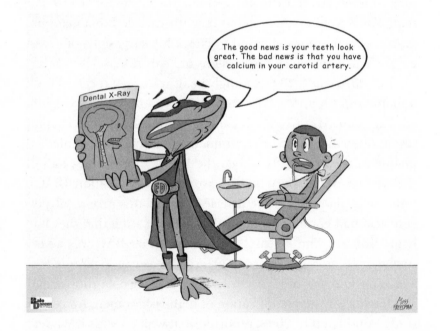

If a careful review of your imaging records, including your dental X-rays, doesn't reveal any plaque, talk to your provider about the pros and cons of having vascular scanning to formally evaluate your arterial health. In the next chapter, we'll provide an in-depth guide to the available imaging options to evaluate blood vessel health. We recommend cardiovascular screening that includes vascular scanning for everyone forty or older, or younger patients with any of the red flags in chapter three or a family history of CVD or diabetes. If you've already been diagnosed with arterial disease, you'll also find information on the best imaging tests to evaluate if your treatment is working.

CHAPTER 7
Tests That Could Save Your Life

"Vision is the art of seeing what is invisible to others."
— JONATHAN SWIFT

Two of our patients, Elaine, sixty-four, and Courtney, seventy-three, have been happily married for decades and have four adult children. However, they have dramatically different health profiles and goals. During her first visit to our center, Elaine said that her top priority was to avoid ending up like her mother, Joan, who had died a few months earlier. "The last three years of her life were a living hell due to vascular dementia," the author from Alberton, Montana, told us. "Some days, she'd seem fine and on others, she'd say, 'I'm cracking up! I'm losing everything!' Watching her deteriorate before my eyes was heartbreaking and knowing that this was the result of small-vessel disease has made me determined to do everything in my power to avoid the same fate."

Elaine has also lost several relatives to heart attacks and strokes. Courtney, on the other hand, has no family history of these events or dementia. "All of my relatives have lived into their late eighties or nineties, and my father was always as healthy as a horse. He died at eighty-six from complications of a fall that occurred while he was fishing," the airline pilot instructor reported. With a note of pride, Courtney added that doctors were often surprised that he wasn't on any medications. Indeed, other than persistently high LDL cholesterol, he'd never been diagnosed with any chronic condition. Therefore, he anticipated that his evaluation at our center would confirm that he was on track to live a long and healthy life.

Conversely, over the previous thirty years, Elaine has been hit with a series of seemingly unrelated health issues, including gallstone disease, high blood pressure, high levels of LDL cholesterol and triglycerides, low vitamin D, gum disease, and an autoimmune disorder called Hashimoto's thyroiditis. She'd also undergone gallbladder removal surgery, ten root canals to treat endodontic disease (infection of the tooth's pulp), and five emergency extractions of severely infected teeth after their root canals had failed.

Almost all the doctors she'd consulted over the years about her various ailments thought that the real problem was pretty obvious. "My endocrinologist only paid attention to my thyroid and everybody else said, 'Just get the weight off and you'll be fine,'" recalls Elaine, who was then carrying 240 pounds on her five-foot-five-inch frame. "I've lost fifty pounds, four different times, on extreme crash diets—and it always came back as soon as I started eating regular food again. My doctors were very disappointed in me for not being able to get my weight under control and I felt very discouraged."

She often wondered *why* it was so hard for her to slim down, despite exercising regularly. After all, Courtney and their four children were all able to maintain healthy weights, mainly through an active lifestyle that included competing in marathons and even ultramarathons. Despite her exercise, Elaine has been battling obesity since she was in her twenties. "At one point, I spent six months training intensively for a marathon and only lost eleven pounds," she reports. "I felt very discouraged and frustrated because I'd tried everything that I could think of to get my weight down and improve my health—and nothing worked. It was like trying to put a jigsaw puzzle together when a bunch of the pieces were missing."

Three years ago, she started seeing a new dental provider who helped her solve the puzzle. "I thought I was getting top-quality care from my old dentist, who is affiliated with a leading medical center, but in all the years when he was treating me with crowns, bridges, root canals, and implants, he never told me about the oral–systemic connection," the link between the health of the mouth and overall health, says Elaine. When she turned to the new provider for follow-up care after one of these extractions, the dentist also checked her for high-risk oral bacteria (the kind that have been implicated as key players in a rapidly expanding list of chronic diseases).

After the test detected high levels of these bacterial villains in her mouth, the dentist, who is a patient of ours, referred her to our center for a comprehensive assessment of her cardiovascular health. During her initial visit, Elaine told us that her mom, a type 2 diabetic, had a long history of terrible dental problems. "In the 1950s, when my mom was in college, she was in a study to see if a change of diet would reduce harmful oral bacteria. At the end of the study, she had even higher levels of these pathogens than she did in the beginning. Several of my siblings also have a lot of dental issues, and I used to think that we were just cursed with bad teeth," she added. "We'd even make jokes about it—not knowing that pathogens in your mouth can lead to the diseases that killed our mom and three of our grandparents."

Do You Have a Ticking Time Bomb in Your Arteries?

Now that we've shared Elaine's and Courtney's medical histories with you, which one do you think has the highest risk for heart attacks, strokes, and dementia? If you guessed Elaine, the AHA/ ACC risk scoring algorithm begs to differ. Based on Courtney's age, gender, and elevated total cholesterol levels, it predicted that there is a 23 percent probability that he'll suffer a major cardiovascular event in the next ten years. That's considered a high risk, warranting treatment with medications, such as a statin and low-dose aspirin, to help him avoid heart attacks and strokes. Elaine's risk, on the other hand, was calculated at 5 percent, suggesting that she's at moderate risk and doesn't need medication, according to the AHA/ACC algorithm.

A large body of scientific research, however, supports the opposite conclusion: that Elaine is at greater cardiovascular risk than her husband is. In fact, studies have linked *all* her medical and dental problems to increased risk for arterial disease and its many complications. For example, a recent analysis of studies that included nearly 1 million patients found that those with a history of gallstone disease are 23 percent more likely to suffer fatal or nonfatal cardiovascular events as those without this digestive disorder.[1] The two conditions share many of the same risk factors, including obesity, high blood pressure, diabetes, abnormal cholesterol levels, an unhealthy diet, and a sedentary lifestyle.

Another study reported that people with Hashimoto's thyroiditis (HT) are up to twice as likely to develop heart disease than those without it, particularly if they also have high blood pressure or high cholesterol, as Elaine does.[2] HT is a disease in which the body's immune system produces antibodies that attack the thyroid (a butterfly-shaped gland at the base of the neck) as if it were a foreign invader, typically leading to an underactive thyroid (hypothyroidism). The cause of this autoimmune disorder, which mainly strikes middle-aged women, is unknown. People who have it tend to have high levels of LDL (bad) cholesterol, which may explain why they're at increased risk for heart problems.

Many studies—including our own landmark research identifying oral bacteria as a contributing cause of arterial disease—also suggest that Elaine's dentist was right to be alarmed by her high levels of periodontal bacteria. People with infected gums have up to twice as much small, dense LDL cholesterol (the most dangerous kind) in their blood as those with healthy gums, according to a recent study. The size of cholesterol particles matters: Some are big and buoyant, so they tend to bound off arterial walls, and others are small and dense, making it easier for them to penetrate the arterial lining and form plaque. Think of the difference between beach balls and bullets. In addition, people with high levels are at up to eight times higher risk for developing metabolic syndrome, even when other risk factors, such as obesity and inflammation, are taken into account, a 2019 study reported.[3]

When we met Elaine, she was already on an excellent home care program to improve her oral health and her dentist was treating her, with considerable success, using the dental therapies we'll discuss in chapter ten. As a result, her mouth was no longer a hot zone of infection, her bacterial load had dropped dramatically, and her gums had stopped bleeding. But had she gotten this superb dental care in time to avoid arterial disease? And was Courtney really in as much danger as his risk score suggested? In the rest of this chapter, we'll take a close look at the best imaging tests to answer such questions, at a cost comparable to what you might spend on a pair of eyeglasses, going to the theater, or having dinner at your favorite restaurant. Certain arterial beds are particularly well suited for imaging studies. The walls of the carotid arteries can be examined directly with the cIMT test, the coronary arteries can be checked for calcified plaque with CACS, and the aorta can be checked for abdominal aortic aneurysm (a weak, ballooning area in the body's largest artery). Here is a guide to these tests and two that are used to check for arterial blockages: the treadmill stress test and carotid duplex.

Ultrasound: The Safest Vascular Scan

One of the most appealing aspects of ultrasound is its inherent safety. Unlike X-rays and CT scans, which use ionizing radiation to create images, ultrasound uses the same principles as the sonar employed by submarines, bats, and fishermen: Images are generated with high-frequency sound waves.

Recently, several radiology societies have launched an international campaign called Image Wisely, in which healthcare professionals pledge to minimize their use of radiation during medical imaging examinations. The goal is to reduce the health risks associated with exposure to medical radiation, particularly from CT scans. One study estimated that twenty-nine thousand future cancers—about 2 percent of the cancers diagnosed annually in the U.S.—could be related to CT scans performed in 2007.[4] In most cases, the lag time between exposure to radiation and cancer diagnosis is one to two decades.[5] To address these risks, many medical groups advocate the use of ultrasound imaging whenever possible to spare patients the hazards of ionizing radiation.

Ultrasound is an inexpensive and painless way to check for vascular disorders, including peripheral artery disease (PAD), aortic abdominal aneurysm (AAA), and plaque that could trigger a heart attack or stroke. Unlike X-rays, which can only detect calcified plaque (plaque that contains flecks of calcium), the carotid intima-media thickness ultrasound scan discussed in this section can also detect soft, vulnerable plaque—the kind that can cause heart attacks and strokes if it becomes inflamed. Because ultrasound images are generated in real time, they can also capture movement, such as blood flowing through blood vessels.

Some of the ultrasound tests discussed below are often marketed to older adults in a direct-to-consumer package deal. Because each patient is unique, we don't support the concept of one-size-fits-all vascular screening. Instead, as you'll see in this chapter and throughout this book, the tests we recommend for one patient can be quite different than those we advise for another, based on the person's age, medical history, and genes.

In addition, as you'll learn later in this chapter, one of the tests that is typically included in these screening packages, carotid duplex, has been shown to be highly unreliable—and potentially dangerous—when used to check symptom-free patients for arterial blockages.

Here is a look at three common ultrasound tests that we recommend for vascular screening, including who should get them, what's involved, the pros and cons, and what the results mean.

Carotid Intima-Media Thickness (cIMT)

What It Checks:

Carotid intima-media thickness is an FDA-approved test that measures the combined thickness of the two inner layers—the intima and the media—of the carotid arteries, the major arteries of the neck, which transport oxygenated blood from your heart to your brain, neck, and face. Abnormal thickness is an early marker of increased risk for arterial disease, alerting your medical provider to potential cardiovascular danger at the earliest—and most easily treatable—stage.[6] A similar, but much less widely available, test called femoral artery intima-media thickness (fIMT) can be used to measure the IMT of the femoral artery, one of the major vessels that supplies the legs with oxygenated blood. Like cIMT, femoral IMT is a highly accurate way to directly check for atherosclerosis.

A cIMT scan can also determine how "old" your arteries are. It's normal for your artery walls to gradually thicken as you age, but in some patients—particularly if they smoke, have high blood pressure, high cholesterol, or diabetes—arterial aging is accelerated. The test compares your arterial age to your chronological age, based on norms for your age and gender derived from large studies of healthy people.

Even more important, cIMT can identify atherosclerosis (plaque lurking in the carotid artery wall, between the intima and the media), which is often undetectable with tests that only examine the arterial "pipes" through which blood flows. In patients with arterial disease, cIMT can also reveal what kind of plaque they have—and if their treatment is working. Some plaque is soft and lipid rich. Known as soft plaque, this type of plaque is echolucent, meaning that sound waves do not bounce off it. In ultrasound images, soft, echolucent plaque does not show any bright white, stable calcium deposits. This type of plaque is the most dangerous: It's like an active volcano that could erupt at any time if it becomes inflamed, potentially leading to a heart attack or stroke.

Other plaque is hard and stable with no lipid core: Known as calcified plaque, these deposits are like an extinct volcano in which the molten lava has cooled into solid stone, indicating stable, effectively treated disease. They are "echogenic" indicating that sound waves do bounce off them, and appear predominantly white in ultrasound images. Due to its calcium content, echogenic plaque can be associated with arterial stiffness (hardening of the arteries).[7] It's also possible to have plaque deposits that contain a mix of soft and hard plaque: This is called heterogenous plaque. The higher the lipid content of these areas, the greater the risk of plaque rupture and associated events.

The Procedure:

A thick gel, similar in consistency to hairstyling gel, is applied to your neck. Then the sonographer glides an ultrasound transducer (a small device that resembles a microphone) over the right and left sides of your neck. During this exam, sound waves are bounced off your carotids, creating echoes that return to the transducer, which turns them into electronic signals.

Computer software then converts the signals into images that are displayed on a video screen. The software also generates measurements of specific locations on the carotid arterial wall. These are analyzed for the mean common carotid wall thickness (which reveals your arterial age) and, most important, for the presence of atherosclerosis. The exam takes about fifteen minutes. Wear a loose-fitting, open-necked shirt or blouse and remove jewelry, such as necklaces or dangling earrings, before the test.

Who Should Get the Test:

We recommend cIMT if you have traditional cardiovascular risk factors or any of the red flags for heart attack, stroke, and dementia risk discussed in chapter three. If you've already been diagnosed with arterial disease, the test is also valuable for monitoring your response to treatment over time to see if your therapy is working. Amy Doneen recently served on a Society of Atherosclerosis Imaging and Prevention expert committee, which developed guidelines for the appropriate use of cIMT, including these applications:[8]

> Patients whose ten-year risk for coronary heart disease (CHD) is moderate (6 to 20 percent).
> Patients thirty or older who have metabolic syndrome.

Patients with diabetes or a family history of early CHD.

People with two or more of the following risk factors: low HDL (good) cholesterol, high LDL (bad) cholesterol, diabetes, age (being over forty-five for a man and over fifty-five for a woman), and a family history of early CHD.

Pros and Cons:

While checking the neck may seem like a surprising way to tell if heart attack or stroke might be looming in your future, the carotids, which are just below the surface of the skin on each side of your neck, offer an easily accessible "window" to blood vessel health, without exposure to X-rays. This test has a long track record of accuracy and success in predicting cardiovascular risk in symptom-free patients. CIMT can also predict risk for memory impairment in apparently healthy older adults, a 2017 study reported, leading the researchers to conclude that early detection and treatment of atherosclerosis may be an effective strategy to slow down cognitive aging.[9]

In 2000, an expert panel of the American Heart Association published a scientific statement describing cIMT as "a safe, non-invasive and relatively inexpensive means of assessing subclinical [asymptomatic] atherosclerosis. The technique is valid and reliable." Since we began using cIMT in our clinical practice in 2001, numerous studies have confirmed that this imaging technology is a highly effective tool for vascular screening and diagnosis.[10] In fact, one recent study found that detecting atherosclerosis in the carotid artery is a better predictor of heart attack and stroke risk than finding disease in the coronary arteries! Several other studies have shown that adding cIMT and the presence of plaque to Framingham Risk Score (FRS) factors significantly improves the accuracy of ten-year risk predictions for these events, as compared to only looking at FRS.

There's also overwhelming scientific proof that if cIMT decreases over time, patients have a corresponding drop in their risk for heart attacks, strokes, emergency procedures to avoid these events, and death from CV causes. Accordingly, risk for these events rises if cIMT increases. Not only does this mean that cIMT is an excellent way for providers and patients to tell if a treatment is working, but this imaging test could also be used to speed up the development and testing of potentially lifesaving new therapies, a 2020 study reported. The researchers analyzed 119 randomized, controlled clinical trials that used cIMT to track the progression of the patients' disease. The study found that these measurements accurately predicted the impact the experimental therapy had on rates of major CV events. Therefore, they concluded that cIMT could help scientists identify effective new therapies faster—and quickly determine if an experimental drug was ineffective.

What's the downside of cIMT? Since this test requires special ultrasound software, it's less widely available than older technologies, such as carotid duplex, and your health plan may not cover the cost. However, a few states have passed or proposed laws mandating insurance coverage of cIMT and coronary artery calcium score (discussed later in this chapter). For example, in 2010, Texas became the first state in the nation to require plans to reimburse up to two hundred dollars each for these screening tests for men forty-five to seventy-five and women between fifty-five and seventy-five. The goal was to prevent more than 4,300 deaths from CVD each year in Texas and save $1.6 billion in healthcare costs annually through early detection and treatment.

What the Results Mean:

Courtney, then seventy-three, was horrified when his cIMT revealed that he had the arteries of an octogenarian. Having arteries that are eight or more years "older" than you are is a sign of trouble, since it's evidence that you're headed for vascular disease in the future, while finding plaque means that you already have atherosclerosis. He also turned out to have several areas of soft, vulnerable plaque, with a combined measurement (called total plaque burden) of 11.2 mm. That meant that he would have been at extremely high risk for a heart attack or stroke if he'd remained untreated.

While all plaque is dangerous, size matters. One recent study found that plaque buildup measuring 1.5 mm or larger significantly raises risk for both heart attacks and strokes, compared to people with less plaque. However, for these events to occur, the plaque must become inflamed, which can occur for a variety of reasons, including dental infections. This explains why Melinda, whom you met in chapter six, suffered a stroke, even though she had two relatively small plaque deposits, while her husband, Casey, had not yet experienced a cardiovascular event, despite having much worse arterial disease than she did. His case and that of Courtney, both of whom were only diagnosed by chance—after their wives persuaded them to come to our center—highlight the potentially lifesaving value of vascular screening, even for people who look and feel healthy.

Armed with the information provided by cIMT, patients with atherosclerosis can work with their healthcare providers— and take action to prevent heart attacks, strokes, and dementia, using the therapies recommended in part three, and fine-tune their treatment as needed to optimize their arterial wellness. For these patients, cIMT should be repeated periodically (usually annually) to evaluate how well their treatment is working. Signs of success include no new areas of soft plaque and the gradual conversion of soft, vulnerable plaque into hard, stable plaque. Studies of our patients indicate that it takes about five years of treatment with the BaleDoneen Method to transform soft, lipid-rich plaque into a totally stable disease that's no longer vulnerable to plaque ruptures and associated events. In many of our patients, however, plaque starts to shrink and stabilize during the first year of treatment, with further improvements in the second year. By year five, all lipid-rich plaque had been converted into hard, stable plaque.[11]

Should you do a happy dance to celebrate if no plaque or signs of accelerated arterial aging are found, as occurred in Elaine's case? Unfortunately, as is true of all medical tests, a normal cIMT result isn't proof that there are no cats lurking in your gutter. While this scan is highly accurate, it only examines one of the body's many arterial beds. It's possible to have *no* plaque in your carotids, but to still have it elsewhere, such as the coronary arteries. Therefore, we advise patients with normal cIMT results to also be evaluated with the coronary artery calcium score test discussed later in this chapter, which uses a different imaging modality to directly check for plaque. Such patients may also be candidates for peripheral artery disease testing along with ultrasound examination of the aortic artery. Both tests are discussed below.

Abdominal Aortic Aneurysm Scan

What It Checks:

An estimated 1.1 million Americans have abdominal aortic aneurysm (AAA, pronounced triple-A), a weak, bulging area in the lower portion of the body's largest artery, which supplies blood to the abdomen, pelvis, and legs.[12] Like a balloon, the bigger the aneurysm grows, the more likely it is to burst, triggering massive bleeding that's fatal in up to 85 percent of cases, according to a 2016 study.[13] Ruptured AAA kills about ten thousand Americans a year.[14]

Although AAA is often stereotyped as a disease of older

male smokers, nearly half of the people who develop it are women, nonsmokers, or people under sixty-five, the study cited above reported. While the exact cause is still under investigation, it shares many of the same risk factors as CVD, including smoking, obesity, diabetes, high cholesterol, high blood pressure, and genetics. A 2020 study and earlier investigations have identified twenty-four genes that play a role.[15] Carriers of the 9P21 gene are at up to a 75 percent higher risk for AAA than noncarriers.

Not only can the AAA scan reliably detect an aneurysm, but it can also identify calcification (atherosclerosis) in the artery wall that signals increased risk for a heart attack or stroke. In a 2014 study, calcification of the aorta was a stronger predictor of CV risk than coronary artery calcification.[16]

The Procedure:

Like the other tests in this section, the AAA scan is an ultrasound scan, performed as you lie on an examination table. To obtain the best images, you must avoid eating or drinking anything for four hours before the test. The scan takes ten to fifteen minutes.

Who Should Get the Test:

We recommend this scan for everyone over fifty, or at forty if you are a smoker, have a family history of AAA, or are a carrier of the 9P21 gene, particularly if you have two copies of the gene (inherited from both your mother and father), which raises risk for AAA by 74 percent.[17]

Sometimes called the heart attack gene, because it's an independent predictor of risk for developing extensive coronary artery disease at an unusually young age, the 9P21 gene also boosts the threat of PAD and AAA. Therefore, we recommended that Casey, Courtney, and Elaine, all of whom have the 9P21 genotype, be screened for both of these disorders.

Pros and Cons:

Screening is painless, noninvasive, and relatively inexpensive. The scan can detect AAA with close to 100 percent accuracy and is equally reliable for determining that you don't have this disorder. In the majority of cases, an aneurysm doesn't cause any symptoms prior to rupture. This condition is often difficult for healthcare providers to detect during a physical exam, unless you are relatively thin, with a large aneurysm, making ultrasound imaging by far a better bet for finding out if you have AAA.

The downside is that Medicare only covers the scan (on a one-time basis, with a 20 percent copay) for men sixty-five or older who have smoked more than one hundred cigarettes in their lifetime and for men and women who have a family history of AAA. Some private plans will only pay for men sixty-five or older to be screened, while women may not be covered at all, regardless of their age or family history.

What the Results Mean:

If an aneurysm is detected, your healthcare provider may advise "watchful waiting" (scanning the aneurysm periodically with ultrasound to see if it's getting bigger) or you may be referred to a vascular surgeon, depending on the size of the bulge. Aneurysms measuring less than 1.6 inches in diameter are classified as small. Medium aneurysms measure 1.6 to 2.2 inches, and large ones exceed 2.2 inches. Surgery generally isn't advised for small aneurysms, since the risks of the procedure outweigh those of rupture.

Finding calcified plaque during a AAA scan means that you have the cat in the gutter and therefore could be at risk for a heart attack, stroke, or dementia. When Elaine, Courtney, and Casey were scanned, all of them had normal results. That meant we still didn't know if Elaine was "innocent" or "guilty" of harboring potentially lethal plaque in her arteries and needed to continue our investigation. Later in this chapter, we'll tell you which imaging test can pinpoint how much calcified plaque (if any) is in your coronary arteries—and what it may reveal about your true heart attack risk, even if you have no outward warning signs or symptoms.

Ankle-Brachial Index (ABI)

What It Checks:

This rapid test is used to diagnose peripheral artery disease (PAD), the circulatory problem that caused Neal to be unable to walk more than twenty-five feet before excruciating leg pain forced him to stop. This disorder occurs when plaque buildup narrows arteries, reducing blood flow to your extremities (usually the legs). If you have heart disease, there is a 42 percent probability that you also have PAD.[18]

Smokers are up to six times more likely to develop PAD.[19] Smoking ten cigarettes a day can magnify your risk for developing PAD by as much as 50 percent.[20] About 90 percent of the people who develop this debilitating disorder are current or former smokers.[21] People with the 9P21 gene and those with a family history of PAD are also at increased risk.

The classic symptom is leg pain or cramps when you're walking that improve with rest. However, up to 40 percent of people with PAD—a serious, but treatable condition—have no symptoms, so the disorder often goes undiagnosed. That's dangerous, since having PAD, particularly if it goes untreated, more than doubles heart attack and stroke danger.[22]

The Procedure:

Ankle-brachial index is a simple, painless exam that compares the blood pressure in your lower legs to that in your arms. After you've been resting on your back for ten minutes, a healthcare provider measures the pressure in your arms, using a standard blood pressure cuff, then measures the pressure in arteries near your ankles using a blood pressure cuff and an ultrasound probe (or stethoscope). Blood pressure readings may be taken while you're at rest and again after you've walked on a treadmill. The test takes about fifteen minutes.

Who Should Get the Test:

We recommend ABI if you are fifty or older, even if you have no symptoms, or at any age if you do. We also recommend starting screening for PAD at forty if you have any of these risk factors: diabetes, high blood pressure, high cholesterol, atherosclerosis, abdominal aortic aneurysm, a family history of CVD, or if you are a carrier of the 9P21 gene. In chapter eleven, you'll learn which potentially lifesaving test can determine if you're a carrier of this extremely common gene or other variants that magnify heart attack and stroke danger, along with the right steps to tailor your personalized prevention plan to your DNA.

Pros and Cons:

ABI can reliably diagnose PAD. Since the disorder often causes no symptoms until it reaches an advanced stage, in many cases, screening is the only way to catch the disease early, before it triggers dangerous or fatal complications. If severe enough, PAD can lead to leg infections and in the most serious cases, gangrene, and lower limb amputation. PAD is frequently a sign of widespread atherosclerosis, signaling that you could be at high risk for a heart attack or stroke without proper treatment. Studies also report that people with PAD are at up to 6.5 times higher risk for dying from CVD, particularly if their circulatory issues go undiagnosed and untreated, compared to people without this circulatory disorder.[23]

Some older adults, or those with a history of kidney disease or diabetes, may develop stiff blood vessels that don't compress easily with a blood pressure cuff. Consequentially, their ABI results may be inaccurate. For these patients, a similar test called toe-brachial index (TBI) is sometimes used instead of the ABI, since the toe's blood vessels rarely become rigid.

What the Results Mean:

To calculate your ankle-brachial index, the doctor divides the highest blood pressure recorded in your ankle by the highest pressure in your arm's brachial artery. The normal range is between 0.9 and 1.4. Casey's, Elaine's, and Courtney's results all fell in this range, indicating that they did not have PAD. In some cases, patients with a normal ABI may be advised to have a repeat scan or other tests to evaluate peripheral blood flow, based on their individual risk factors or symptoms.

Any number lower than 0.9 indicates some degree of compromised blood flow to the feet, signaling that you have PAD, while a measurement above 1.4 indicates stiff arteries (often due to buildup of calcified plaque, a condition known as calcified atherosclerosis). If you have PAD, it can often be treated with lifestyle changes, including quitting smoking, exercising more, and eating a healthy diet. You may also need medication, such as anti-clotting drugs. These include low-dose aspirin or clopidogrel bisulfate (Plavix). For severe blockages, such as those that affected Neal, treatment may also include balloon angioplasty and/or stents to reopen the obstructed arteries.

Tests That Check for Arterial Blockages

Unlike cIMT, which directly examines the arterial wall and can therefore detect plaque, some imaging tests, such as carotid duplex and the treadmill stress test discussed below, look for indirect evidence of disease (reduced blood flow to the brain or heart). In other words, some tests can tell if you have the cat in the gutter (and are therefore at increased risk for heart attacks, strokes, and dementia) and others can only tell if there *might* be a cat.

As we will explain more fully when we discuss each of these tests, the U.S. Preventive Services Task Force, a group of public health experts that issues evidence-based guidelines, has specifically recommended *against* the use of carotid duplex or treadmill stress tests for screening purposes. In some medical scenarios, as you'll learn in this section, these tests can provide valuable diagnostic information when used to evaluate patients with symptoms that might be caused by obstructed arteries.

Carotid Duplex Ultrasound

What It Checks:

Unlike cIMT, which directly examines the arterial walls for plaque, the carotid duplex test looks for indirect signs of disease by measuring blood flow through the carotids. In other words, it's based on the plumbing concept of CVD and checks for blockages in the pipes, a condition that's known as carotid artery stenosis in the medical world.

The Procedure:

Performed in a similar manner to cIMT, carotid duplex uses two types of ultrasound: A conventional, or B-mode, ultrasound bounces sound waves off blood vessels to generate images of their structure, and a Doppler ultrasound bounces high-frequency sound waves off circulating blood cells to determine the velocity of the blood as it travels past the ultrasound transducer. It's similar to the highway patrol using a radar gun to find out how fast vehicles are moving.

Who Should Get the Test:

As noted earlier in this chapter, public health guidelines issued in 2014 recommend *against* using carotid duplex to screen patients for atherosclerosis. It is appropriately used as a diagnostic test for patients with symptoms of reduced blood flow to the brain, such as temporary blindness in one eye or the brief loss of the ability to talk, understand speech, or move. It can also be a valuable test for stroke survivors like Nikki and Melinda to see if these events were caused by blockages, and is also useful to evaluate the effects of surgical procedures to improve blood flow through the carotids, such as stent placement.

Pros and Cons:

Like all ultrasound tests, it's safe, painless, and noninvasive. Carotid duplex can determine if life-threatening blockages are present in the carotid arteries in people with symptoms of reduced blood flow. However, if performed inappropriately as a screening tool, patients like Casey and Courtney, whose plaque was not obstructing their arteries, could be lulled into a false sense of security since their arterial disease would have been completely missed.

In February 2021, the United States Preventive Services Task Force reaffirmed its longstanding recommendation against using carotid duplex for screening purposes, stating that the test yields many false positives (test results indicating that patients have arterial blockages when they don't). That can lead to invasive tests or treatments that are unnecessary and potentially dangerous. Nor did the task force find any evidence that screening symptom-free patients for carotid artery stenosis helps prevent strokes or deaths from CV causes.

What the Results Mean:

Carotid duplex results are expressed as percentages, indicating the extent to which the diameter of the artery is narrowed (stenosis). Each lab sets its own range of normal results. For example, the University of Massachusetts's clinical vascular service defines 1 to 29 percent stenosis as the normal range, while higher numbers are considered increasingly abnormal. One hundred percent stenosis (also called occlusion) means that the vessel is completely blocked, with no blood flow. Severely obstructed carotid arteries are usually treated with surgery, such as endarterectomy, an operation to remove plaque buildup, or angioplasty and stenting to reopen the clogged artery.

Treadmill Stress Test

If you think you don't need cIMT or CACS because you've already been screened with a treadmill stress test, here's some news that may make your heart skip a beat: when used for screening, this test is so unreliable that it misdiagnoses up to 40 percent of patients, with the highest error rate in women.[24] Like the carotid duplex test, the stress test checks for arterial blockages. There are several variations of the test, some of which include imaging, such as echocardiography, which uses ultrasound to capture images of the heart before the patient starts exercising and at various points during the test.

Treadmill tests are often included in annual physicals to screen seemingly healthy people for atherosclerosis. What most patients don't know, however, is that in order to "fail" this test, their arteries must be at least 70 percent obstructed. What's more, this test rarely detects nonobstructive heart disease — the culprit in about 86 percent of heart attacks.[25] In 2018, the United States Preventive Services Task Force published a recommendation *against* using stress tests and EKG to screen low-risk, symptom-free patients for heart disease, stating the potential harms outweigh the benefits in asymptomatic adults at low risk for heart disease. The rationale is that the high risk of getting false positive results means that many healthy people will be needlessly subjected to additional testing, including invasive procedures that could have potential complications.

Several other medical groups, including the American College of Physicians, the American College of Preventive Medicine, and the American Academy of Family Physicians, have issued similar recommendations. The ACC has concluded that exercise stress tests are "rarely appropriate" for such patients, but may be appropriate for people at intermediate or high risk for heart attacks and strokes.[26]

What It Checks:

Stress tests, also called exercise stress tests or treadmill stress tests, look at how well the heart works during exertion and helps healthcare providers evaluate patients with symptoms that only emerge when the heart is forced to pump harder and faster than usual, such as angina, a type of chest pain triggered by reduced blood flow to the heart. Later you'll meet a patient who had such severe angina that he was unable to walk across our exam room during his first visit to our center without stopping to take nitro-glycerine to temporarily quell the agonizing pain in his chest.

Angina, also known as angina pectoris, is often described as a sensation of squeezing, tightness, pressure, or heaviness in the chest, and can also affect the shoulders, arms, neck, or jaw, and tends to occur during physical exertion. A stress test can also detect irregular heartbeats or blood pressure abnormalities during exercise.

The Procedure:

There are four types of stress tests, all of which aim to "stress" the heart and examine it while it's not at rest:

The *exercise stress test* usually involves exercising on a tread-mill or pedaling a stationary bike, with electrodes attached to your chest, legs, and arms. These sensors are connected to an electrocardiogram (EKG or ECG) machine that monitors your heartbeat, while a cuff measures blood pressure during the test. You begin by walking or bicycling slowly, then the exercise grad-ually becomes more strenuous. Most patients will be asked to walk or pedal for ten to fifteen minutes. The healthcare pro-vider overseeing the test will tell you to stop when you reach the target heart rate, you become too tired to continue, or you develop symptoms that concern the provider, such as chest pain or blood pressure changes.

In a *nuclear* or *thallium* stress test, as in the exercise stress test, you exercise on a treadmill or bike. In this version, however, thallium is injected into a vein before the test and, after a fifteen-to-forty-five-minute wait, a special camera scans your chest. Then you use the treadmill or bike while your heart is moni-tored. While it's working hard, thallium is again injected and another scan taken. Comparing the two sets of images may reveal blockages that reduce the flow of oxygenated blood to the heart.

Pharmacological stress testing is designed for people who are unable to walk on a treadmill. You'll be hooked to an IV, which delivers a small amount of a short-lived radioactive chemical into the vein. After a forty-five-to-sixty-minute wait, you'll be asked to lie on your back for about twenty minutes while an imaging camera takes pictures of your heart. During the stress portion of the test, you'll be hooked up to an EKG machine. Then you will receive an IV medication that makes your blood vessels expand as additional images are taken of your heart. Pharmacological stress testing is typically used for patients who are unable to exercise; they rest during the entire test.

Stress echocardiography improves on the basic exercise stress test by adding ultrasound imaging to the process. Images are taken before you begin exercising and at various points during the test. Your blood pressure and EKG are monitored throughout the test.

Who Should Get the Test:

A number of studies indicate that the stress test is a highly inaccurate vascular screening tool, prompting the US Preventive Services Task Force to recommend against using it to check the heart health of low-risk people who lack symptoms. The test can be helpful to evaluate people with chest pain, cardiovascular disease (to assess severity or response to treatment), irregular heartbeats (arrhythmias), heart failure, congenital heart disorders, and to check the cardiovascular health and fitness of sedentary people prior to participating in exercise or sports programs.

Pros and Cons:

One of the biggest benefits of this test involves measuring physical fitness, as determined by analyzing the intensity and amount of exercise performed, along with heart rates during the workout and the heart rate recovery during rest. If there is a narrowing of 70 percent or more in one of the coronary arteries, stress test results may indicate that a portion of the heart is inadequately perfused with blood during the exercise portion of the exam.

The downside is that stress tests have a high rate of false positives (healthy people being told they have disease), leading to anxiety, fear, and unnecessary additional tests, as well as false negatives (missing disease). This occurred with one of our patients, who was extremely physically fit and always passed his annual stress test with flying colors despite having 100 percent blockage in one area of his coronary arteries, and 70 percent blockage in another! Overall, the stress test misdiagnoses up to 40 percent of patients, with the highest error rate in women.

The stress test is relatively expensive, but very well covered by insurance, a combination that contributes to its inappropriate use for screening low-risk people, while depleting healthcare resources that would be more wisely allocated to screening tests better supported by scientific evidence, such as cIMT.

What the Results Mean:

Abnormal results may indicate arrhythmia or a possible blockage in your arteries. However, a normal result may not be as reassuring as it sounds, since a study published in *Journal of the American Academy of Cardiology* reports that "Patients who have normal imaging stress tests frequently have extensive atherosclerosis."[27] In the next section of this chapter, we'll tell you which imaging test can accurately pinpoint how much calcified plaque is in your coronary arteries—and what it may reveal about your true heart attack risk, even if you have no outward warning signs or symptoms.

Calcium in the Crosshairs

Atherosclerosis (also called hardening of the arteries) starts with fatty streaks that develop very early in life. Astonishingly, studies of premature babies have revealed that fatty streaks can even form before birth, particularly if the mother had high cholesterol.[28] As cholesterol and other fatty materials continue to accumulate in the arteries, they initially form soft plaque. In a study in which teenagers' arteries were scanned with ultrasound, 17 percent of adolescents studied already had small plaques.[29]

One way the body tries to repair the damage from plaque is by removing the lipid (cholesterol) and replacing it with collagen and calcium. These substances are denser than lipid, so as the plaque "heals," it shrinks and becomes calcified. In fact, calcium can comprise up to 20 percent of the volume of some plaque deposits.[30] Calcium is what creates the hardness in hardening of the arteries.

Coronary Artery Calcium Score

What It Checks:

Also known as cardiac calcium score or coronary calcium scan, coronary artery calcium score (CACS) uses an electron beam tomography (EBT) or computed tomography (CT) scanner to look for flecks of calcium in coronary artery walls. The reason EBT or CT—rather than standard X-rays—is needed to find them is that the heart is in constant motion, so the images must be taken very quickly. This challenge has been compared to trying to photograph spaghetti as it shimmies in rapidly boiling water, since the coronary arteries are relatively small and take many twists and turns as they travel through the beating heart muscle.

The amount of calcium found in your coronary arteries is called a calcium score and is a powerful predictor of heart attack risk, regardless of your risk factors.[31] A 2012 study of patients with no symptoms of heart disease (average age, fifty-four) found that those with calcium in their arteries (as diagnosed by CACS) had more than double the risk for a heart attack or stroke—even if their cholesterol levels were low, compared to people without calcium in their arteries. Data from the ongoing Multi-Ethnic Study of Atherosclerosis (MESA), published in 2016 and 2018, has also linked a high CACS to increased risk for developing several chronic diseases of aging in initially healthy participants, including chronic kidney disease, cancer, dementia, and such respiratory disorders as chronic obstructive pulmonary disease and pneumonia.[32]

For younger adults, having *any* calcified plaque in the coronary arteries quintuples risk for heart-related events, such as heart attacks, and triples it for all cardiovascular events, such as strokes, according to a 2017 study. In other words, if you are under fifty, having a CACS above 0 (indicating no calcified plaque) is a very big deal! The study included more than three thousand men and women thirty-two to forty-six who were tracked for up to 12.5 years. The study also found that risk for heart problems rose as CACS increased, so people with the highest scores were in the greatest danger.[33]

The Procedure:

Before the scan, a technician hooks you up to electrodes, which are placed on your chest while you lie on a moveable examining table. These sensors are connected to an electrocardiogram (EKG or ECG) machine, which monitors your heart. As the table slides into a tunnel-like scanner, you will be asked to hold your breath briefly while the CT or EBT machine rotates around your body, capturing extremely rapid images at certain points during your heartbeat.

Calcium shows up as white spots in the arteries of the heart. The technician is in the room next door, but can see and hear you; since your head remains outside of the machine throughout the scan, it's unlikely that you'd feel claustrophobic during the test. The procedure takes ten to fifteen minutes.

Who Should Get the Test:

Evidence-based guidelines developed by the Society for Heart Attack Prevention and Eradication (SHAPE) task force advise vascular screening with either CACS or cIMT for almost all men forty-five or older and almost all women fifty-five or older.[34] The only exception is men or women in these age groups who are at extremely low risk for heart attack or stroke because they meet *all* of the following criteria: they don't smoke, have total cholesterol below 200 and blood pressure below 120/80, don't have diabetes, and have no family history of CVD.

Among the studies the SHAPE task force reviewed are findings from the MESA study, which reported that the predictive power of traditional risk-scoring algorithms, such as FRS, is greatly improved with the addition of CACS, particularly in people deemed at intermediate risk for cardiovascular events. The SHAPE strategy, which the BaleDoneen Method recommends, is designed to identify people who might otherwise go undiagnosed until they've already suffered heart attacks.

Pros and Cons:

The value of detecting calcium is that it can diagnose plaque and therefore can help your healthcare provider determine if you are at higher risk for a heart attack or stroke—and if so, initiate therapies to help you avoid these events. A 2012 study also linked buildup of calcified plaque in arteries outside of the brain with an elevated risk for dementia, suggesting that this screening could also help healthcare providers identify and treat people with the best available therapies to protect their brain function and memory, such as those we recommend in part three. CACS is painless, noninvasive, and relatively inexpensive. As of this writing, it costs about a hundred dollars. Because CACS involves exposure to a low level of radiation, pregnant women should avoid taking the test.

Health plans usually don't cover CACS if it's used as a screening test. However, as noted earlier, a Texas law that took effect in 2010 requires plans to reimburse up to two hundred dollars of the cost of vascular screening with cIMT or CACS for men forty-five to seventy-five and women between fifty-five and seventy-five. Private plans and Medicare will often pay for the test if it's used for diagnostic purposes in people with symptoms of CVD, such as chest pain or chronic, unexplained shortness of breath. It may also be covered if you have high cholesterol, since recently updated AHA/ACC guidelines advise the use of CACS in cases in which healthcare providers are having difficulty deciding if a patient needs statin therapy.

The key takeaway is that CACS is an excellent one-time screening test to check for plaque that may have been missed by other imaging modalities. For example, this test revealed that despite her low AHA/ACC risk score and completely normal cIMT results, Elaine did have atherosclerosis and needed treatment to ward off heart attacks, strokes, and dementia. Since Casey, Melinda, and Courtney had already been diagnosed with plaque using cIMT, they didn't need CACS. Instead, we are monitoring their arterial health with cIMT and will discuss their outcomes later.

What the Results Mean:

If your calcium score is above 0, you have arterial disease and greater danger of a cardiovascular event. The higher the score, the more calcified plaque has been detected in your coronary arteries, with a score of 400 or more indicating extensive coronary artery disease.

Elaine had a score of 120. Many medical providers consider a score that's above 0 (no calcified plaque detected) and below 101 to be "mild heart disease" and scores of 101 to 400 to be "moderate heart disease." To us, both of these terms are as much of an oxymoron as saying that someone is "a little bit pregnant." *Again, having any plaque in your arteries means that without aggressive prevention, you could have a heart attack or stroke. And without the optimal medical care recommended in this book, you could also be at increased risk for dementia and many other chronic diseases.* It is also important to realize that having a CACS of 0, however, doesn't rule out CAD, since you could have uncalcified (soft) plaque that this test is unable to detect. CACS is less reliable in younger patients than older ones.

Patients are often surprised to learn that if they have soft plaque that is successfully treated, their levels of calcified plaque are likely to rise, sometimes dramatically. As a result, if they have repeat CACS tests, their results may seem increasingly alarming. Here's why: In 1995, a landmark study reported that in untreated patients, the calcified deposits that CACS is able to detect may only account for about 20 percent of the person's total plaque burden.[35] The rest is soft plaque, which is invisible to this technology. In other words, in these patients, the deposits that this test picks up may be like icebergs in a shipping lane, with most of their mass—and danger—hidden from sight.

Coauthor Brad Bale is a case in point. In the late 1990s, soon after he started treatment for atherosclerosis that had previously gone undiagnosed until he detected it by scanning himself, his CACS was 208, seemingly putting him in the "moderate" category. Based on the study cited above, we theorized that this might only represent 20 percent of his coronary plaque, with the other 80 percent being the soft, dangerous kind. Therefore, we predicted that over time, if treatment with the BaleDoneen Method was effective, his score would eventually rise to about 1,800 when the lipid-rich soft plaque in his coronary arteries had been transformed into hard, stable plaque that posed no heart attack or stroke risk.

Brad's most recent CACS proved our hypothesis to be correct: That test, performed in 2013, showed a level of 1,756 (a level deemed so high that researchers recently did a study of these extreme outliers, as discussed in chapter six). While that might sound like numerous lions are prowling his arteries, ready to pounce, in reality, this result shows that these fearsome predators have been captured and put in very strong calcium cages. To help our patients with CVD live well, free of the fear of heart attacks, strokes, and dementia, our next step, once this condition has been diagnosed, is to find and treat all its root causes. These will be discussed in part three, along with the best ways to find out if you have them.

If vascular screening shows that you are "innocent" of atherosclerosis, congratulations! In chapter nine, we'll show you how to stay that way by alerting you to two extremely common, but often undiagnosed disorders that can greatly increase your risk for developing arterial disease if they go undetected and untreated. If you already have atherosclerosis, there is a 70 percent probability that you also have one or both of these conditions, which are easily treatable with simple lifestyle changes. Early detection and treatment of these disorders, which affect about 1 billion people worldwide, can also greatly reduce your risk for many other chronic diseases.

Action Step

Step 1: Gather and Organize Your Medical and Dental Records

Collecting and studying your medical and dental records is a crucial part of being an empowered patient. You'll need them if you change healthcare providers, consult a specialist, want a second opinion, or face a medical crisis. Having a complete set of your records can also help you avoid having to needlessly repeat a medical test because your provider was unable to access your previous test results. You'll also avoid losing important information about your diagnoses, treatment plans, prescriptions, and test results if a medical practice or healthcare facility closes or decides to destroy older records that it is not legally required to save for more than ten years.

In addition, having a complete set of your medical and dental records can also be helpful for quickly resolving issues that may come up with insurance claims. It's also important to check your records for errors that might affect your health or life insurance coverage—such as listing your diagnosis as kidney cancer when you were treated for kidney stones—and mistakes that could put your life at risk, such as failing to include your medication allergies. If you spot an error, contact the provider or facility to see if they have a form that they require for making corrections to your record. If not, send them a letter describing the error and the correction needed. Attach a copy of the record with the error.

Under the federal Health Information Portability and Accountability Act (HIPAA), you are legally entitled to copies of your records, including copies of heart and other tests you've had, hospital and emergency room discharge summaries, and radiology reports. And whenever you have an imaging study (such as a mammogram, ultrasound, medical or dental X-ray, MRI, CT, or PET scan), always ask the technician for a copy of the film or a digital copy on a CD or flash drive. Providers don't have an easy way to access imaging done at other facilities, so having your own copies can save you time and money if you need to be evaluated again for the same condition or want a second opinion.

The easiest way to start compiling your healthcare history is to ask your providers for copies of your test results and treatment summaries during your next visit, then build a file of your current records. You may also be able to access your medical data via online patient portals offered by hospitals and medical practices where you've been treated. Although these sites don't typically contain your complete medical records, you can usually find lab results, imaging reports, discharge summaries, and medications that have been prescribed.

After you've compiled your current records, work backward to gather older ones. Also tuck a personal medical information card in your wallet, listing such key information as the names and dosages of your medications, any adverse reactions you've had to drugs, the medical conditions with which you've been diagnosed, and your emergency contact's information. There are also "in case of emergency" apps you can use to store this data on your phone and digital tools that help you compile medical records from multiple providers and facilities.

Step 2: Get Your Test Results

Although patients often assume that no news is good news, it could mean that your healthcare provider hasn't checked your test results, has lost them, or has misinterpreted them. A horrifying study published in *Archives of Internal Medicine* reports that in more than 7 percent of cases, primary care doctors failed to inform patients of medically significant abnormal test results, including those that revealed potentially life-threatening conditions.[36] Scarier still, some of the providers studied made this dangerous mistake more than 26 percent of the time. Make sure that your healthcare providers tell you the result of every test performed and ask for a copy of the results for your personal medical records.

CHAPTER 8
Are Your Arteries on Fire?

"A spark neglected makes a mighty fire."
— ROBERT HERRICK, SEVENTEENTH-CENTURY POET

As a certified nurse-midwife, Catherine has brought more than 1,250 babies into this world. Working seventy or more hours a week, mostly on the night shift, she was too busy to pay much attention to her own health. With no time to exercise and a diet that mainly consisted of meals grabbed on the go from hospital vending machines, her weight climbed to 165 pounds on her five-foot, two-inch frame. At fifty-seven, she became concerned about her chronic exhaustion and low energy level.

She consulted her primary care provider and discussed her alarming family history. Both of her parents—and her fifty-nine-year-old sister—had died from heart attacks. All three of them—as well as her twin brother and her daughter—were insulin-dependent type 2 diabetics. She received a standard medical checkup that included measurements of her cholesterol and blood pressure, both of which were elevated. Despite these abnormalities, when her doctor calculated her Framingham Risk Score, it predicted that her chances of having a heart attack or stroke in the next ten years were only 2 percent.

She was also checked with the carotid duplex ultrasound scan we discussed in chapter seven. Like most patients—and some healthcare providers—Catherine was unaware that this test can only detect an indirect sign of arterial disease: reduced blood flow through the neck's largest arteries due to large blockages. Nor did she know that the U.S. Preventive Services Task Force has long recommended *against* using this test to screen symptom-free patients for arterial disease due to its high error rate.

The duplex scan didn't detect any obstructions, and her provider wrote five reassuring words in her medical record: "No carotid artery plaque found." Then Catherine was advised to "lose some weight and get more sleep." But would these measures be enough to prevent a fatal heart attack, like those that had killed her parents and older sister? A friend recommended that she consult us for a comprehensive risk assessment. "Other than being about 25 pounds overweight, I didn't think I had anything to worry about, but my friend convinced me that it was all about prevention," Catherine recalls.

During her initial evaluation at our center, she was scanned with the highly accurate carotid intima-media thickness (cIMT) test that you learned about in chapter seven. The results horrified her: "Not only did I have arterial plaque that the duplex scan had completely missed, but what really stood out was finding out that my arterial age was twenty years older than my chronological age," she says. "That was truly scary and such a wakeup call. I realized that if I didn't start taking better care of my health, I wouldn't have any health at all, because I must have been on the verge of keeling over."

The Root of All Diseases?

To find out if Catherine was in imminent danger of having a heart attack or stroke, our next step was to find out if her arteries were inflamed, using the Fire Panel of simple blood and urine tests described in this chapter. Each of them can save your life by alerting your medical provider if there is a tiny spark — or a mighty flame — in your arteries that could ignite a heart attack or stroke. Studies dating back to the early 2000s have shown that even subtle changes in these inflammatory biomarkers can predict future cardiovascular events, including heart attacks, strokes, sudden cardiac death, and the development of peripheral artery disease, in seemingly healthy people.[1]

Detecting and treating arterial inflammation, which we call fire, has been the keystone of the BaleDoneen Method since its inception in 2001. Initially, our goal was to prevent heart attacks and strokes by keeping our patients' arteries as "cool" as possible, so the cat in the gutter wouldn't leap out. However, an ever-expanding body of scientific evidence suggests that the benefits of preventing and treating chronic inflammation go far beyond warding off cardiovascular events. This fiery process has been implicated in a long list of debilitating or fatal illness, including CVD, arthritis, diabetes, depression, chronic kidney disease,

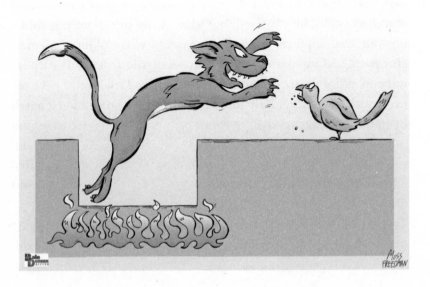

dementia, heart failure, erectile dysfunction, non-alcoholic fatty liver disease, macular degeneration, neurodegenerative disorders (such as Alzheimer's and Parkinson's disease), autoimmune conditions, and various cancers.[2]

In a medical version of physics' "unified field" theory, some scientists have even theorized that chronic systemic inflammation—driven by such factors as obesity, a large waistline, insulin resistance, lack of exercise and periodontal disease—may be at the root of *all* chronic diseases. Indeed, these lifestyle-linked maladies now rank as the world's leading killers, with a 2019 study reporting that globally, more than 50 percent of all deaths are attributable to inflammation-related diseases.[3] Why is chronic inflammation so dangerous? Here is a look at some of the most important discoveries and why almost everything patients—and most doctors—believe about how plaque attacks is completely wrong.

Old thinking: High cholesterol is the leading cause of heart attacks.

Like most patients and many medical professionals, Catherine assumed that the cause of her arterial plaque was pretty obvious, given her high levels of total and LDL cholesterol. For decades, LDL, the notorious "bad" cholesterol, has been demonized as the leading threat to heart, brain, and arterial health. First proposed in the 1950s, the lipid hypothesis holds that high levels of cholesterol circulating in the blood are the underlying cause of plaque formation.[4] So entrenched is this concept in the medical mindset that cardiology guidelines have long emphasized reducing LDL as the primary goal in heart attack and stroke prevention.

Yet studies have shown that only about 50 percent of heart attacks happen to people with elevated levels of bad cholesterol, creating a scientific conundrum: If high LDL is the instigator of these life-threatening events, why do the other 50 percent occur in people with normal or even "optimal" levels of bad cholesterol?[5] A rapidly growing body of scientific evidence has zeroed in on another culprit. "The four horsemen of the medical apocalypse—coronary artery disease, diabetes, cancer, and Alzheimer's—may be riding the same steed: inflammation," a Harvard Medical School report theorized in 2006.[6] Since then, several landmark studies have shown that chronic systemic inflammation, which we call fire, is both a cause of heart attacks and strokes and an important treatment target to help prevent them.

Old thinking: If your artery walls are healthy, cholesterol can't invade.

Until very recently, doctors, including us, thought that the endothelium (blood vessel lining) acted as a smart barrier that blocked cholesterol from entry unless this membrane became diseased, inflamed, or otherwise dysfunctional. We call the endothelium the tennis court because if it was taken out of your body and flattened, it would cover six tennis courts. This membrane, which is only one cell thick, acts as the "brains" of your blood vessels, releasing substances that regulate blood clotting, blood pressure, immune function, and other vital functions.

The latest evidence has revealed an amazing fact that most physicians still don't know: In people with healthy arteries, cholesterol particles, which are extremely tiny, routinely flow through the tennis court and all three layers of the artery wall—the intima, the media, and the adventia—*without* causing disease, even in people who have high cholesterol.[7] This surprising discovery explains why some people with extremely high cholesterol never develop plaque, enabling them to avoid heart attacks and strokes, despite having one of the leading risk factors for these events. Conversely, even low levels of LDL can spell trouble in people with an unhealthy lifestyle, the primary driver of chronic inflammation.

Here's what happens in people with healthy arteries: After passing through the arterial layers, cholesterol particles normally exit on the advential side, where they are picked up by the veins and lymph vessels. After that, these waxy particles are recirculated throughout the body, where they perform many essential functions, from waterproofing cell membranes to helping produce vitamin D, bile acids that help you digest fat, and many types of hormones, including the sex hormones testosterone, estrogen, and progesterone. It also helps form synapses, the wiring that lets nerve cells communicate with one another. In fact, without cholesterol, you couldn't survive!

It is now recognized that arterial disease results from a triple whammy called the atherogenic triad. Inflammation, driven by such factors as obesity, insulin resistance, a poor diet, lack of exercise, a high stress level, sleep deprivation, and gum disease, is the key culprit in each step of the disease process, which begins when contractile smooth muscle cells in the media undergo a genetic transformation that turns them into migratory smooth muscle cells. These cells move to the deep layer of the intima and produce a Velcro-like substance that latches on to apolipoprotein B-100 molecules (ApoB), a major component of all the dangerous cholesterols we discussed in chapter four, including LDL and lipoprotein (a).

When ApoB gets stuck in the intima, it becomes oxidized, which in turn sparks a fire in the arteries by activating the immune system. The tennis court releases proteins that trap white blood cells and allows them to pass through to the intima, where these Pac-Man-like compounds try to clean up the mess by gobbling them up. If the inflammatory triggers for the genetic transformation persist, more and more ApoB gets trapped, oxidized, and engulfed by the white blood cells. Eventually, they get so engorged with cholesterol that they become foam cells that form fatty streaks and evolve into the cats in the gutter.

Old thinking: Chronic inflammation is equally harmful to everyone's arteries.

In 2012, two groundbreaking genetic studies were the first to prove that atherosclerosis is an inflammatory illness. In one of the studies, researchers analyzed 82 previous studies that included more than 200,000 people and demonstrated a cause-and-effect relationship between an inflammatory biomarker called interleukin 6 (IL-6) and the creation of the cat in the gutter. The study focused on people with a common variant of the IL-6 gene that dials down the body's inflammatory response. People with this variant have a smaller-than-usual number of receptors for IL-6, a signaling molecule involved in the first step of the inflammatory response.

This response, known as the inflammatory cascade, evolved about 500 million years ago to help our primordial ancestors survive injuries and infections.[8] If one of them (or you) stepped on a jagged, slimy clam shell, cells in the affected area would release signaling molecules, such as IL-6, as a biochemical call to arms to summon immune system soldiers to battle the invading pathogens. These troops, which resemble video game monsters, swarm to the area and blast the interlopers with toxins until they explode, then Pac-Man-like macrophages surround and gobble up the invaders. Once the enemy was dispatched by an army of more than twenty white blood cell components, increased blood flow to the wounded area would result in the familiar signs of warmth, redness, and swelling as the injury began to heal.

Chronic inflammation harms, rather than heals, because the immune system attack never stops. Think of it as similar to being shot by "friendly fire" during a never-ending war raging inside the body, ignited by the disorders discussed earlier in this chapter. In people with the IL-6 variant, however, the malignant effects of arterial fire are dampened because these men and women have relatively few IL-6 receptors, which act as molecular switches to turn on the inflammatory cascade. As a result, people with this variant have significantly lower rates of arterial disease and associated events, as compared to people without this variant, even when numerous risk factors are taken into account. In other words, their genes act as natural firefighters.

The second 2012 study found that people with two copies of the IL-6 variant get twice the reduction in CVD risk as those with one copy (a 10 percent drop, as compared to a 5 percent drop).[9] Although that reduction may sound modest, reducing the annual death toll of CVD in the US by 10 percent would save eighty thousand lives each year and would also prevent about 150,000 heart attacks and strokes. The researchers also suggested that drugs that block IL-6 and other inflammatory signaling molecules might offer a revolutionary new approach to preventing these catastrophic events.

Old thinking: Medication is the most effective way to quell arterial fire.

To find out if anti-inflammatory medication is safe and effective for people with arterial disease, another team of researchers launched a landmark clinical trial called CANTOS (Canakinumab Anti-Inflammatory Thrombosis Outcome Study). In 2017, the trial's results generated massive media coverage around the world by reporting that a drug that blocked inflammation—with no effect on cholesterol—reduced risk for heart attacks, strokes, and cancer.[10] Gushing media reports hailed the medication used in the study, canakinumab, as "a new wonder drug," "a magic bullet," and "the biggest breakthrough since statins."[11] Sold under the brand name Ilaris, canakinumab is an anti-inflammatory medication that's FDA approved for the treatment of a few rare conditions, but not for heart disease.

Sponsored by the drug company Novartis, the trial was designed to find out if reducing inflammation in heart attack survivors would lower their risk for repeat events. The researchers randomly assigned 10,061 patients, all of whom had high levels of the inflammatory biomarker high-sensitivity C-reactive protein (hs-CRP) to either receive canakinumab (given in either 50, 150, or 300 mg doses) or a placebo. All patients also received standard cardiovascular care, including cholesterol-lowering statins.

The team tracked the participants' health for nearly four years and reported in 2020 that those who received canakinumab were 15 percent less likely to suffer cardiovascular events—including fatal or nonfatal heart attacks and strokes—or need invasive procedures, such as bypass surgery or angioplasty to reopen blocked arteries.[12] The drug reduced their risk by lowering their levels of hs-CRP, without reducing cholesterol at all. The canakinumab group also had a nearly 50 percent lower rate of cancer death, but a slightly higher rate of fatal infections, as compared to the placebo group.

So exciting did the medical community find these results that world-renowned cardiologists proclaimed the findings "revolutionary." Cleveland Clinic's cardiovascular medicine chair, Dr. Steven Nissen (who was not involved in the study), opined on national television, "For the first time, we have this new target—inflammation. It's sort of the dawning of a new era. I really think it's that big."[13] Dr. Paul Ridker, who led the CANTOS research team, was equally enthused, telling reporters that the study leveraged "an entirely new way to treat patients" with "far-reaching implications."

After the CANTOS results were published, Novartis asked the FDA to expand canakinumab's approved uses to include cardiovascular risk reduction in heart patients. In October 2018, however, the drug maker announced that its application had been declined because the FDA didn't consider the CANTOS data sufficient to support this proposed use. Sold at a staggering list price of $200,000 a year, it's a monoclonal antibody—a type of drug that acts like a smart bomb—that selectively targets an inflammatory substance called interleukin-1 beta (IL-1B). As we'll discuss more fully in chapter eleven, some people carry IL-1A or IL-1B genes that heighten their response to inflammation, greatly raising their risk for CVD. In fact, their lifetime risk equals that of a smoker!

Although excitement about canakinumab has faded after it failed to win FDA approval as a new treatment for heart patients, the CANTOS trial remains an extremely important proof of concept: Quelling arterial fire helps save lives, hearts, and brains. Not only are other anti-inflammatory drugs now in clinical trials, potentially offering new treatment options for high-risk patients, but numerous studies have revealed that when it comes to "fireproofing" your arteries, an optimal lifestyle is the ultimate wonder drug![14] In part three, we'll show you how the right personalized diet and exercise plan is your best bet to prevent heart attacks, strokes, and other inflammation-driven chronic diseases—without a $200,000 medication!

The Fire Panel: Simple Tests to Check for Heart Attack and Stroke Risk

In chapter one, we told you about the written guarantee that we offer to all our patients stating that if they have a heart attack or stroke while under our care, they'll receive a refund of 100 percent of the fees they paid during the year. The Fire Panel of six simple blood and urine tests discussed in this section is the secret that allows us to make this guarantee with confidence, even though most of our patients have many risk factors for cardiovascular events or have already suffered one or more heart attacks or strokes. These inflammatory biomarker tests have four important goals:

1: Identifying patients who are at risk for developing athero-sclerosis, so their arterial inflammation can be treated *before* plaque develops (primary prevention).

2: Finding out if people with arterial disease, such as Cathe-rine, have dangerously "hot" arteries, so they can be put on the right therapies to prevent heart attacks, strokes, dementia, and other chronic diseases (secondary prevention). As it turned out, her results were quite alarming since she had elevated levels of several of the biomarkers we checked, revealing a very high level of cardiovascular peril and immediate need for treatment.

3: Checking patients like Camille and J.P., who had already survived one cardiovascular event, for arterial fire, so the blaze can be extinguished before they suffer another event (tertiary prevention). In all three cases, these patients' initial lab results revealed that their diseased arteries were severely inflamed, indicating that without immediate changes in treatment, they would be at high risk for another heart attack or stroke. Neal is another example of a patient who needed tertiary prevention, since he had repeatedly needed emergent procedures, such as bypass surgery and stent placements, to avoid heart attacks and strokes. Needing invasive procedures to treat blockages and restore blood flow to the heart or brain is also a CV "event."

4: Monitoring patients' response to treatments, to find out if the therapies that have been prescribed have successfully "cooled" inflammation in their arteries. In Neal's case, our ini-tial treatment plan included tweaks in his heart and diabetes medications and improving every aspect of his lifestyle, using the strategies in chapter thirteen. When we tested him again a year later, his levels of inflammation had dropped dramatically, as had his blood sugar and lipid levels. Unable to take more than ten steps without pain when we met, Neal reported that after following our prevention plan for twelve months, he could walk for two hours on the beach (with frequent stops to rest) and felt great. In fact, he was so excited about the rapid improvement in his lab results that he told us he was looking forward to the next round of testing—because he was confident that he'd get even more good news!

The Fire Panel

Just as firefighters have several ways to tell if a hidden blaze is raging inside the walls of a building—such as feeling heat, smelling smoke, or seeing the lights go out if the wiring catches fire—we use a combination of six lab tests to check for arterial inflammation. Each of them provides important information about your arterial health. These inexpensive blood and urine biomarker tests can all be done in the same medical visit. This panel of tests is available through Boston Heart Diagnostics, Cleveland HeartLab, Quest Diagnostics, LabCorp, and many other medical laboratories. Although the cost can vary, it's often covered by insurance plans and is usually less than $150 for the entire panel of tests.

The testing should be repeated at least annually even if the results are normal, since adverse changes in your lifestyle (such as increased stress, less exercise, lack of sleep, a poor diet, or weight gain, particularly in the belly) or in your health (such as dental infection, developing an inflammatory disorder like rheumatoid arthritis, or any of the other red flags discussed in chapter three) can cause a flare-up of inflammation, which we call sparking.

If you're at increased risk for cardiovascular events, your medical provider may recommend more frequent testing. We retest high-risk patients every three months, and medium-risk patients every six months.

If you have abnormal results on any of the six tests discussed in this section, it's extremely important to identify and treat *the root cause* of the inflammation. For example, our evaluation revealed that along with an extremely unhealthy lifestyle, Catherine also had several previously undiagnosed disorders that were sparking arterial fire, including full-blown type 2 diabetes, vitamin D deficiency, and elevated levels of lipoprotein (a), which has been shown in a 2020 study to be highly predictive of both the presence of new-onset coronary artery disease and its severity in postmenopausal women.[15] She also had almost all of the lifestyle factors that lead to chronic inflammation: obesity, lack of exercise, skimping on sleep, a poor diet, insulin resistance, and a wide waistline. However, she also had excellent oral health and was determined to make improving her arterial wellness a top priority.

Ask your healthcare provider if the conditions that are sparking fire in your arteries are being adequately addressed by your current treatment, since a rise in inflammatory biomarkers suggests that you may need different therapies or additions to your current prevention plan.

Typically, the first line of defense to extinguish fire in the arteries is lifestyle changes to combat the abnormalities that usually trigger inflammation, such as getting more exercise if you've slipped into a sedentary lifestyle, losing weight to combat insulin resistance and the toxic effects of belly fat, quitting smoking, managing stress, and eating a diet that's rich in antioxidants (found in many healthy foods, particularly fruits and vegetables) and fish (which has also been shown in studies to reduce inflammation in general and hs-CRP in particular). You'll find detailed advice on the best diet to protect your heart in chapter thirteen, including specific foods that help add years to your life, as well as those to avoid or limit.

Should these healthy changes not be enough, you may also need some of the medications and supplements discussed in chapter fourteen. Statins are one of the best medications to combat inflammation and also have powerful antioxidant and anti-clotting properties. All these attributes explain why statin therapy powerfully reduces heart attack and stroke risk in people with *normal* cholesterol levels. For example, the landmark 2008 JUPITER (Justification for the Use of Statins in Primary Prevention: an Intervention Trial Evaluating Rosuvastatin) clinical trial reported that when seemingly healthy people with normal or even low cholesterol—and high levels of hs-CRP—were treated with the statin drug rosuvastatin, their rate of cardiovascular complications (including heart attacks and strokes) was 50 percent lower than that of a group of similar patients who received a placebo, and their hs-CRP levels fell by nearly 40 percent.[16] Conducted in twenty-six countries around the world, the study included more than seventeen thousand men fifty and older and women sixty and older who have no prior history of coronary artery disease.

Niacin (vitamin B), vitamin D, fish oil, and the other supplements we recommend in chapter fourteen can also be valuable therapies. And the good news is that with the right treatment, elevated inflammatory biomarkers typically drop quickly, signaling that you're no longer on the fast track to a heart attack, stroke, or chronic disease. Here is a guide to the six Fire Panel tests, which are designed to answer four crucial questions about your arterial and overall health.

How fast is your body aging?

The test that can tell: F2 Isoprostanes

What the Test Checks for:

We've dubbed this blood test the Lifestyle Lie Detector because it can reveal whether our patients are practicing heart-healthy habits. Recently, a CEO we're treating claimed he'd been following our lifestyle advice to the letter, boasting that he'd kicked the nicotine habit, worked out daily, ate a healthy diet high in fruits and vegetables, and made sure to get eight hours of sleep a night.

However, his abnormal level of F2 isoprostanes suggested that he was lying. When confronted with his test results, he admitted that he'd been burning the midnight oil to work on an important business project, had let his fitness slide, and was mainly eating junk food from the local greasy spoon. Overwhelmed with the stress of this project, he'd also been sneaking cigarettes. By the end of the visit, he was apologizing profusely for trying to deceive us. "I just can't get away with anything with you," he remarked, before vowing to mend his ways.

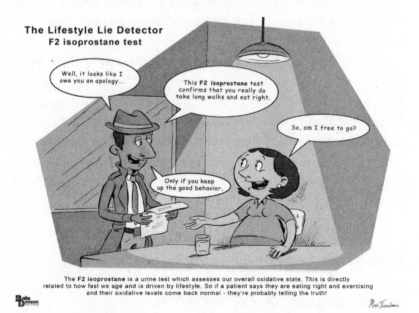

The F2 isoprostane is a urine test which assesses our overall oxidative state. This is directly related to how fast we age and is driven by lifestyle. So if a patient says they are eating right and exercising and their oxidative levels come back normal - they're probably telling the truth!

Since lifestyle is the most important therapy for chronic disease prevention, this test helps motivate patients to practice healthy habits, rather than just pretending they do, in the hope of avoiding a scolding from their healthcare provider. However, the test is much more than a lifestyle lie detector: It also reveals how fast your body is aging on a cellular level—and if you might be on the fast track to CVD and other chronic illnesses. Catherine, who was completely honest with us about her unhealthy lifestyle, was right to be alarmed about having arteries that were twenty years "older" than she was, because this test revealed that her cells were also aging much faster than normal.

The test measures F2 isoprostanes, a biomarker of oxidative stress, an imbalance between the formation of free radicals and protective antioxidant defenses. Oxidative stress increases platelet-derived growth factor—one of the strongest "sparks" of arterial disease.[17] Think of it as akin to lightning igniting a raging wildfire. As you learned earlier in this chapter, oxidation is one of the main triggers that causes contractile smooth muscle cells to go rogue, migrate into the intima, and form Velcro to capture cholesterol. This is what turns on the immune system's inflammatory response, which can lead to the formation of cats in the gutter.

Oxidative stress is also pro-inflammatory in another way that may surprise you: It can lead to premature cellular senescence, in which stressed cells can no longer divide to make new cells. When this occurs in endothelial cells, they can die, which can lead to plaque erosion and subsequent heart attack or stroke. Cellular senescence rises with aging and plays a pivotal role in many chronic age-related afflictions, including diabetes, chronic kidney disease, arthritis, erectile dysfunction, vision disorders, cancer, and such fatal brain disorders as Alzheimer's disease, Parkinson's disease, and amyotrophic lateral sclerosis (ALS), a neurodegenerative disorder that is also known as Lou Gehrig's disease.[18]

Essentially, the goal of the F2 isoprostanes test is to find out how fast your body is oxidizing, or breaking down. Although oxygen is essential for our survival, it also can be corrosive. When a freshly cut apple turns brown, a copper penny turns green, or a wrought-iron railing gets rusty, the culprit is oxidation, a reaction between oxygen molecules and substances they touch. As you may recall from high school chemistry, oxidation is the process of removing electrons from a molecule or atom.

Your body generates energy by burning fuel (nutrients from digested food) with oxygen. One by-product of normal metabolism—as well as smoking and other unhealthy habits—is the formation of free radicals, highly unstable atoms or molecules that are missing one of their electrons. To achieve stability, they steal an electron from nearby molecules, leading to a chain reaction in which the attacked molecules become free radicals and then rob their neighbors.

As a free radical chain rips through cells like a firestorm, it can cause extensive injury to crucial components. If DNA, the cell's blueprint, is damaged, mutations that might lead to cancer could result, while damage to proteins, the cell's workhorses, can make the cells dysfunctional and more susceptible to disease. The F2 isoprostanes test measures a marker of free radical damage to lipids (blood fats, such as cholesterol).

However, the body also has antioxidant defenses to protect against free radical damage, including physical barriers to cage free radicals, enzymes to neutralize dangerously reactive forms of oxygen, antioxidants in our diet (found in fruits and vegetables, among other foods) that donate electrons and defuse free radical chain reactions, repair processes to fix damaged DNA, a garbage disposal system to sweep up these destructive scavengers, and other responses, such as programmed cell suicide if the damage is too extensive.

Therefore, the key to slowing down aging and protecting your cardiovascular health is achieving a balance between destructive oxidation and antioxidant defenses. Among the ways you can strengthen your antioxidant defenses—and slow the rate at which your body is "rusting"—is by following healthy habits, including avoiding smoking, eating a Mediterranean-style diet that's high in fruits and vegetables and low in saturated fat, managing the stress in your life, and exercising regularly. Many of our patients report that they look and feel much younger after following the personalized lifestyle recommendations in part three.

What the Results Mean:

As is true of other biomarker tests, there is a continuum of risk. One study found that people with the highest levels of F2 iso-prostanes were *nine times more likely* to develop coronary artery disease than those with the lowest.[19] Although labs have established "cut points" for risk, the reality is that the lower your number is, the better, since some people will be sparking to some degree when their number is between normal and optimal. Therefore, if your other fire markers are elevated, and your F2 isoprostanes are normal, you may still be advised to make lifestyle changes to protect your heart, brain, and arterial health.

A normal F2 isoprostanes level is less than 0.86 ng/L, while an optimal result is less than 0.25 ng/L. Although abnormal levels typically signal an unhealthy lifestyle that could cause premature aging, as was true in Catherine's case, an important caveat is that some professional athletes or very dedicated amateur fitness buffs may also have increased oxidation, due to the extreme stress they're putting on their bodies.

With exercise, as with other healthy behaviors, it's crucial to find the sweet spot between doing too little and doing too much. A 2012 study published in *Mayo Clinic Proceedings* found that extreme endurance training may cause long-term heart damage in some marathoners, professional cyclists, and ultra-marathon runners, prompting the researchers to recommend moderate exercise or interval training (mini-bursts of high-intensity exercise that will be discussed later in the book) as healthier for the heart.[20]

Is your blood vessel lining inflamed?

The tests that can tell:

Fibrinogen, high-sensitivity C-reactive protein, and microalbumin/creatinine urine ratio are biomarkers of endothelial (tennis court) inflammation.

"Tennis court"

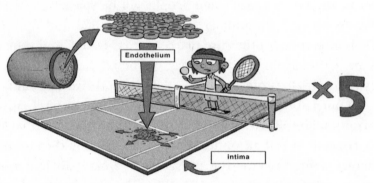

The endothelial cells which line our arteries are so numerous that, if taken out of your body, they would cover the surface of five tennis courts. These endothelial "tennis court" cells create a vital protective wall against heart attacks and strokes.

Fibrinogen

What the Test Checks for:

This blood test measures your level of fibrinogen, a sticky, fibrous protein produced by your liver. Fibrinogen helps stop bleeding and heals wounds by causing your blood to clot.

While fibrinogen's clotting effects can be lifesaving after an injury, abnormally high levels in the bloodstream can be dangerous, by contributing to the clotting cascade that leads to heart attacks and strokes. Fibrinogen is also a marker of inflammation, but other factors can boost levels, so this test shouldn't be used as the sole method of checking for fire in the arteries.

The higher your blood level of fibrinogen, the greater the risk of cardiovascular events. In a meta-analysis that pooled results of thirty-one studies that included more than 154,000 patients, risk for heart disease and stroke rose by 82 percent for each 100 mg/dL increase in fibrinogen levels above 250 mg/dL, even when the results were adjusted for the participants' ages, genders, and numerous major cardiovascular risk factors, including smoking, diabetes, high blood pressure, high cholesterol, and obesity.[21]

Another large study called the EUROSTROKE project reported that "fibrinogen is a powerful predictor of stroke," including both fatal and nonfatal strokes, as well as first-time strokes, ischemic strokes, and hemorrhagic strokes (those caused by a torn or ruptured blood vessel).[22] The researchers found that people with the highest fibrinogen levels were nearly seven times more likely to suffer a hemorrhagic stroke than those with the lowest levels, and had double the risk of a fatal stroke. The study also found that high blood pressure plus high fibrinogen packed a double whammy, magnifying risk even more than high fibrinogen alone. That's probably because fibrinogen and its by-products, such as fibrin, contribute to vascular disease by damaging the blood vessel lining, while high blood pressure further increases wear and tear that makes it easier for plaque to burrow inside. Plaque often contains large amounts of fibrin.

High fibrinogen has also been linked to other diseases, including diabetes, cancer, and high blood pressure, and is frequently elevated in people with insulin-resistant conditions, such as metabolic syndrome, which will be discussed in depth in the next chapter. And for people with coronary artery disease, elevated fibrinogen increases the risk that a clot will form if plaque ruptures or erodes, setting the stage for a heart attack.

What the Results Mean:

The normal value is less than 370 mg/dL. In one study, having a fibrinogen level of 600 mg/dL was associated with a 200 percent increase in the risk for cardiovascular events, compared to people whose fibrinogen level was normal.[23]

High-Sensitivity C-Reactive Protein (hs-CRP)

What the Test Checks for:

This inexpensive blood test uses a technology called laser nephelometry to rapidly measure very small amounts of C-reactive protein (CRP) with high sensitivity (accuracy). CRP, a protein produced by the liver, rises in the bloodstream when there's inflammation throughout the body, which may indicate fire in the arteries that could ignite a heart attack or stroke.

However, the downside of the test is that it's possible to have high levels of CRP *without* arterial disease, because infections, injuries, having a fever, or inflammatory disorders (such as rheumatoid arthritis) can also cause a spike in levels. Despite this limitation, large studies have consistently shown that abnormally high CRP levels can be a strong predictor of cardiovascular danger. For example, in a pooled analysis of data from about 250,000 people without CVD, adding hs-CRP and/or fibrinogen levels to conventional factors significantly improved risk assessment for a first-time CV event.[24] In the Physicians Health Study, which tracked about eighteen thousand apparently healthy doctors, elevated levels of CRP were linked to triple the risk of heart attack, compared to doctors with normal levels.[25] In a similar study of about twenty-eight thousand women, results of the hs-CRP test were *more* accurate than cholesterol levels in predicting risk for cardiovascular events. The researchers reported that women with the highest levels of CRP were 4.4 times more likely to suffer a heart attack or stroke than were women with lowest levels.[26] Elevated CRP is even more dangerous if you also have a large waist, the leading sign of insulin resistance, which further magnifies heart attack and stroke risk.

What the Results Mean:

One strength of hs-CRP and fibrinogen testing is that if either one of them is normal, it's extremely unlikely that your arterial lining is inflamed. A score of under 1.0 mg/L is normal, while a score of 0.5 is optimal, indicating that short-term risk for cardiovascular events is very low. However, it's important to have the test repeated periodically since even a slight elevation could be an early warning sign of increased heart attack or stroke risk.

While it's comforting to have a normal or optimal level of CRP, a high level, as discussed above, isn't conclusive evidence of heart attack, stroke, or CVD risk. Therefore, if your hs-CRP results are abnormal, and there's no other apparent reason for inflammation, your healthcare provider will probably advise repeating the test a week later to confirm the results.

To find out if arterial wall inflammation is the reason for persistently elevated hs-CRP, it's helpful to compare hs-CRP results with those of the test described below, microalbumin/creatinine urine ratio (MACR). Since the two tests measure completely different biomarkers that may signal fire in the arteries, if both are elevated—as was the case with Catherine—there's a very strong probability that blood vessel inflammation is the culprit. If MACR is normal and hs-CRP and/or fibrinogen are high, this is most likely due to some other health issue, such as insulin resistance, diabetes, an infectious illness, or an inflammatory disorder, such as arthritis.

Microalbumin/Creatinine Urine Ratio

What the Test Checks for:

This test detects small amounts of albumin, a blood protein, in the urine. The term "microalbumin" refers to amounts of albumin that are too small to detect in the urine dipstick test used for routine urinalysis during annual physicals. Having protein in the urine is abnormal, because albumin is a large molecule that circulates in blood and shouldn't spill from capillaries in the kidney into your urine. Therefore, the test checks for a biomarker of endothelial dysfunction, as an indication of arterial disease. The urine ratio compares the amounts of microalbumin with those of creatinine (CR), a waste product produced by muscles.

Although this simple urine test costs just pennies, is covered by virtually all health plans, and provides valuable information about arterial wall health, healthcare providers rarely use it for this purpose, even though it's an extremely cost-effective way to check for evidence of arterial disease. Instead, MACR is most commonly performed to screen people with diabetes, high blood pressure, or kidney disorders for kidney damage.

The ongoing Framingham Offspring study found that UACR is an independent biomarker that predicts risk for cardiovascular events in seemingly healthy patients, while hs-CRP and fibrinogen were not independent predictors in that study. Therefore, *an abnormal UACR is an important warning sign of cardiovascular danger, even if your hs-CRP and fibrinogen levels are normal.* The researchers found that people with an elevated UACR had 20 percent higher rate of CV events, even when other risk factors were taken into account.[27]

Another insight from research is that MACR is more accurate than the conventional albumin urine test often used in routine annual physicals because MACR considers how much water the patient has consumed and calculates the concentration of albumin in the urine accordingly.

What the Results Mean:

Recent evidence from the large Framingham Offspring study shows that MACR results that have traditionally been considered normal can signal greatly increased risk for cardiovascular events. Specifically, women whose MACR was above 7.5 and men with a ratio above 4 had *nearly triple* the risk for heart attacks, strokes, and other cardiovascular events during six years of follow-up in that study.[28] Therefore, ratios of 7.5 or lower for women and 4 or lower for men are optimal, rather than the much higher numbers that are still considered normal by standard care.[29]

Based on the Framingham Offspring study results, Catherine's MACR of 15 was quite alarming, since these numbers put her in the highest risk group for a heart attack or stroke. Yet practitioners of standard care would have patted her on the back and assured her that the test results were perfectly normal, had these healthcare providers even ordered this extremely valuable and cost-effective but rarely used inflammatory biomarker test in the first place.

Do you have arterial plaque that is "hot" and growing?

The test that can tell: Lipoprotein-Associated Phospholipase A-2 (Lp-PLA2)

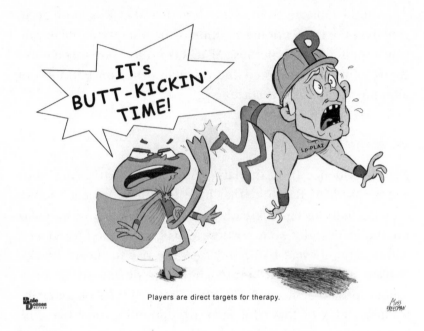

IT's BUTT-KICKIN' TIME!

Players are direct targets for therapy.

What the Test Checks for:

This blood test measures lipoprotein-associated phospholipase A-2, a blood vessel–specific enzyme that's mainly attached to LDL (bad) cholesterol. Levels of Lp-LPA2 rise when arterial walls become inflamed, which may indicate that plaque is more likely to rupture, which could lead to a heart attack or stroke. In December 2014, the Lp-PLA2 test was FDA approved as a screening test to predict a patient's future risk for heart disease–related

196

events. In December 2014, the FDA cleared this test to screen all adults for risk for future cardiovascular events, whether or not they have a history of CVD.

This enzyme is now emerging not only as a biomarker of arterial wall inflammation, but also a direct *player* in the atherogenic triad. Why is that important? A biomarker of risk serves only as a warning that arterial disease may be in progress. However, treatments that reduce levels of that biomarker have no effect on the end disease. For example, if your car's "check engine" light went on, removing the light bulb wouldn't solve the mechanical problem. Biomarkers that are players in the disease serve both as warnings of risk and direct targets for therapies to halt and reverse the disease. For example, if your car's temperature gauge went into the red zone, you could add coolant to the engine to prevent catastrophic damage from overheating.

A 2012 study suggests that Lp-PLA2 plays a key role in cholesterol plaque formation and vulnerability (risk that the plaque may rupture explosively and trigger a heart attack or stroke). In a series of lab experiments, they demonstrated that exposing Pac-Man-like macrophages to oxidized LDL cholesterol for forty-eight hours induced the production of foam cells and a sharp rise in Lp-PLA2, indicating that it was marking an active atherosclerotic disease process. The researchers note that their findings support reducing Lp-PLA2 as a strategy for preventing CHD.

Large studies have also shown that people with elevated Lp-PLA2 levels are up to twice as likely to suffer heart-related events as those with normal levels and that this biomarker independently predicts CV risk as accurately as a person's blood pressure or cholesterol levels.[30] Research has also revealed that people with periodontal disease (PD) are nearly twice as likely to have elevated Lp-PLA2 levels than those with healthy gums.[31]

The good news, however, is that treating this chronic oral infection significantly decreases Lp-PLA2 levels—and helps patients avoid tooth loss and other complications of PD.[32]

Evidence-based guidelines from the American Heart Association, the Centers for Disease Control and Prevention, and other groups also endorse the test for screening symptom-free people who are at intermediate risk for heart disease or increased risk for stroke.[33] Other research indicates that elevated levels of Lp-PLA2 and hs-CRP are also strong, independent predictors of risk for developing metabolic syndrome, a gang of heart attack, stroke, and diabetes risk factors that we'll discuss more fully in the next chapter.[34]

Unlike the MACR test, which evaluates the health of the endothelium (by checking if the blood vessel lining had become so dysfunctional that large molecules of albumin are spilling from the bloodstream in the kidneys into the urine), the Lp-PLA2 test is designed to answer a different, but extremely important question: How hot is it *under* your tennis court? In other words, is there fiery plaque hidden inside the artery wall that might erupt like a volcano?

What the Results Mean:

Lp-PLA2 values of less than 200 ng/mL are considered normal. In the Mayo Heart Study, 95 percent of patients with scores under this threshold did *not* have a heart attack or stroke in the next four years, even though they had coronary artery disease (CAD).[35] The researchers also found that the higher Lp-PLA2 levels, the greater the risk for a first attack, stroke, or major CV event. Compared to patients with normal levels, those with scores of 200 to 266 ng/mL had a 70 percent higher risk of these events over the next four years, while a level of 267 or above more than doubled risk.

For Camille, whose MACR was in the optimal range, the

Lp-LPA2 test sounded a potentially lifesaving alarm by revealing that several weeks after her heart attack, the plaque inside her arterial wall remained dangerously inflamed, even though her tennis court looked normal. Her score of 257 ng/mL meant that the treatments her doctors had prescribed weren't good enough to prevent another heart attack, because they'd failed to put the fire out.

To illustrate just how dire the young mom's risk would have been without changes in her treatment, in the KAROLA heart study, which looked specifically at people who had already experienced cardiac events, participants with this score were *2.3 times* more likely to suffer a recurrent event—or sudden cardiac death—over the next 4.5 years than those with lower scores.[36] And the main clue that her arteries were still on fire was the Lp-PLA2 test results, since almost all of her other inflammatory biomarkers were in the normal range.

Are you in imminent danger of a heart attack or stroke?

The test that can tell: Myeloperoxidase (MPO)

What the Test Checks for:

This FDA-approved blood test measures myeloperoxidase, a white blood cell–derived inflammatory enzyme that the immune system uses to fight infection. Normally, MPO is only found at elevated levels at the site of an infection. In our patients, we find that elevated MPO frequently occurs in tandem with dental infections, a topic we will discuss more fully in chapter ten. We call MPO the joker because if it's elevated throughout the body—as occurs in about two in fifty people, a similar distribution to the jokers in a deck of cards—all bets are off. Of all the inflammatory biomarkers, it's the worst: If this wild card, which appears to be genetically influenced, gets played, without the right treatment your game of life might be over.

Elevated levels of MPO strongly predict future risk for coronary artery disease in healthy people, regardless of all other known risk factors.[37] One reason that this malevolent joker is so dangerous is that it produces numerous oxidants that make *all* cholesterol compounds more inflammatory. This includes HDL, the good cholesterol that normally helps clean the arteries, protecting against plaque buildup. If your blood levels of MPO are high, HDL goes rogue and joins the gang of inflammatory bullies. The joker also interacts with hydrogen peroxide in the bloodstream to produce hypochlorous acid (the active ingredient in bleach).

Another of MPO's nasty tricks is reducing the body's production of nitric oxide (NO), the best "food" to nourish the endothelium and protect its health. Lowering NO weakens the

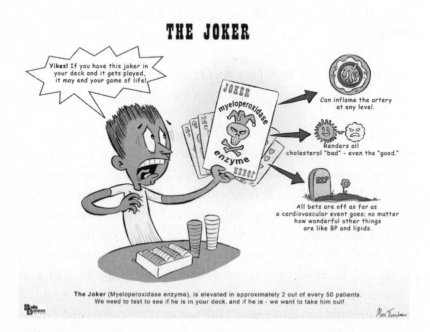

THE JOKER

Yikes! If you have this joker in your deck and it gets played, it may end your game of life!

JOKER
myeloperoxidase
enzyme
JOKER

Can inflame the artery at any level.

Renders all cholesterol "bad" - even the "good."

All bets are off as far as a cardiovascular event goes; no matter how wonderful other things are like BP and lipids.

The Joker (Myeloperoxidase enzyme), is elevated in approximately 2 out of every 50 patients. We need to test to see if he is in your deck, and if he is - we want to take him out!

integrity of the tennis court, which can either promote atherosclerosis, or for people who already have plaque in their arteries,
magnify the risk that the cat will leap out of the gutter and cause
a heart attack or stroke. The joker contributes to creating vulnerable plaque in two ways: It can make the normally protective
fibrous cap that covers plaque more prone to rupturing explosively or it can eat holes in the tennis court, leading to plaque
erosion and a subsequent CV event. On average, serum levels of
MPO are higher in people who suffer erosive events, a 2018
study found.[38]

What the Results Mean:

The normal value is less than 480 pmol/L. Unlike hs-CRP, levels of MPO in the blood are not likely to be elevated due to
infections or illness: This enzyme is a *specific* biomarker of blood
vessel inflammation and vulnerable plaque (the dangerous kind
that can lead to heart attacks and strokes). Elevated MPO predicts future risk for coronary artery disease and cardiovascular
events, including fatal heart attacks and strokes. In a recent
study, people with high levels of the joker were 2.4 times more
likely to die from heart disease over the next thirteen years.[39]
Elevated MPO has also been shown to be an important independent risk factor for having a major cardiovascular event in the
next one to six months.[40]

One of the most common culprits for a spike in MPO is dental infections. If untreated, these can trigger heart attacks or
strokes in people with vulnerable plaque. For example, as you
read in chapter six, shortly after Melinda's seemingly inexplicable stroke, she was treated for a severely infected tooth, which
required extraction. If you have elevated MPO, ask your dental
provider to check you for tooth and gum infections, both of
which are highly treatable, using the therapies in chapter ten. If
you're being treated for atherosclerosis, elevated MPO can be a

warning that your current therapies are not doing enough to cool and stabilize your disease. Ask your medical provider about additional treatment options. In chapter fourteen, we'll tell you about the most effective medications and supplements to halt, stabilize, or even reverse arterial disease.

Action Step: Use These Easy, Natural Ways to "Fireproof" Your Arteries

Study after study has proven that an optimal lifestyle is the most powerful defense against chronic inflammation and the devastating diseases it can spark, as we will discuss more fully in chapter thirteen. Here are four proven strategies to fight arterial fire—without a $200,000 a year drug:

Practice mindfulness daily.

A 2017 study published in *The Lancet* used PET imaging to show that when the brain's amygdala is over-activated by stress or anxiety, bone marrow produces more white blood cells, leading to arterial inflammation, which in turn magnifies heart attack, stroke, and chronic disease risk.[41] Mindful meditation, however, appears to have the opposite effect, the researchers reported. Not only can it boost heart health, but mindfulness also improves sleep and mood. We recommend devoting *ten* minutes a day to mindful meditation. Sit in a relaxed position, close your eyes, and focus on your breathing and the present moment as you let stressful or upsetting thoughts float away. Prayer is another great way to soothe the mind and spirit, enhancing cardiovascular wellness.

Step up physical activity.

Why does regular exercise greatly reduce heart attack and stroke risk? While you might guess that physical activity keeps the heart healthy by lowering cholesterol, blood pressure, and body weight—all of which help protect against cardiovascular (CV) events—the well-known Women's Health Study found that the number one cardiovascular benefit of regular exercise is reducing inflammation.[42] Aim for at least thirty minutes of aerobic exercise, such as brisk walking, jogging, or biking, daily. Check with your healthcare provider before starting a new fitness regimen to make sure it's right for you.

Eat the rainbow.

Consuming a variety of colorful fruits and vegetables has amazing cardiovascular benefits, including lower risk for heart attacks, strokes, diabetes, high blood pressure, and several forms of cancer. What's more, people who eat a diet that is high in fiber (found in most produce) are nearly 60 percent less likely to die from CV causes, according to a study of nearly 400,000 people ages fifty and older.[43] Stock up on leafy green veggies, tomatoes, citrus fruit, fresh berries, and cruciferous vegetables (such as broccoli, cabbage, and Brussels sprouts), all of which have been shown in studies to boost heart, brain, and arterial wellness.

Ditch sweet drinks.

Consuming just one or two sugar-sweetened beverages daily— such as energy drinks, fruit drinks, soda, or coffee drinks—raises risk for a heart attack or dying from CVD by 35 percent, diabetes risk by 26 percent, and stroke risk by 16 percent, according to a 2015 study in the *Journal of the American College of Cardiology*.[44] Sometimes called liquid candy, sweet drinks are the top source of added sugar in the U.S. diet. Excessive sugar intake also magnifies the threat of developing chronic inflammation, cancer, insulin resistance, and obesity. Sugary beverages also increase the likelihood that you'll develop a disorder that's been called the deadly pandemic that you've never heard of. Yet this cluster of heart attack and diabetes risks, which affects nearly 40 percent of U.S. adults, is so easy to diagnose that you can do it yourself, without any medical tests. In the next chapter, you'll learn why this cardio-vascular villain is at the root of most chronic diseases, how to find out if you have it, and the best ways to prevent it.

CHAPTER 9

The Deadly Pandemic You've Never Heard Of

"Our separation from each other is an optical illusion of consciousness."

— ALBERT EINSTEIN

Dwayne thought he was in pretty good health—until he applied for life insurance. "They did a blood test and none of the numbers meant anything to me, so I showed them to my family doctor," says the retired truck driver from Cheney, Washington. "He was absolutely floored by my lab results and said, 'And they gave you *life insurance?*' Throughout the visit, he kept looking at the numbers and shaking his head in disbelief. That's when I found out that my triglycerides were through the roof: It sounded like there was more fat than blood flowing through my arteries."

A few years later, Dwayne, then forty-seven, was one of the first people to be treated at the Heart Attack & Stroke Prevention Center. During the two decades that he's been our patient, he's astonished and inspired us with one of the most remarkable health turnarounds that we've ever witnessed. When we did our initial assessment, it was easy to see why his family doctor deemed him a questionable candidate for life insurance. Not only were his lipid numbers abnormal, but he also had hypertension (blood pressure of 130/80 mm Hg or higher).

High blood pressure, which affects nearly half of U.S. adults, is often called a silent killer, because if untreated, it's a stealthy assassin that gives few clues to its presence as it wreaks slow havoc on its victim's arteries and vital organs, including the heart, brain, and kidneys. In Dwayne's case, persistently high blood pressure was putting his life and his livelihood at risk. Then employed as a long-distance truck driver, he feared that if he didn't get his hypertension under control, he'd fail the Department of Transportation's (DOT) annual physical, which required truckers to have a systolic pressure (the top number in a blood pressure reading) below 140 mm Hg.

"Even on the blood pressure medication my doctor had prescribed, I was struggling to pass the physical," recalls Dwayne, who was also worried about his weight, which had climbed to 285 pounds on his five-foot-eleven frame. In addition, he'd developed a spare tire around the middle and our testing revealed that he was prediabetic. This combination of disorders meant that Dwayne had metabolic syndrome, a gang of cardiovascular bullies that attack in tandem, tripling risk for a heart attack and more than quintupling it for type 2 diabetes.[1]

"I'd never heard of this syndrome and was shocked to learn how serious it is," he says. "Finding out that I had it was scary because my mom had a long battle with diabetes and cardiovascular problems—including high cholesterol, peripheral artery disease, and a stroke—and passed away when she was sixty-four," adds Dwayne, whose father died at seventy-one from complications of heart surgery. However, he was relieved to learn that the syndrome is highly treatable and can often be reversed with the optimal lifestyle and personalized therapies advised by our AHA for Life plan.

Only One in Eight American Adults Is Metabolically Healthy

Eighty-five percent of Americans have never heard of metabolic syndrome, a national health survey reported.[2] And of the more than 211,000 people polled, only 0.6 percent thought they had the condition themselves. While that may make it sound extremely rare, metabolic syndrome affects *1 billion people* worldwide, including 66 million Americans.[3] Although it's most common in older adults—affecting about half of those over sixty—rates of this lifestyle-linked malady are on the rise in people of all ages, particularly among those in their twenties and thirties, according to a 2020 study published in *Journal of the American Medical Association*.[4] Millions of them are undiagnosed and unaware of their peril.

These are "very alarming" trends, because the disease can have a snowball effect if it goes undetected and untreated, study coauthor Dr. Robert Wong told *HealthDay*.[5] "Young adults have so many years for damage and impact from metabolic syndrome." Among the many perils they face, according to other recent studies, are atherosclerosis, strokes, fatty liver (fat buildup in the liver), obstructive sleep apnea (OSA), polycystic ovary syndrome, gallstones, diabetes, cancers of the liver, colon, bladder, breast, uterus and pancreas, heart attacks, and Alzheimer's disease, which is *twelve times more likely* to strike people with the syndrome as those without it.[6] If untreated, metabolic syndrome has been shown to double or even triple the risk for early death due to heart attacks, strokes, sudden cardiac death, cancer, and other causes.[7] Another frightening finding: If you have metabolic syndrome and catch COVID-19, your risk for severe or fatal illness is *seven times higher* than that of a metabolically healthy person.[8]

Only one in eight Americans, however, is achieving optimal

metabolic wellness, according to another new study.[9] Researchers from the University of North Carolina at Chapel Hill defined optimal metabolic health as meeting guideline-recommended targets for five factors — blood pressure, blood sugar, triglycerides, HDL (good) cholesterol, and waist circumference — and not taking any medications related to these factors. To determine how many Americans were at high versus low risk for chronic illness, the team examined data from nearly nine thousand adult participants in the National Health and Nutrition Survey. The analysis found that only 12.2 percent of them were metabolically healthy, suggesting that nationally, only 27.3 million adults are meeting optimal goals to protect their cardiovascular health and ward off chronic illness. The study also reported that only one percent of the obese people they studied were metabolically healthy.

Dwayne's story highlights some of the perils of obesity paired with poor metabolic health. Our initial evaluation revealed that he had arterial plaque and high levels of inflammation, the dangerous duo of disorders that can ignite heart attacks and strokes. What's more, he was then in the early stages of non-alcoholic fatty liver disease, an obesity-linked disorder that affects about 25 percent of U.S. adults. Marked by buildup of fat and triglycerides in liver cells, this disorder, which is also known as fatty liver, can sometimes progress to liver inflammation, scarring (cirrhosis), and end-stage liver failure, if untreated.[10] A recent study also reported that people with fatty liver were up to six times more likely to develop diabetes in the next five years than those with healthy livers.[11] If caught early, fatty liver can often be reversed with weight loss.

Our evaluation also revealed that Dwayne had previously undiagnosed OSA, which occurs so frequently in people with metabolic syndrome that some scientists have proposed that it be added to the diagnostic criteria.[12] One study reported that people with OSA are 40 percent more likely to have the syndrome than those without this sleep disorder, even if they are not obese.[13] OSA also increases risk for fatty liver disease, heart attacks, strokes, and diabetes. And as you learned in chapter two, this sleep disorder is a frequently overlooked root cause of hard-to-control high blood pressure, as turned out to be the case with Dwayne. In addition, since he was already prediabetic, the combination of metabolic disorder, obesity, fatty liver, and OSA was putting him at extreme risk for progressing to full-blown type 2 diabetes, a disease that had contributed to the deaths of his mother and other relatives.

Horrified by all the ways that metabolic syndrome was robbing him of his health, the trucker decided to embark on a different journey, one that would lead to wellness and healing. "I stopped doing the things that were killing me and switched to habits that would help me," he says. "Instead of eating fatty foods like hamburgers, bacon, and brisket at truck stops, I ate from the salad bar and also brought healthy foods with me, such as fruit, nuts, and canned tuna fish. At that time, I was driving for twelve to sixteen hours a day and got almost no exercise, so I began parking my truck for thirty minutes and taking a brisk walk every day."

After implementing these healthy changes, Dwayne's health metrics and inflammatory markers gradually began to improve. We also made adjustments in his medications and advised him to use a CPAP machine at night to treat his OSA, both of which, along with an improved lifestyle, helped get his hypertension under control. Regular exercise helps treat or prevent more than forty diseases, including diabetes, cancer, CVD, obesity, Alzheimer's disease, and arthritis—with effects comparable or even superior to medication, according to a 2018 American Heart Association scientific statement.[14] Conversely, physical inactivity kills more than 5.3 million people around the world prematurely each year—more than the toll from smoking![15]

A Surprising Risk Factor Most Doctors Don't Check

Given the many deadly dangers of metabolic syndrome, which have been documented in numerous large studies dating back to the 1980s, why is public awareness of this disorder so stunningly low? Part of the problem is that over the years, it's gone by many monikers, including Syndrome X, insulin resistance syndrome, obesity syndrome, and hypertriglyceridemic waist.[16] Another issue: Some people confuse metabolic syndrome with better-known conditions linked to metabolism, like diabetes or obesity.

Now there's a movement afoot to rename metabolic syndrome yet again. Some medical providers deem cardiometabolic syndrome a more descriptive moniker since the condition damages the cardiovascular system *and* impairs metabolism (how the body burns and stores energy from food). Others have suggested it be dubbed sitting disease, since the syndrome is most common in obese people with a sedentary lifestyle and/or occupation, such as Camille, Dwayne, and Neal. This term has been coined by the scientific community and the media to refer to both metabolic syndrome and the myriad maladies linked to spending most of the day parked in a chair.

Prolonged sitting often leads to abdominal obesity (too much belly fat), which is one of the driving forces behind metabolic syndrome, along with insulin resistance and, in some cases, genetic factors. Our patients are often surprised when we measure their waists, since many healthcare providers fail to include this essential vital sign in the physical examination. However, they should: A large waistline is the leading indicator of both metabolic syndrome and a closely related condition, insulin resistance, which we'll discuss more fully later in this chapter.

Numerous studies have shown that a large waist circumference is a stronger predictor of increased risk for a heart attack or stroke than the patient's weight or body mass index (BMI), a number calculated from the person's height in inches and weight in pounds, using a mathematical formula: weight is divided by height squared, then multiplied by 703. One long-term study found that even women with normal weights and BMIs were three times more likely to die from heart disease if their waist was above thirty-five inches, as compared to normal-weight women with waists that were smaller than thirty-five inches.

The researchers also reported that the women with the largest waists had a similarly increased risk for early death from cancer and other diseases than those with the smallest waists—and that risk rose with each additional inch around the middle.[17] Another study of nearly 500,000 older adults linked having a spare tire to increased risk for dementia in older adults.[18] Studies show that waist size alone can also accurately predict risk for type 2 diabetes, especially in women.[19] Later in this chapter, we'll tell you about two surprising lipid numbers that can also reveal if you have IR or are on the fast track to arterial disease and its many complications. If so, partnering with your provider to halt or reverse these maladies could save your life.

Since it takes just seconds to measure a patient's waist—and gain immediate, actionable, and, in some cases, potentially life-saving insights into the person's cardiovascular and metabolic health—why do so few doctors check this important metric? Has any medical provider ever measured *your* waist? Some psychologists theorize that medical bias against overweight patients may play a role in their getting substandard care. For example, in a recent presentation at the American Psychology Association, Joan Chrisler, PhD, professor of psychology at Connecticut College, reported that some doctors are reluctant to touch obese patients and also shortchange them on necessary diagnostic tests and treatments. "Research has shown that doctors repeatedly advise weight loss for fat patients, while recommending CAT scans, blood work, or physical therapy for other, average weight patients," she stated.[20]

All too often, providers attribute a fat patient's symptoms to obesity, as Elaine's doctors did, or brush off their health concerns with patronizing, dismissive advice. She was repeatedly told, "just get the weight off and everything will be fine," while Catherine was counseled to "lose weight and get more sleep." Actually, both had potentially lethal arterial plaque and high levels of inflammation that were completely missed. Similarly, Camille's metabolic syndrome, prediabetes, and arterial disease went undiagnosed until she'd already had a heart attack! What's more, her early warning signs—and those of J.P., who was also overweight at the time of his widow-maker heart attack—were mistakenly attributed to psychological issues, a medical misjudgment that could have cost both of them their lives.

Tragically, research indicates that obese patients face a much higher threat of medical misdiagnosis or neglect than normal-weight patients, even when they have life-threatening disorders: In one study of more than three hundred autopsy records, obese patients were 1.65 times more likely to have serious undiagnosed medical conditions—including cancer, heart attacks, ruptured aortic aneurysms, blood clots in the lung, and other blood-vessel disorders—that led to their death than other patients.

Although medical bias, fat-shaming, and doctors' microaggressions—such as a headshake, wince, or *tsk-tsk* when recording an obese patient's weight in the chart—can lead some overweight people to avoid seeking healthcare at all, one of our major goals in writing this book is to help patients of all ages, weights, and sizes learn how to navigate the medical system successfully and empower them with the knowledge required to demand the top-quality care they need to ward off serious health threats.

Later in this chapter, you'll learn which blood-sugar test provides the most accurate screening for IR and diabetes and what to do if you have either of these maladies.

A Dangerous Disorder You Can Diagnose Yourself

Although metabolic syndrome may not be on your medical provider's radar, you can find out if you have it simply by looking at a few basic numbers that should be in everyone's health record. You should also be aware that it's possible to have this condition even if you are not overweight, since the key driver is abdominal obesity, not overall fat. To make the diagnosis, check the following five warning signs. Making the call is a little like baseball: Three strikes and you're out, since having at least three of these factors means that you have metabolic syndrome. If so, we've included some action steps to address the various risk factors.

1: A large waist.

Up to 70 percent of people with the syndrome are saddled with excessive belly fat, giving them an apple shape.[21] Sometimes called middle-age spread, this type of fat is metabolically active, releasing compounds that contribute to chronic inflammation, insulin resistance, and high blood pressure, all of which increase your risk for CVD and other chronic diseases. A waist measurement of thirty-five or more inches for a woman, or forty or more inches for a man, is one strike, according to the standard definition of the disorder. Recently, however, researchers have reported that the numbers vary by ethnicity as follows: For Africans and Middle Easterners, the abnormal numbers are 37 and 31.5 inches respectively for men and women; for most Asians and people from Central South America, 35.5 (men) and 31.5

(women); and for the Japanese, the abnormal number for men, 33.5 inches, is *smaller* than the number for women: 35.5 inches.[22]

To tell if you might be at risk, wrap a tape measure around the top of your pelvic bones (where the love handles grow) and exhale before measuring. Don't assume that your belly button marks your waistline, as its location can vary. And here's an important note for men: Don't be tempted to substitute your pants size for your waist measurement—it's highly inaccurate!

What to do if you have this cardiometabolic disorder risk:

Combine aerobic exercise, such as walking, jogging, cycling, or swimming, with muscle strengthening activities, such as lifting weights or resistance training. Both types of exercise help dieters avoid regaining belly fat after weight loss, suggesting that regular workouts are essential for maintaining a healthy weight and waistline.[23] Aim for at least thirty minutes of exercise daily, using the personalized diet and fitness plan in chapter thirteen. Check with your provider before starting a new fitness regime to make sure it's right for you. Also ditch sodas and other sugary drinks: Drinking even one per day boosts risk for metabolic syndrome and diabetes by up to 20 percent![24] Coffee, on the other hand, *lowers* risk by about 13 percent, according to an analysis of studies that included nearly 160 million people.

2: High blood pressure.

Recently, the American Heart Association and American College of Cardiology updated their blood pressure guidelines, with 130/80 mm Hg as the new threshold for a hypertension diagnosis, while systolic pressure (the top number) between 120–129 and diastolic pressure (the bottom number) below 80 is classified as "elevated."[25] Based on this definition, nearly half of U.S. adults—116 million people—have hypertension.[26] Medical criteria for metabolic syndrome, however, use a different blood pressure number: If your pressure is 130/85 mm Hg or higher, you have a strike. Decades of data show this level of pressure (or higher) damages arteries, heightening risk for heart attacks, strokes, kidney failure, vascular dementia, and many other debilitating conditions.

What to do if you have this risk factor:

Have your blood pressure checked regularly and talk to your provider if even one of your numbers is abnormal (a reading of 120/80 or above). About 75 percent of people with hypertension—91 million Americans—don't have their disorder under control, even though most of them are under the care of a medical provider and take medication, according to an alarming 2019 report from the CDC.[27] If you fit this profile, ask your provider if it's time to consider additional medications or intensifying the dosage. In chapter fourteen, we'll tell you about a new genetic test that helps ensure that you get the most effective medications—at the right dosage.

Although medication is usually necessary to treat hypertension, there are also some natural ways to lower blood pressure. These include mindful meditation to reduce stress (an important contributor to elevated blood pressure), eating foods that are rich in magnesium (which helps regulate blood pressure), such as dark green leafy vegetables, unrefined grains, and legumes, and getting seven to eight hours of sleep a night (skimping on slumber is linked to increased risk for hypertension).

3: Low HDL cholesterol.

HDL (high-density lipoprotein) is the good cholesterol. An HDL level below 50 mg/dL for women, and under 40 mg/dL for men, is another strike for metabolic syndrome. Many people who are headed for arterial disease and diabetes will have low HDL levels. If you are being treated for low HDL, you have a strike even if the levels are above 50 and 40 mg/dL. Along with measuring your HDL level, the standard cholesterol test also provides a number that ranks as one of the top predictors of heart attack risk: your total-cholesterol-to-HDL ratio (TC/HDL).[28]

For decades, TC/HDL ratio has been the *only* cholesterol number that most life insurance companies look at, since they stand to lose millions of dollars if they rate applicants' risk incorrectly. Although they typically consider a ratio of 5 or below acceptable — explaining why Dwayne (whose ratio was 5) qualified for a policy — research shows that a lower number is much safer. Based on scientific evidence from multiple studies, we consider a ratio of 3.5 to be a desirable target and a number below 3 to be optimal.[29] If this number doesn't appear on your cholesterol results, doing the math yourself is simple. For example, if your total cholesterol is 180 mg/dL and your HDL is 60 mg/dL, you'd divide 180 by 60 to get your TC/HDL ratio of 3 (good).

What to do if you have this risk factor:

If you use tobacco or nicotine in any form, here's yet another reason to kick this deadly habit: Several studies link quitting to a rise in HDL levels. Eating oily fish (such as salmon, tuna, and sardines) or other foods that are high in omega-3 fatty acids helps boost levels of good cholesterol, while reducing inflammation. Olive oil is also a healthy fat that helps raise HDL and contains heart-healthy antioxidants.[30] For an added benefit, use it to dress a salad that contains purple produce, such as red cabbage, blueberries, black raspberries, or blackberries. These tasty foods contain disease-fighting antioxidants called anthocyanins, which fight inflammation, reduce disease-inducing free radicals, and have been shown to increase HDL by up to 19 percent in small clinical trials (using an anthocyanin supplement, not fresh produce).[31]

4: High triglycerides.

Like cholesterol, triglycerides are a type of fat (lipid) found in your blood. When you consume more calories than you burn, the extra calories are converted into triglycerides and stored in fat cells until they're needed for energy. In other words, when fat accumulates on your thighs or belly, that's where excess triglycerides end up. If your triglyceride level is 150 mg/dL or above, you have acquired another strike. If you are being treated for high triglycerides, it is a strike even if the level is below 150 mg/dL. In Dwayne's case, it was his eye-popping triglycerides (nearly triple the normal number) that astonished his doctor, not his cholesterol levels, which were only mildly abnormal.

A Harvard-led study reported that having high triglycerides alone magnifies heart attack danger by nearly threefold, while *people with the highest ratio of triglycerides to HDL had nearly sixteen times the risk of heart attack than those with the lowest.*[32] The researchers concluded that TG/HDL ratio is "a strong predictor" of heart attacks. The optimal ratio is less than 3.5 mg/dL if you're Caucasian, less than 2.0 mg/dL if you're African American, and less than 3 mg/dL if you're Hispanic.[33] TG/HDL ratio is calculated by dividing your triglyceride level by your HDL level. For example, when we divided Dwayne's initial triglyceride level of 412 mg/dL by his HDL level of 39 mg/dL, his TG/HDL ratio was 10.5 mg/dL (one of the most abnormal ratios we've seen in our practice).

What to do if you have this risk factor:

If you're overweight, losing 5 to 10 percent of your body weight (ten to twenty pounds if you weigh two hundred) can lower your triglycerides by 20 percent, according to a scientific statement from the American Heart Association.[34] Limiting or avoiding sugar, and increasing the fiber in your diet, also are helpful. Also ask your healthcare provider to check you for vitamin D deficiency. Among the many benefits of the sunshine vitamin is supporting healthy triglyceride levels. Multiple studies have linked low levels of vitamin D to increased risk for high triglycerides, other lipid abnormalities, and metabolic syndrome.[35]

5: High fasting blood sugar.

Fasting means you have not consumed anything with calories for at least ten hours. A level of 100 mg/dL or higher counts as a strike. Fasting blood sugar levels of 100 mg/dL to 125 mg/dL indicate that you're prediabetic, while a level above 125 mg/dL is diagnostic of diabetes. About 88 million Americans have prediabetes and 84 percent of them don't know it because they haven't had their blood sugar checked. That's dangerous, because if it goes undetected and untreated, prediabetes can often progress to full-blown type 2 disease in four to seven years. If you don't know your blood sugar numbers, ask your provider for the two-hour oral glucose tolerance test discussed in the next section of this chapter. Prediabetes is now considered a reversible disease.

What to do if you have this risk factor:

To prevent or reverse prediabetes, the treatment that surpasses all others is aerobic exercise, such as running, brisk walking, biking, and swimming. Working out thirty minutes daily, five or more times a week, has been proven to prevent prediabetes from progressing to full-blown diabetes 60 percent of the time, while the success rate rises to 70 percent if regular exercise is combined with moderate weight loss (5 to 7 percent of your body weight), large studies report.[36] Even low-intensity exercise, such as walking slowly, substantially improves insulin sensitivity for the next twenty-four hours, according to a position statement from the American Diabetes Association.[37] Research also indicates that weight loss plus boosting physical activity is far more effective than medication at preventing prediabetes from progressing to full-blown diabetes.[38]

The Hidden Cause of Most Heart Attacks, Many Chronic Diseases, and Memory Loss

It's extremely common for people to be diagnosed with diabetes shortly after they suffer a heart attack or stroke. Patients often chalk this up to bad luck, assuming that they've been inexplicably hit with two seemingly unrelated diseases. Actually, there is a very strong link between insulin resistance—the disorder that leads to type 2 diabetes—and heart attack risk.

A groundbreaking 1999 study published in *The Lancet* was the first to reveal that arterial damage starts at the onset of IR and continues to silently progress as long as this prediabetic condition remains untreated.[39] As soon as someone becomes resistant to their own insulin, a perfect storm of dangerous events occur at the cellular level, affecting all the body's arteries. Fundamentally, IR is an inflammatory disorder and a key player in all three steps of the atherogenic triad: the disease process that creates cats in the gutter.

In addition, people with IR tend to have complex cholesterol issues, including high triglycerides and low levels of heart-protective HDL, and are more prone to forming blood clots that can lead to heart attacks and strokes. Recently, this inflammatory disorder, which is the precursor to type 2 diabetes, has also been shown to drive the development of Alzheimer's disease (AD). In fact, a 2017 study reported that 80 percent of people with AD also have insulin resistance or type 2 diabetes.[40]

Despite the mountain of evidence that IR is extremely damaging to the body's arteries, most medical dictionaries ignore these devastating complications, perhaps explaining why healthcare providers are doing such a poor job of detecting and treating this potentially reversible condition. Instead, IR is typically defined solely as the beginning of a long, slow march toward type 2 diabetes, the form that affects 90 percent of people with diabetes.

Unlike people with type 1 diabetes—an autoimmune disorder in antibodies that attack and destroy the pancreas's insulin-producing beta cells, irrevocably halting insulin production—people with type 2 do produce insulin, but their bodies don't use it properly. Normally, this hormone helps cells in the body use glucose (blood sugar) for energy. When people develop IR, their cells become insensitive to insulin, forcing the pancreas to crank out higher and higher amounts, trying to keep up with demand. Very often, people with IR have both high levels of insulin and glucose circulating in their bodies.

Think of this scenario as similar to a factory in which the workers are forced to toil longer and longer hours on the assembly line to meet ever increasing production quotas. Eventually, the workers will grow so exhausted that they either collapse or go on strike, forcing the assembly line to grind to a halt. Similarly, as insulin resistance progresses, the beta cells eventually become fatigued and blood sugar rises. By the time someone crosses the line into type 2 diabetes, arterial damage has typically been happening for at least ten years and, in some cases, twenty or more. This explains why people with diabetes are at greatly increased risk for cardiovascular events.

In a study of patients treated in the ER for a heart attack, researchers found that, after excluding known diabetics, 66 percent of the remaining patients had abnormal blood sugar levels that met criteria for diabetes or prediabetes, an earlier stage of the disease.[41] In one of the most egregious failures of the

American medical system, both conditions frequently go undiagnosed until serious complications have occurred, a situation comparable to walking blindfolded through a minefield of unexploded ordnance.

As you learned earlier, a person with untreated diabetes is at as high a risk for a heart attack as a nondiabetic person the same age who has already suffered one! Yet even people with known diabetes, such as Neal, are often not warned about their cardiovascular danger. Other patients with obvious diabetes risk factors, such as obesity and a family history of the disease, such as Camille, Elaine, Catherine, and Dwayne, can also be missed, simply because their medical providers either haven't ordered the most accurate diabetes screening tool, the two-hour oral glucose tolerance test (OGTT), or didn't check their blood sugar at all.

The CDC reports that of 34 million U.S. adults with diabetes, more than 7 million are unaware of their condition, putting them at high risk for heart attacks, strokes, peripheral artery disease, Alzheimer's disease (which is so closely linked to IR that some scientists think it should be renamed type 3 diabetes), and a wide range of diabetic complications, such as nerve damage, vision and hearing impairment or loss, and lower limb amputations.[42] The statistics are even more appalling for prediabetes—a dangerous but usually reversible disease that affects 88 million Americans, more than 84 percent of whom don't know they have it.[43]

Here are three important things to know about screening for IR and diabetes:

In the time that it takes to watch a movie, you can get the best screening test for diabetes, prediabetes, and IR— and it's covered by almost every health plan.

The American Diabetes Association (ADA) advises screening if you're forty or older, or at a younger age if advised by your medical provider because of such factors as obesity or family history. The ADA rates the two-hour oral glucose tolerance test, in which you drink a sugary liquid after an overnight fast, as the gold standard in accuracy. Blood samples are drawn at the one- and two-hour marks to check glucose levels.

Some people with "normal" blood sugar results may be in the early stages of insulin resistance.

Historically, the ADA has defined an OGTT two-hour sugar level of less than 140 mg/dL as normal, a level of 140 to 200 mg/dL as marking prediabetes, and a level above 200 mg/dL as diagnostic of diabetes. Recent research by one of the world's top diabetes experts, Dr. Ralph DeFronzo, however, suggests that the danger zone for IR starts when two-hour blood sugar reaches 120 mg/dL or higher, a point at which 60 percent of the beta cells are exhausted. When 90 percent of the cells are fatigued (a situation also known as beta cell function loss), you are diabetic. Dr. DeFronzo has also published excellent data in peer-reviewed journals showing that if one-hour blood sugar results exceed 125 mg/dL, the patient should be considered prediabetic.[44]

Other widely used diabetes screening tests often yield misleading results.

Several studies show that the A1c test, which doesn't require fasting, is not very reliable for detecting IR/prediabetes. For example, a 2011 BaleDoneen study presented at the Fourth International Congress on Prediabetes and Metabolic Syndrome found that of 547 patients checked with various blood sugar tests, the A1c test, which reports results as a percentage, missed 63 percent of those with IR/prediabetes. This test can also miss full-blown diabetes, as occurred in Catherine's case. Her A1c measured in the prediabetic range (5.7 to 6.4 percent), when the highly accurate OGTT showed that she was diabetic, with a two-hour sugar level of 228 mg/dL. Moreover, our study found that 27 percent of the patients who were classified as prediabetic by the A1c had normal blood sugar when checked with the highly accurate OGTT. An A1c below 5.7 percent is considered normal, and a level of 6.5 percent or higher indicates diabetes.

An Astonishing Health Turnaround

Now sixty-seven and retired, Dwayne has totally revamped his lifestyle. Six years ago, he began going to the gym daily, where he spends thirty-five to forty-five minutes a day running on the treadmill, lifting weights, boxing, and using the elliptical machine. "I used to love barbecued ribs, but I've cut out red meat, simple carbs like rice and potatoes, and all sweets and desserts completely," adds the grandfather of three. Instead, he eats a low-carb diet based on his DNA that's high in fruits, vegetables, nuts, and fish with moderate amounts of healthy fats, such as olive oil. Thanks to these lifestyle changes, he's lost forty-five pounds.

"When I went to have my Department of Transportation physical two years ago," he says, "I was in such good shape that the doctor told me that physically, I was like a fifty-five-year-old man—ten years younger than my actual age at that time!" Recent tests at our center confirm that Dwayne's hard work to turn his health around has paid off in a variety of ways. His triglycerides levels, which were nearly triple the normal number during his initial evaluation twenty years ago, are now in the healthy range, as are his cholesterol numbers. His blood pressure has improved so much that he's gone from needing three medications to control it to just one, and inflammation testing revealed that his arteries are no longer on fire.

"There's no doubt in my mind that without the BaleDoneen Method, I wouldn't be here today, given my genetic predisposition for heart attacks and strokes," says Dwayne. "I found out what was killing me and got the guidance I needed to take action that has saved my life. Instead of being a heart attack or stroke waiting to happen, I can walk into a room with other sixty-seven-year-olds and feel confident that nobody else is in as great shape as I am."

Action Step: Move More to Trim Your Risk for Insulin Resistance.

Taking short activity breaks from sitting helps prevent insulin resistance, researchers recently reported. The study found that even among people who spent most of the day parked in a chair, those who took the most activity breaks—even ones as brief as a minute at a time—had, on average, thinner waists (by nearly two inches) and lower levels of inflammatory markers, triglycerides, and blood sugar.[45] Try taking a five-minute break every hour to get up and move around.

To optimize cardiovascular health, we advise cutting down on TV and other screen time and spending a minimum of thirty minutes daily working out. Exercising in the morning before you go to work is a great way to set a positive, healthy tone for the rest of the day. Another easy way to build more movement into your day and get your heart pumping is to take the stairs instead of the elevator. If you have a desk job, try scheduling "walking meetings" in which you discuss projects while taking a lap or two around the block. Also, pace while you are on the phone and consider using a standing desk.

CHAPTER 10

Healthy Gums and Teeth Help You Live Longer

"Every tooth in a man's head is more valuable than a diamond."

— MIGUEL DE CERVANTES

One of our patients, Robert, was in such poor cardiovascular health when we met him that he later told us that he was shocked we didn't start the visit with the question that his other doctors always asked: "Did you bring your nitroglycerin tablets?" Our initial assessment revealed that he was suffering from twenty-six different disorders and symptoms, including such severe coronary artery disease that he'd undergone an emergency stenting procedure three years earlier to treat a 90 percent blockage in his left ascending anterior artery that was putting him in imminent danger for a widow-maker heart attack. Eleven months later, he was rushed back to the operating room after his symptoms—excruciating chest pain and shortness of breath—returned. Two of his heart's other major arteries were also obstructed, requiring additional stents to prop them open.

Then sixty-six, the rancher and cattleman from Texas also had chronic kidney disease, uncontrolled high blood pressure, gout, vision disorders, prediabetes, metabolic syndrome, obstructive sleep apnea, obesity, gastroesophageal reflux disease (GERD), a persistent cough, swollen legs, and elevated levels of lipoprotein (a), the "mass murderer" inherited cholesterol disorder you read about in chapter four, among other conditions. Despite his many maladies, which had left him so debilitated that he was no longer able to ride his quarter horses—his favorite hobby—Robert told us that he was more concerned about the arterial wellness of his second wife, Kellee, than his own.

Speaking in a slow, deep, and sometimes breathless voice, he explained that five years earlier, his first wife, Debbie, had suffered a massive heart attack at fifty-nine. "She was a wonderful Christian wife and a real little firecracker," he recalled. "On our last night together, she woke me at 4:20 a.m. with terrible pain in her arm." He gave Debbie two baby aspirin and helped her to the car. Then he floored the accelerator and set off to the nearest ER. On the way, Debbie—his childhood sweetheart, wife of forty years and mother of their two sons—died. Robert paused, as if reliving events that were too painful to describe further, then added that less than three months earlier, Debbie had gotten a clean bill of heart health at a well-known medical center.

Fingering his wedding ring, Robert told us that he'd been blessed to find love again with Kellee, who was employed as an interior decorator. Then he asked us to evaluate her. "I can't lose another wife to this disease," he said grimly, then beckoned Kellee, who had been sitting in the waiting room, to join us in our office. Then fifty-three, she looked like a very unlikely candidate for a heart attack. Not only did she appear much younger than her true age, but she was slender and extremely fit. Initially, Kellee was bracing herself for more bad news about Robert. "I didn't think this was about me, because it had taken everything I had to get my husband to this appointment: He could hardly breathe or talk, was very tired and lethargic, had chills, and looked ashy white," she says. "I thought I was going to hear that his heart had deteriorated further."

Kellee was very relieved to learn that although Robert's

cardiovascular issues were serious, we'd already come up with a comprehensive treatment plan that will be discussed in part three. "We'd already been to many doctors and this was the first time anyone had given us hope that the wonderful, heartbroken man I love so much could recover and heal," says Kellee. "He was so impressed by the care and advice he received during the initial evaluation—including immediate changes in his medications and many adjustments in his lifestyle—that he felt confident that this plan could save his life. And he convinced me that getting checked out might save mine, too."

Robert's intuition turned out to be on target: Our testing revealed that Kellee was in the early stages of atherosclerosis. "I was leaner and fitter than I'd been for many years and had never felt healthier, so I was very deflated to find out I had heart disease," says Kellee, who turned out to be a carrier of the 9P21 gene. "Even though heart disease runs in my family, especially on my mother's side, hearing that I had the heart attack gene really played with my mind," she adds. "At first, I was terrified, then I felt blessed to have found wonderful doctors who knew the secret of curing this disease and had already helped two of our friends who had much worse problems than I did."

The Dangerous Health Threat in Your Mouth

As part of our initial evaluation, we referred Kellee and Robert to an excellent Texas dentist who is trained in the BaleDoneen Method. His thorough assessment of the couple's oral health identified a culprit in their arterial disease that truly shocked them. Even though they have beautiful white teeth, are extremely diligent about brushing and flossing, and got annual dental checkups, both of them turned out to have previously undiagnosed periodontal disease (PD), a chronic bacterial infection of the gum tissue and bone supporting the teeth.

Also known as gum disease or periodontitis, PD is one of the world's most common—and preventable—chronic diseases. In the U.S., this dental disorder affects nearly 65 million Americans, including 50 percent of those thirty and older and 70 percent of those sixty-five and up.[1] Many people don't know they have it because, in the early stages, the disease is painless and may not cause any obvious symptoms.

Even when patients do have symptoms of PD, they may go unrecognized. For example, Kellee used to think it was normal for her gums to bleed a little after brushing and flossing. That's an extremely common misconception. In reality, it's *not* normal to experience any bleeding, even slight amounts, when you brush or floss. Any sign of bleeding—such as a pink-tinged toothbrush or spitting out blood or pink saliva—after cleaning your teeth is the number one warning sign of gum disease. Other symptoms include red, swollen, or tender gums, receding gums that make your teeth look longer than normal, sensitive or loose teeth, changes in your bite, uncomfortable chewing, and persistent bad breath.

Gum disease starts with gingivitis, a potentially reversible disorder marked by inflammation of the gums (gingiva). If untreated, gingivitis can lead to periodontitis. Without treatment, this dental disorder causes slow, progressive destruction of the alveolar bone around the teeth that can eventually lead to tooth loss. Studies have also linked gum disease, the bacteria that cause it, and poor oral health to an ever-expanding list of debilitating or life-threatening conditions, including:

Heart attacks and strokes

People with periodontitis are 2.5 times more likely to suffer heart attacks than those with healthy gums, according to a pooled analysis of studies that included more than seven thousand people.[2] Another study found that people with infected gums are nearly

50 percent more likely to suffer strokes or angina (chest pain due to narrowing or blockages in the heart's major arteries), compared to people without PD.[3] Later in this chapter, we'll tell you a surprising discovery we made that explains these findings—and offers a new way to protect yourself from CV events.

Diabetes

There is a two-way relationship between PD and diabetes: People with diabetes are three times more likely to have infected gums than nondiabetics. Having gum disease also raises the risk of developing diabetes in the first place, by contributing to insulin resistance and rising blood sugar levels.[4] In addition, people who have diabetes and severe PD have triple the risk for fatal cardiovascular or kidney complications, compared to diabetic people with healthy gums. The good news, however, is that treating PD greatly reduces these threats.[5]

Cancer

A long-term study found that people with severe gum disease have an 80 percent higher risk for colorectal cancer and double the risk for lung cancer than people with mild PD or healthy gums.[6] In a study of nearly seventy-four thousand women, those with PD faced a 14 percent higher threat of breast cancer. Among former or current smokers, breast cancer risk was 36 percent higher.[7] Any form of nicotine use is the leading risk factor for gum disease, offering yet another powerful motivation to kick this deadly habit.

Erectile dysfunction

Men who struggle with erectile dysfunction are three times more likely than other men to have periodontal disease.[8]

Studies have also shown that treating PD rapidly improves the quality and duration of men's erections, as well as enhancing both their oral and heart health.[9]

Frailty

A study of more than 1,200 older men found that those with poor oral health were twice as likely to develop signs of frailty, such as a weak grip, slow walking speed, and exhaustion.[10] Frailty raises risk for hospitalization, disability, physical and mental decline, and a shorter life span.

Obesity

Excess weight is the second biggest risk factor for gum disease, doubling or even tripling the likelihood of developing it. In an intriguing study, researchers analyzed oral bacteria collected from about 550 women of various weights. Simply by checking the bacterial samples for high levels of a periodontal bug called *Selenomonas noxia*, the team was able to identify the overweight women with greater than 98 percent accuracy. Research is needed to explore the possibility of *Selenomonas noxia* being a contributory cause of obesity.

Rheumatoid arthritis

While the initial trigger for this chronic inflammatory disease of the joints is still under investigation, studies have reported very high rates of PD in people with rheumatoid arthritis (RA). In one recent study, patients with RA were *more than twenty times more likely* to have PD than a control group of age- and gender-matched patients without RA.[11] *Treating gum disease has been shown to reduce pain, number of swollen joints, and morning stiffness—and researchers are now investigating if optimal oral care could help people at high genetic risk for RA avoid getting the disease.*[12]

Alzheimer's disease and dementia

As we will discuss more fully in chapter twelve, a wave of recent studies has linked gum disease with increased risk for cognitive impairment and memory loss. For example, a large study found people with PD are up to 70 percent more likely to develop Alzheimer's disease and other memory-robbing conditions, especially vascular dementia.[13] "That really scared us, because my husband's mom had a horrible seventeen-year battle with dementia and I lost to my father to vascular dementia. He was a very brilliant man with multiple college degrees who used to read five or six books a week," says Kellee. "It was heartbreaking to see that disease rob him of everything, particularly in the last year and a half of his life, when his eyes were blank and he could no longer recognize us."

How Gum Disease Harms Your Heart and Arteries

Your mouth is home to more than seven hundred species of bacteria, most of which are harmless or even beneficial.[14] Along with these bacteria, your mouth also contains other microbes, such as fungi, viruses, and protozoa, forming a community of microorganisms known as the oral microbiome. If it's healthy, the oral microbiome plays a key role in food digestion and disease prevention, by helping to regulate your immune system, maintain a balance between pro-inflammatory and anti-inflammatory processes, detoxify environmental chemicals, and repel invading pathogens.[15] Many factors, including smoking, poor oral hygiene, stress, obesity, IR, and an unhealthy diet, can adversely affect your oral microbiome, leading to increased growth of the bacteria that cause periodontal disease.

What's the link between the health of your mouth and diseases that affect other parts of your body, such as the heart or the brain? A landmark 1954 study was the first to show that oral germs, such as those that cause gum disease, frequently enter the bloodstream and quickly spread throughout the body.[16] Among the ways this can happen are chewing food, brushing, flossing, periodontal cleaning, and tooth extractions.[17] The spread of these pathogens throughout the body can result in chronic inflammation, the fire that ignites arterial disease. Research suggests that the harmful cardiovascular effects of PD are due to a gang of five high-risk oral bacteria: *Aggregatibacter actinomycetemcomitans (A.a.)*, *Porphyromonas gingivalis (P.g.)*, *Tannerella forsythia (T.f.)*, *Treponema denticola (T.d.)*, and *Fusobacterium nucleatum (F.n.)*.

As you learned in chapter eight, CVD results from a triple whammy known as the atherogenic triad. In 2011, after an extensive review of the literature, an American Heart Association scientific statement reported that PD is independently associated with arterial disease, based on Level A evidence (the highest standard of scientific proof).[18] In 2017, we conducted our own rigorous analysis and made a landmark discovery of our own, drawing on Level A evidence: Gum disease isn't just a risk factor for developing arterial plaque: it is a potentially preventable *cause* of the disease, as we demonstrated in a peer-reviewed study published in *Postgraduate Medical Journal*.

Why is this distinction important? There is a key difference between a condition being *associated* with another disease and being *causal*. Optimal treatment of an associated condition may have no impact on risk of developing the end disease, while such management of a causal condition for CVD would not only have a beneficial effect, but could be potentially lifesaving, by helping to prevent heart attacks and strokes. Our paper was the first to show that these bacterial villains can intensify *each* component of the arterial disease–inducing triad as follows[19]:

People with gum disease have up to twice as much small, dense LDL cholesterol (the most dangerous kind) in their blood. When LDL is converted to small, dense LDL, levels of ApoB also rise.[20] As you learned in chapter four, ApoB is a major component of *all* the bad cholesterols circulating in your blood. People with gum disease take large LDL particles and convert them to small dense particles. If the person had X number of large particles they end up with 2X the number of small dense particles. Since ApoB is woven into all LDL particles, the person doubles the amount of ApoB they possess. ApoB is the most predictive lipid (cholesterol) measurement for risk of heart attack, partly because it gets electrostatically attached in the wall of the artery to proteoglycans. Small dense LDL has two potential points for that attachment. This basically doubles the risk of it building up in the artery wall. This is one of the reasons people with gum disease have increased risk for forming arterial disease.

Chemicals produced by high-risk oral bacteria make the walls of the artery more permeable, so it's easier for bad cholesterol to invade. Since people with PD due to these pathogens also have higher blood concentrations of small, dense LDL cholesterol and ApoB, this creates a one–two punch on the arteries, much like a gang assault on a house with broken windows or doors.

Substances produced by high-risk bacteria can also make the inner layers of the arterial wall (where plaque forms) stickier, much like Velcro, so bad cholesterol is more likely to get trapped there and create plaque deposits, resulting in a triple threat to arterial health.

Watch Out for This New Dental Danger

New and recent research has shown that endodontic disease (tooth decay) can also drive heart attack and stroke risk. For example, in a study of 101 people who were in the throes of an acute heart attack, Dr. Tanja Pessi and colleagues removed the culprit blood clots and used DNA analysis to check for oral pathogens.[21] They also analyzed arterial blood samples from the same patients and found that the concentration of these bacterial villains was sixteen times higher in the clot than the arterial blood, revealing that the pathogens came from the ruptured plaque deposit that had caused the heart attack. The DNA analysis also revealed that 75 percent of the clots contained the strep bacteria that cause endodontic disease and 35 percent contained periodontal bacteria.

Thirty of the patients studied received panoramic CT scans and of this group about 50 percent had periapical abscess, pockets of pus at the root of a tooth, typically caused by a bacterial infection. That meant they had endodontic disease, which also appears to play a role in deep vein thrombosis (DVT), according to a 2018 study.[22] DVT is a serious disorder that occurs when a blood clot forms in the deep veins of the body, most commonly those in the thigh or lower leg. Symptoms can include swelling, discoloration, or cramping pain in the affected leg. If undiagnosed and untreated, DVT can put people at risk for pulmonary embolism: a blood clot in the lung that can be potentially life-threatening if untreated.

The 2018 study also found that strep bacteria from endodontic disease may also contribute to ischemic stroke risk. The researchers analyzed blood clots removed from stroke patients, nearly 80 percent of which tested positive for DNA from strep bacteria, and those removed from DVT patients, more than 50 percent of which also tested positive for strep bacteria DNA.

The key takeaway from these groundbreaking studies is that regular dental care should be a crucial component of your heart attack, stroke, and chronic disease prevention plan. In chapter twelve, we will also show you how maintaining optimal oral wellness is one of the keys to safeguarding your memory and achieving a health span that matches your life span.

An Easy Four-Step Plan to Optimize Your Oral-Systemic Health

By now we hope we've convinced you that your dental provider is a potentially lifesaving member of your chronic disease prevention team! Here are some proven tips that will help you combat bacterial villains and achieve a perfect ten in oral-systemic wellness from Doug Thompson, DDS, FAAMM, ABAAHP, founder of the Wellness Dentistry Network, and Cris Duval, RDH, who has served as the BaleDoneen Method's oral wellness liaison.

Step 1. Partner with your dental provider and set goals to take your oral health to the next level of excellence.

With study after study linking poor oral health to higher risk for life-threatening conditions, says Dr. Thompson, "dentists and dental hygienists are increasingly attuned to the oral-systemic connection and our important role in chronic disease prevention. My colleagues and I like to say, 'On a good day, we save a smile and on a great day, we'll save a life.'" Patients are also taking a more active role in their oral care. Make the most of your next dental visit by preparing a list of your oral health goals, concerns, and questions, such as these:

How do you rank my oral health on a scale of 1 to 10?
What are my risk factors for periodontal disease?

How can I work with my dental team to get my oral health to a 10?

Are you willing to partner/coach me on how to achieve my oral health goals?

How do you rank my overall health on a scale of 1 to 10, and are there any red flags in my medical history that stand out?

How can I partner with my dental team to get my overall health to a 10?

Step 2. Ask your dental provider to screen you for periodontal and endodontic disease and check you for high-risk oral bacteria.

Our landmark study discussed earlier in this chapter could transform how dental providers diagnose and manage periodontal disease (PD), since the research shows it's important to find out if patients have the high-risk bacteria that are now known to be a contributing cause of atherosclerosis. Dr. Thompson recommends that your exam include these three components:

X-rays to check for signs of gum disease, such as bone loss

Ask your dental provider if you are at risk for endodontic disease, which mainly affects people who are prone to tooth decay, says Dr. Thompson. "If you have a lot of fillings or other dental work, such as root canals, your dental provider may recommend that you be evaluated for endodontic disease with an imaging test called 3-D cone beam tomography [CBCT], which may require being referred to a specialist since not all general dentists have this equipment." In a recent analysis of studies, CBCT was 96 percent accurate for finding periapical abscesses and other signs of endodontic disease, as compared to a 73 percent accuracy rate for conventional dental X-rays.[23] Adds Dr. Thompson, "If you've never had a cavity in your life, it's very unlikely that you'd need cone beam CT since your risk for endodontic disease would be extremely low."

A periodontal exam

This painless exam involves using a thin instrument called a periodontal probe to measure the depths of the pockets between your teeth, with each of these measurements recorded on your dental chart. Pockets are spaces around each tooth where it connects to your gums, and the deeper the pockets, the greater the probability that you have PD. A healthy pocket typically measures 1–3 millimeters, and a depth of 4 millimeters or more suggests gum disease. Having pockets that bleed during the exam is another common symptom. "Periodontal disease is now staged the same way cancer is, with stage one indicating gingivitis and stage four indicating advanced periodontitis with substantial loss of bone support (very loose or missing teeth) and deep pockets of infection," says Dr. Thompson.

An oral salivary test for high-risk periodontal bacteria

To find out which patients harbor the dangerous oral bacteria discussed earlier in this chapter, the BaleDoneen Method recommends using diagnostic tests that measure oral pathogens through DNA analysis, including OralDNA, OraVital, Direct Diagnostics, and Hain Diagnostics. Because people without gum disease can also harbor these dangerous bacteria, Duval recommends this painless oral testing for all dental patients: "I'll even test children if one of their parents has a high load of oral pathogens, since the bacteria can spread easily between family members through kissing or sharing food. Dogs are another potential source of bacterial infection, so avoid letting your pet lick you or your kids on the face. Always wash your hands after handling objects your dog has licked or chewed, such as their toys or food bowl."

Step 3. Disinfect your entire mouth daily.

In the study of older adults, those who brushed and flossed daily outlived people with neither habit, which prompted Duval to strongly recommend both practices to her patients, as does the American Dental Association. However, a 2015 review of the scientific evidence published in the *Journal of Clinical Periodontology* concluded that "the majority of available studies fail to demonstrate that flossing is generally effective in plaque removal."[24] Dr. Thompson advises his patients to clean between their teeth with a water flosser device, such as Water Pik or Oral-B Water Flosser, instead of using dental floss, but adds that his recommendations for home care are personalized for each patient. "The most important thing is a thorough daily method of removing bacteria from between the teeth that you're comfortable with, whether it's water flossing or using dental floss," he says.

If you use dental floss, be sure to employ the proper technique: Avoid snapping the floss up and down, which irritates your gums and does a poor job of cleaning. Instead, glide it gently up and down in zigzag motion as you clean the tooth surface and under the gum, with the floss contoured in a C-shape to wrap around the tooth. Also be sure to floss the back surface of the last teeth on each side of your lower and upper jaw. Use a clean section of floss for each tooth. Along with water or dental flossing, Dr. Thompson and Duval also recommend the following ways to safeguard your smile and overall wellness:

To reduce harmful bacteria in your mouth, don't just brush your teeth and gums. Also brush your cheeks, the roof of your mouth, and the vestibule (the area between the teeth, lips, and cheeks).

Use a tongue scraper—not a toothbrush—to clean your tongue.

After dental or water flossing, also use dental picks (such as GUM Soft-Picks) to efficiently remove debris between teeth that floss doesn't reach.

Fight bacterial buildup by using a high pH (alkaline) toothpaste, such as CariFree or CloSYS. These companies also have high pH mouthwashes.

Choose dental products that contain xylitol, a compound with an antimicrobial effect. Xylitol products, such as toothpaste, chewing gum, and lozenges, help prevent cavities and may reduce risk for gum disease. *Important warning: If you have pets, keep all xylitol products out of their reach—xylitol is extremely toxic or even fatal to dogs, even in small amounts.*

Go to bed with a clean mouth. Since your mouth makes less saliva when you are sleeping to wash your teeth and gums, it's particularly important to disinfect your mouth thoroughly at bedtime.

Avoid mouthwashes that contain sugar or alcohol.

Step 4. Get a dental cleaning at least twice a year or as advised by your dental provider.

Doing so could save your life! In the study of older adults, those who hadn't seen a dentist in the previous year had a 50 percent higher death rate than those who went multiple times a year. "One of our goals is to keep all of our patients in what I call the safety zone, as opposed to the danger zone where gum disease and high-risk bacteria create a perfect storm of inflammatory responses that leave people susceptible to heart attacks and strokes," says Duval.

To stay in the safety zone, it's crucial to get dental checkups and any necessary treatments on the schedule advised by your dental provider. If you have gum disease, treatments include nonsurgical periodontal therapy, a daily program of self-care to follow at home, prescription mouthwashes, dental trays with antibacterial gel (Perio Protect), and in some cases, a short course of antibiotics. Regardless of which treatment is prescribed, the DNA testing should be repeated to make sure the treatment was successful, says Dr. Thompson. "Unlike gingivitis, which can be reversed, periodontitis is not curable, but with the right treatment, it can be halted and stabilized to prevent further damage, usually with three to six months of active treatment, followed by maintenance care to keep the disease from reactivating."

Action Step: Take Excellent Care of Your Teeth and Gums

A habit that takes five minutes a day can add years to your life and may also lower your risk for many dangerous health threats, including heart attacks, strokes, diabetes, chronic kidney disease, cancer, Alzheimer's disease, erectile dysfunction, pneumonia, and other debilitating or life-threatening conditions. One study of more than 5,600 older adults also found that one of the easiest—and cheapest—keys to a longer life is brushing and flossing daily.[25] Conversely, neglecting your teeth and gums can be fatal, the researchers reported. The team tracked the participants for seventeen years and reported that:

> Never brushing at night elevated risk for death during the study period by 20 to 25 percent, compared to brushing every night.
>
> Never flossing upped mortality risk by 30 percent, versus daily flossing.
>
> Not seeing a dentist in the previous twelve months raised mortality risk by up to 50 percent, compared to getting dental care two or more times a year.

Another startling finding from the study: One major predictor of early death was missing teeth, even when other risk factors were taken into account. A subsequent study of these participants also found that older adults who neglected their teeth were up to 65 percent more likely to develop dementia than those with excellent oral health!

Healing Your Arteries

CHAPTER 11
Mining Your DNA for Actionable Health Insights

"[Decoding the human genome] is the most significant undertaking that we have mounted so far in all of science. I believe that reading our blueprints, cataloguing our own instruction book, will be more significant than even splitting the atom or going to the moon."
— Francis S. Collins, MD, PhD,
sixteenth director of the National
Institutes of Health

Diane H. has one of the most tragic family histories that we've ever heard. During her initial evaluation at our center seventeen years ago, she told us that in her family, fifty is considered old, because almost none of her maternal relatives ever reached that age. "Genetically, we are kind of cursed," said the then thirty-seven-year-old system analyst from Liberty Lake, Washington. "My mom and her two brothers were the first people on that side of the family to live past forty-two. Everyone else died before that from heart attacks." What's more, two of her relatives were battling dementia and such severe coronary artery disease (CAD) that both of them had undergone multiple stenting and bypass procedures.

In addition, her parents, Babs and Paul, have CAD, and

Babs also suffers from peripheral artery disease (PAD)—an often-debilitating disorder that can make such everyday activities as climbing stairs or even walking extremely painful. At one point, Babs had so little blood flow to her lower legs that she needed a stent procedure to reopen severely narrowed arteries. Babs also has atrial fibrillation (AF), an irregular heartbeat that can lead to blood clots, heart failure, and increased risk for death from cardiovascular causes. Later in this chapter, we'll tell you about a new genetic test that can reveal if you're at risk for this dangerous disorder, which affects about 6 million Americans.[1] We'll also alert you to the best ways to avoid AF, which is now on the rise, especially among people over forty. It's also highly treatable and to date, Babs has not suffered any AF complications.

During another visit to our center, Diane H. looked us in the eye and blurted out a question that had been haunting her. "How do I avoid becoming my mom with her vascular disease? Her greatest fear is that she'll end up with dementia." Getting a little choked up, Diane H. added that she'd recently lost her fifty-two-year-old sister, very unexpectedly, due to surgical complications during a hysterectomy. "She had a fibroid tumor, and during the operation, a piece of the tumor broke off and went to her heart. The doctors actually brought her back after forty-five minutes of CPR, but she didn't survive the night."

After pausing to wipe a tear away, Diane H. continued, "Although her death was unrelated to our family history, it made me think, 'Am I doing enough to stay healthy, when I have heart disease on both sides of my family?'" At thirty-seven, she was a nonsmoker with normal blood pressure and cholesterol levels. Other than being a little overweight, she looked and felt healthy. Our testing, however, revealed that she had soft, vulnerable plaque (the most dangerous kind) and her inflammatory markers were elevated, putting her at risk for a heart attack or stroke. She was also in the early stages of insulin resistance.

"I thought I was being extremely proactive by getting checked for cardiovascular disease when I was in my thirties, so it was quite a shock to learn that I already had it at such a young age," says Diane H., who turned out to be homozygous for the 9P21 heart attack gene. That means she has inherited two copies of this gene, one from each of her parents. "My family jokes that I got all the bad genes. A lot of people think that's morbid, but it's my parents' way of saying, 'This is the hand you've been dealt and it just means you need to more proactive about preventive care.'" Determined to break the family "curse," she persuaded her parents, her husband, and her brothers to plug into our AHA for Life plan.

Diane H. and Paul launched a friendly competition to see which one of them could get their inflammation numbers down fastest, using the genetically guided therapies recommended in this chapter. A few years ago, both had sudden spikes in their levels of myeloperoxidase (MPO), the inflammatory marker we call the joker. Since elevated MPO often occurs in tandem with dental infections—and warns of imminent heart attack and stroke danger—we advised them to get an immediate oral health evaluation. Paul credits this advice with saving his life. "I had no symptoms and nothing showed up in the regular dental X-ray, but when I went to a specialist and had 3-D cone beam tomography, there were two abscesses," he says. "That scared me because if they'd gone undetected and untreated, I could have had a fatal heart attack."

After Paul and Diane H.'s dental infections were successfully treated, they resumed their competition, which ultimately ended with a tie, since their arteries are no longer on fire and their plaque is completely stabilized. Thanks to the genetically guided therapies discussed in this chapter—and the medications discussed in chapter fourteen—Babs's arterial disease is also under control and she's no longer in pain from her PAD. She and Paul are now eighty-six and enjoy an active lifestyle that includes swimming, exercise classes at their assisted living facility, and golf.

Unlocking the Secrets of the Human Genome

In 1990, the National Institutes of Health launched one of the most monumental research projects in history: a collaboration between thousands of scientists around the world to perform the first full sequencing of the human genome. Dr. Francis S. Collins, then director of the National Human Genome Research Institute, compared the genome to a book, written in genetic letters called bases. "It's a history book — a narrative of the journey of our species through time. It's a shop manual, with an incredibly detailed blueprint for building every human cell. And it's a transformative textbook of medicine, with insights that will give health care providers immense new powers to treat, prevent and cure disease."

Our genome has about 3 billion letters, and if they were printed out as words in a book, it would be 25,000 times longer than *War and Peace*. Another fun fact: Your genome is only about 0.1 percent different than that of any other person, but that equates to 3 million differences in your DNA. These differences hold important clues to health threats that might loom in your future, as well as the best personalized therapies and lifestyle moves to avoid them. Originally estimated to cost $3 billion, the Human Genome Project (HPP) was completed in 2003 for $400 million less than that, thanks to technological breakthroughs, Dr. Collins told Congress at the time.[2]

Hailing this wondrous achievement as a "true dawning of the genomic era," he forecast a future in which "predictive genetic tests will exist for many common conditions in which interventions can alleviate inherited risk, so that each of us can learn of our individual risks for future illness and practice more effective health maintenance and disease prevention." He also predicted that pinpointing the identity and location of every gene in our bodies would transform care for common conditions like diabetes and lead to new gene-based designer drugs for disorders such as Alzheimer's, which lacks a cure or effective treatments.

Since then, the cost of genetic testing has rapidly plummeted—and an explosion of scientific studies has demonstrated its enormous potential to transform patient care. In 2016, the American Heart Association launched an unprecedented initiative inspired by six simple words: "One size does not fit all." Acknowledging that too many people are still suffering and dying prematurely from arterial disease, despite numerous major breakthroughs in early detection, treatment, and prevention, the American Heart Association founded the Institute for Precision Cardiovascular Medicine. One key goal of the institute is to use specific genes that put patients at higher risk for CVD and stroke to revolutionize cardiovascular treatment and care.[3]

More than 50 percent of Americans carry one or more genetic variants (also known as polymorphisms) that dramatically increase risk for heart attacks, strokes, Alzheimer's disease, atrial fibrillation, and related disorders. However, cardiovascular events are *not* inevitable, even for people with high-risk genes. While it's very common for people to assume that there's nothing they can do about their DNA, in reality, genetic testing offers powerful, *actionable* insights to guide medical and lifestyle decision-making. By harnessing this knowledge to turn around their health, patients like Camille, Dwayne, and Diane H. have successfully overcome arterial disease, even though all three are homozygous for the 9P21 gene (the riskiest genotype).

If you have diabetes, you'll want to know about an inexpensive blood or saliva test discussed in this chapter that checks for a variant of the haptoglobin gene that raises heart attack and stroke danger in diabetics as much as smoking does. This genotype also magnifies the threat of other serious complications of diabetes, such as heart failure, end-stage kidney disease, and diabetic retinopathy (damage to the retina, the light-sensitive part of the eye), a condition that can cause vision problems or even blindness. If you have this variant, the wonderful news is that an inexpensive vitamin supplement, sold over the counter at every drugstore, can almost completely eliminate the added cardiovascular menace that this variant would otherwise pose.

Surprisingly, the same supplement that can be lifesaving for people with this haptoglobin variant appears to be downright dangerous for everybody else. In fact, studies suggest that this supplement *raises* the threat of heart attacks and even early death from cardiovascular causes for people *without* this polymorphism.[4] This is a powerful example of one of the biggest benefits of genetic testing: lifesaving and easy-to-implement insights from inexpensive, one-time testing. If you are not diabetic, this haptoglobin test can also reveal if you have a genotype linked to increased risk for intestinal, autoimmune, and inflammatory disorders—and if you'd benefit from a gluten-free diet and probiotics to ward off these threats.

If you are one of millions of Americans who have already had direct-to-consumer DNA tests, we'll also show how to use genetic data you may already have to personalize your diet and fitness plan to protect and improve your arterial health. Many of our patients who had been struggling with obesity—including Neal, Catherine, Camille, Dwayne, and Elaine—also report that following this genetically guided approach enabled them to finally get their weight under control, after years or even decades of frustration with every weight-loss plan they'd tried.

Later in this chapter, we'll reveal the surprising reason why some people *gain* weight on low-fat or low-carb diets. Neal, for example, was shocked to learn that the keto diet he was following was the worst possible eating plan for his genotype. You'll also learn how your genotype can influence your response to commonly prescribed medications and even nutrients in your food—and which easy actions to take if you have any of the potentially harmful variants discussed in this chapter.

Genetics

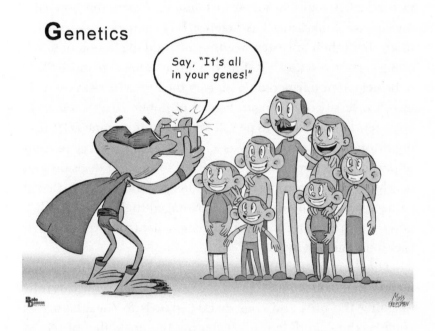

Should You Get At-Home Genetic Testing?

It's never been easier—or more affordable—to mine your DNA for hidden health threats and to discover the best personalized strategies to avoid them. When the first direct-to-consumer (DTC) genetic tests hit the market more than a decade ago, they cost up to $2,500.[5] Now dozens of companies sell at-home genetic testing kits at prices ranging from $100 to $500, often without any involvement of a medical provider to help people interpret the results. In 2017, after years of controversy about the quality and safety of home tests for disease risk, 23andMe was the first company to receive FDA authorization to sell a personal genomic test directly to consumers. The test checks for genes linked to increased risk for ten disorders, including Alzheimer's disease and blood-clotting disorders.

The popularity of personal genomic testing has soared. An October 2020 national survey by *Consumer Reports* reported that one in five Americans has taken a DTC genetic test to learn more about their ancestry, health traits, and likelihood of developing certain diseases.[6] To find out if consumers are more likely to be helped or harmed by exploring their genetic risks on their own, University of Michigan School of Public Health researchers recently studied 1,648 people who had undergone DTC testing through such companies as 23andMe.[7] Ninety-three percent of participants said getting the test was the right decision and nearly 60 percent reported that the genetic insights they'd gained would influence how they managed their health. Only 2 percent regretted receiving their genetic data and 1 percent felt they were harmed by it.

The Centers for Disease Control and Prevention recommends that consumers "think before you spit," by carefully weighing the pros and cons of DTC panels for health threats (such as the 23andMe test), including the possibility of receiving incomplete or even devastating results without a healthcare provider to interpret the results. We think that's excellent advice. Although these home health panels are not part of the BaleDoneen Method, if our patients wish to get this testing on their own, we are happy to review the results with them. Very often, we find, users of these tests receive a plethora of data on myriad diseases and conditions, many of which are not actionable in terms of specific steps to improve their health. All too often, the results end up being filed away, instead of guiding heart-smart treatment and lifestyle choices.

The University of Michigan study identified another potential pitfall of these home health tests: About 40 percent of the consumers they studied were disappointed because their genetic test results were less informative than they'd hoped, particularly about risk for cardiovascular disease, which ranked as the leading health concern of the study participants. One important limitation of the DTC health panels currently on the market is that they don't include all five of the genes now known to be the most powerful predictors of lifetime risk for cardiovascular disease and related conditions: 9P21 (the heart attack gene), 4q25, variants of the apolipoprotein E (Apo E), KIF6, and haptoglobin (Hp) genes.

Since we began using genetic testing for cardiovascular risk in our practice more than a decade ago, the cost has rapidly dropped, from nearly $1,000 in 2011 to less than $350 today for all five of these tests, putting this potentially lifesaving information within reach of most Americans. In most cases, these tests are not covered by health insurance plans unless you have a family history of cardiovascular disease. However, that trend is starting to change as some plans are starting to recognize the value of genetic testing and support this testing. Unlike most medical tests, genetic testing never needs to be repeated, because your genes don't change. In addition, as new discoveries about the cardiovascular impact of these genes are made, they can be filtered through your genetic matrix to improve your healthcare.

Some of the tests we recommend in this chapter used to be hard to get. Now all five are widely available. Your medical provider can order blood or saliva tests for these genes through several American genetic diagnostics laboratories, including Quest Diagnostics, Boston Heart Diagnostics, and Cleveland Heart-Lab. There are additional companies offering these tests and we anticipate home testing availability.

If you've already had DTC testing through 23andMe, Helix, Futura Genetics, or similar companies, you may already know your Apo E genotype, which predicts risk for CVD and Alzheimer's disease. As you'll learn in the next section of this chapter, the results of this blood or saliva test can also guide the optimal lifestyle to help ward off these threats to your brain and heart health. We'll also show you how information from the five genetic tests discussed on the pages that follow can guide potentially lifesaving changes in treatment for arterial disease, diabetes, and other chronic disorders.

Should you also get genetic testing for other diseases and conditions? In a 2020 scientific statement, the American Heart Association noted that the natural temptation for patients and medical providers might be to test for more genes—or even all genes—with the reasoning that more data are better, now that large gene panels or even complete genomic sequencing has become relatively affordable. However, the downside of this scattershot approach is that the more genes you have checked, the more likely that the test panel will include genetic variants of uncertain significance, leading to confusion about what, if anything, to do with this knowledge.

Therefore, the American Heart Association advises clinicians to focus on genetic tests that meet two criteria: 1) There is strong scientific evidence that the gene in question is linked to specific diseases, and 2) identifying carriers of this gene will yield actionable insights, such as changes in the management of the patient's care, improved preventive care, or confirming the diagnosis of a suspected condition. All five of the genetic tests discussed below meet these criteria and are supported by the latest peer-reviewed science.

Do You Have the Heart Attack Gene?

Genetic testing is a rapidly evolving field. More than seventy-five thousand tests for various diseases and conditions are now available and an average of ten new ones reach the market every day, a recent study found.[8] Therefore, we anticipate that additional tests will become available in the future that allow an even more comprehensive cardiovascular threat assessment. *Currently, we recommend that all patients get tested for the 9P21 (the heart attack gene), 4q25, variants of the apolipoprotein E (Apo E), KIF6, and haptoglobin (Hp) genes described in this section. If your total cholesterol level is very high (above 290 mg/dL), we also recommend that you be screened for familial hypercholesterolemia (FH), an inherited cholesterol disorder that affects about one in 200 to 250 people.*[9]

Should any cardiovascular threats be detected, it is essential to discuss a personalized prevention plan with your provider. Although the American Heart Association issued a scientific statement in 2012 recommending that *all* healthcare professionals be trained in genetics and genomics—and issued similar recommendations again in 2016—it is possible that your provider may not be familiar with these tests and the rapidly expanding knowledge about their immense value in guiding treatments and lifestyle choices.[10] If that's the case, the laboratories that provide these tests have extensive clinical information on their websites for both patients and providers, including scientific evidence from peer-reviewed journals. We suggest that you print out this material and show it to your provider.

9P21 Genotype: Identifies Carriers of the Heart Attack Gene and Offers Insight into the Safest Blood Sugar Management Strategy for People with Type 2 Diabetes

This blood or saliva test checks for the 9P21 gene, often called the heart attack gene, because it's an independent predictor of increased risk for cardiovascular events even when such factors as family history, diabetes, high blood pressure, elevated levels of the inflammatory marker C-reactive protein, and obesity are taken into account.[11] People with this genetic variant have an impaired response to interferon, a signaling protein that helps protect against the formation of arterial plaque.

Produced by a variety of cells, interferons are one of our

natural defenses against threats to our health. Best known for their ability to fight viral infections and treat certain cancers, these proteins are produced by many cells of the body, where they serve a variety of roles. In the arteries, interferons usually help block the initial stage of the disease process: cellular changes in the inner layers of the arterial wall that make them stickier, like Velcro, increasing the risk that cholesterol will get stuck there and form plaque. In people with the 9P21 gene, interferons appear to offer little protection against this vascular danger. Recent research suggests that a diminished response to interferons is one of the main reasons why 9P21 carriers often develop severe coronary artery disease (CAD) at a relatively young age, even if they have "normal" cholesterol levels.[12]

About 25 percent of Caucasians and Asians are homozygous for 9P21, meaning they have inherited the gene from both of their parents, as is the case with Camille, Neal, Casey, Robert, and Kellee. Studies link this genetic profile to a:

102 percent rise in risk for suffering a heart attack or developing heart disease at an early age, compared to non-carriers of the gene[13]

56 percent overall increase in lifetime heart attack and heart disease risk[14]

47 percent rise in risk for ischemic (clot-induced) stroke and 60 percent rise for hemorrhagic (bleeding) stroke[15]

200 percent rise in risk for death from cardiovascular causes[16]

74 percent jump in risk for aortic abdominal aneurysm, a weak, ballooning area in the heart's largest blood vessel that's often fatal if it ruptures[17]

Type 2 diabetics with this genotype have persistent poor glycemic control. If they have an HgbA1c greater than 7.0 per cent for ten years, their risk of a heart attack increases 400 percent and their risk of death doubles.[18]

About 50 percent of Caucasians and Asians are heterozygous for 9P21. Since they only carry one copy of the gene (inherited from one parent), studies calculate that they have half the risk of each of the outcomes above. The frequency of this gene in African Americans and other populations has not yet been determined.

As we emphasize to our patients, DNA does not have to be destiny. Regardless of their genotype, no one has to feel like a heart attack or stroke waiting to happen. Diane H., Camille, Catherine, and Dwayne are all homozygous for 9P21, yet have overcome their arterial disease by following our AHA for Life plan. Recently, Camille celebrated sixteen years of being heart attack and stroke free while under our care—and Diane H., Catherine, and Dwayne have *never* experienced either of these events despite their very high-risk genotypes. Dwayne, whose family doctor used to deem him a questionable candidate for life insurance, has also reversed a wide range of chronic diseases linked to poor arterial health. At the start of his treatment, he was suffering from metabolic syndrome, high blood pressure, fatty liver, obesity, prediabetes, arterial disease, and one of the highest levels of triglycerides we've ever seen in our practice. Now sixty-eight, he's already outlived his mother (who was also a 9P21 carrier) and is in the best shape of his life.

About half of Americans carry at least one copy of the heart attack gene, yet by managing their risks with proven prevention strategies and optimizing their lifestyle, they can still avoid heart attacks, strokes, dementia, and other chronic diseases. For example, a recent study revealed that Dwayne was on the right track by dramatically stepping up his activity level. In the study, which included more than 500,000 people who carried genes that put them at high risk for developing CAD, including 9P21, those who got the most aerobic exercise had a 49 percent lower rate of CAD than those who worked out the least, helping them avoid heart attacks, strokes, dementia, and other serious complications of arterial disease.[19] Participants were tracked for ten to fifteen years and asked to log how often they worked out. They also wore activity trackers and measured their grip strength (how hard they could squeeze an object, an indication of the person's overall strength). In chapter thirteen, we'll take a closer look at the best workouts to boost your heart and brain health, including fun ways to get strong and fit.

If you have diabetes, knowing your 9P21 and haptoglobin genotypes can guide important—and even lifesaving—changes in treatment, as occurred in Neal's case. As you learned earlier, a person with type 2 diabetes has the same heart attack risk as a nondiabetic person the same age who has already had one. People who have diabetes and the 9P21 gene are in even greater peril if their blood sugar isn't properly managed. For example, Neal had poorly controlled diabetes when he started treatment at our center. As mentioned earlier, diabetics who are homozygous for 9P21 with poorly controlled blood sugar for ten years were *four times more likely to have heart attacks, and twice as likely to die during that time period,* as those whose blood sugar was well managed.[20]

Medical providers used to think that everybody with diabetes would benefit from intensive treatment to lower their blood sugar as much as possible (tight glycemic control). The goal was to help diabetics avoid the many serious complications of their disease, including heart attacks, strokes, and deaths from cardiovascular causes. However, clinical trials comparing tight glycemic control with less stringent control have demonstrated that tight control didn't improve cardiovascular outcomes for many patients and could be harmful to some.[21] Providers then shifted to advising looser control for everybody, which didn't work very well, either.

In 2021, the American Diabetes Association (ADA) issued new guidelines, calling for blood sugar control to be personalized according to certain factors, including the patient's ethnicity, life expectancy, and patient and provider preferences.[22] Unfortunately, these guidelines, while an improvement on earlier one-size-fits-all recommendations, fail to discuss two genes that recent studies have shown to be extremely important in guiding diabetic care: 9P21 and variants of the haptoglobin gene. Neal's 9P21 status revealed that he needed tight glycemic control to avoid serious or fatal complications of his disease. We adjusted his medication accordingly and not only is his blood sugar under excellent control, but Neal—who had previously undergone quadruple bypass surgery and eighteen stenting procedures before starting treatment with our method—has avoided the need for any further trips to the OR.

Here are some other steps we advise if you have the 9P21 genotype:

At forty, get an abdominal aortic aneurysm (AAA) scan.

If the results are normal, have the test repeated every five years, while abnormal results will require more frequent follow-up, as advised by your healthcare provider, to see if the aneurysm is growing. Typically, only large aneurysms require treatment to prevent rupture. Ruptured AAA kills about ten thousand Americans a year.[23] This ultrasound test is described more fully in chapter seven.

Avoid smoking.

Not only is smoking the leading risk factor for heart attacks and strokes, but it also greatly increases the threat of developing an aneurysm. Other aneurysm risk factors include obesity, diabetes, high cholesterol, high blood pressure, and genes.

Make exercise a daily habit.

A recent scientific statement from the American Heart Association reports that regular exercise can help prevent or manage more than forty diseases besides CAD, including diabetes, cancer, depression, arthritis, osteoporosis, and obesity. Conversely, physical inactivity kills 5.3 million people prematurely each year—more than the toll from smoking![24] The American Heart Association and the BaleDoneen Method recommend getting at least thirty minutes of aerobic exercise at least five days a week, plus muscle strengthening exercises (such as weight-lifting or resistance training) at least two days a week. For optimal cardiovascular benefit, aim for at least three hundred minutes of exercise per week, with the intensity gradually increasing over time. Always consult your provider before starting a new workout regimen to make sure it's right for you.

Maintain healthy cholesterol levels.

Genetic factors, such as elevated levels of Lp(a), may make it necessary to set more aggressive targets for lowering your LDL than are typically advised by standard care. As you learned in chapter eight, it's also key to pay attention to your total-cholesterol-to-HDL ratio—the best predictor of heart attack risk in the Women's Health Study—and your ratio of triglycerides (TG) to HDL. In chapter fifteen, you'll find a list of the optimal treatment targets we recommend, plus tips on how to achieve them.

Apo E Genotype: Predicts Heart Disease and the Best Diet to Avoid It

This blood or saliva test analyzes your Apolipoprotein E (Apo E) genotype, which predicts lifetime risk for CAD and Alzheimer's disease, and also influences how your body metabolizes nutrients in your diet, including fats and carbs. As Neal and many of our other patients have discovered, certain Apo E genotypes make common foods that are healthy for people with other Apo E genotypes potentially harmful.

For example, Neal, who was struggling with obesity at the start of his treatment, was baffled and frustrated because the numbers on his scale hadn't budged, even though he was then following a strict ketogenic (low-carb, high-fat) diet that had helped other people he knew slim down. Nor had this eating plan improved his heart health — instead, he kept getting sicker and sicker. A recent study comparing various low-fat and low-carb diets found wildly varying results: Some people lost as much as thirty pounds with each of these diets, while others *gained* ten pounds. These contradictory findings not only highlight the frustration that many dieters feel when trying to find the optimal eating plan, but provide further proof that the one-size-fits-all approach doesn't work. In chapter thirteen we'll take a closer look at the optimal personalized eating plan for weight loss and arterial wellness.

The Apo E gene has three variants (E2, E3, and E4), resulting in six possible genotypes: Apo E 2/2, Apo E 2/3, Apo E 2/4, Apo E 3/3, Apo E 3/4, and Apo E 4/4. Here are a few insights from research:

The Apo E 2/2 and 2/3 genotypes, which occur in 11 percent of the population, are associated with the lowest risk for CVD. If you have one of these genotypes, your best bet for disease prevention is a moderate-fat diet containing about 35 percent fat from heart-healthy sources, such as omega-3 rich oily fish or olive oil. Some people with these Apo E genotypes have high triglycerides and often get dangerously flawed advice, since providers often tell everybody with this disorder to cut down on fat. However, this seemingly heart-healthy advice can *raise* heart

attack and stroke risk in people with Apo E 2/2 or 2/3 genotypes! That's because, paradoxically, their levels of small, dense
cholesterol (the dangerous kind that can triple heart attack
risk) *increase* if they eat less fat. Instead, people with this genotype get the best cardiovascular perks by cutting down on
carbs, which helps lower LDL and the amount of small, dense
particles.

People with the Apo E 2/4 and 3/3 genotypes, which are
found in 64 percent of the population, have an intermediate cardiovascular disease risk and benefit from the conventional
Mediterranean-style diet that's typically advised to protect heart
health. This diet should contain about 25 percent fat. We also
recommend "eating the rainbow" by including colorful fruits
and vegetables in your diet. Colorful produce is a great source of
heart-healthy micronutrients and disease-fighting antioxidants.

For people with the Apo E 2/2, 2/3, and or 3/3 genotypes,
moderate alcohol consumption (a maximum of one drink a day
for women and two for men) is beneficial to heart health. In
chapter thirteen we'll take a closer look at the latest findings
about moderate drinking and heart health, some of which may
surprise you. However, it's important to remember that even
though alcohol is good for some people's hearts, it can have
health risks. For example, having even one drink a day increases
the risk for breast cancer in women.

About 25 percent of people, including Neal, have the Apo E
3/4 or 4/4 genotypes, which are linked to the highest lifetime
risk for CVD. This group can trim the threat by following a very
low-fat diet (no more than 20 percent fat) and limiting or avoiding alcohol consumption. That meant Neal's low-carb, high-fat
keto diet was the worst possible choice for his Apo E genotype,
explaining why this popular weight-loss plan was of no benefit
to his arterial health or his waistline.

Compared to people who don't have the Apo E 4/4 genotype, those with one copy of this gene (such as Casey) have three

to five times higher risk for late-onset Alzheimer's, the most common form of the disease. Those with two copies are at fifteen to twenty times higher risk.[25] However, the memory-robbing disorder also occurs in people with other genotypes, while many people with the 4/4 genotype never develop AD.

Even if you have the Apo E 4/4 genotype, there's a lot you can do to keep your memory sharp as you age. In the next chapter, you'll find a three-step plan to safeguard your memory. It draws on landmark new research by the world's leading experts on AD and dementia, including the first guidelines for the prevention of these disorders, issued by the World Health Organization in 2019. We'll also tell you how the right lifestyle can clobber AD risk—reducing it by as much as 60 percent!

KIF6 Genotype: Predicts Statin Response and Heart Attack Risk

This blood or saliva test checks for a variant of the KIF6 (Kinesin family member 6) gene. The KIF6 gene's job is to make a protein that transports other substances, such as protein complexes and messenger RNA, within cells. Which version of the gene you carry influences both your risk for a heart attack and whether you'll get any benefit from the statins most likely to be prescribed for heart attack prevention.

Here's scary news: If you're on Lipitor (atorvastatin)—the most commonly prescribed statin—or Pravachol (pravastatin)—as your sole therapy, there's a 40 percent chance that you're getting *no* cardiovascular protection at all, even if your cholesterol numbers look great. Three large randomized clinical trials found that these drugs *only* reduce the risk for heart attacks, strokes, and mortality from cardiovascular causes in the 60 percent of Americans who have the KIF6 variant. These statins had no effect on rates of these events in patients who didn't carry the variant. About 40 percent of European Americans are noncarriers. Few studies have examined carrier and noncarrier rates among people of other ancestries.

Thirty million Americans take statins, which rank among the most widely prescribed drugs in the world. If you have high cholesterol or coronary artery disease, you're probably on a statin. Since these cholesterol-lowering medications also combat the inflammation that drives heart attacks, almost all patients who have suffered cardiovascular events are put on a statin to help prevent recurrence. It's essential to find out your KIF6 status so you can get the most effective treatment. For example, our testing revealed that Camille, who was sent home from the hospital after her heart attack with a Lipitor prescription, was a noncarrier of KIF, so was getting zero protection from her medication.

Because Lipitor and Pravachol are so commonly prescribed—usually without checking the patient's KIF6 status—we wonder if ineffective treatment explains why 33 percent of heart attacks and 25 percent of strokes occur in people who have already survived one or more of these events. Had we not used genetic testing, Camille might well have fallen into that group. To get the best protection from these events, it's essential to learn your KIF6 status so your healthcare provider can tailor your treatment to your DNA.

In addition, women should be aware that in a very large clinical trial, taking Lipitor *raised* women's heart attack risk by 10 percent while reducing risk by 42 percent in men.[26] While the researchers concluded that the increased risk in women was not statistically significant, because the study included fewer women than men, the findings suggest that Lipitor may not be an effective treatment choice for women. In chapter fourteen, we'll tell you about a new genetic test that can help your medical provider identify the most effective medications for your genotype and avoid ineffective or harmful treatments.

There's controversy about the effect of the KIF6 variant on lifetime CVD danger. In five large studies, untreated carriers of the variant had up to a 55 percent higher risk for heart attacks, strokes, or death from cardiovascular causes, compared to untreated participants without the variant. In two clinical trials, carrying the variant had a bigger impact on raising heart disease risk than being over fifty-five, having abnormal levels of LDL or HDL cholesterol, or having high blood pressure. Only smoking and diabetes ranked above the KIF6 polymorphism for boosting disease risk.

4q25: Predicts Increased Risk for Atrial Fibrillation

Available at labs all over the U.S., this blood test checks to see if you are a carrier of the 4q25 gene. Compared to noncarriers of this gene, those who have it are at 140 percent higher risk for atrial fibrillation (AF), the most common type of irregular heartbeat (arrhythmia). It occurs when rapid, disorganized electrical impulses cause the heart's upper chambers (atria) to beat rapidly and chaotically, getting out of sync with the lower chambers (ventricles). As a result, the ventricles don't fill properly and blood may pool in the heart, raising risk for blood clots, heart failure, and other complications.

AF quintuples the risk for strokes and doubles it for heart attacks or dementia.[27] More than 454,000 people are hospitalized with AF each year and it contributes to about 158,000 deaths each year, according to the CDC, which predicts that the number of Americans with AF will double from 6 million in 2021 to 12 million in 2050. Although early detection and treatment can help save lives, this dangerous disorder often goes undiagnosed until the patient has suffered serious complications, such as a stroke. Most common in older adults, AF strikes 20 to 33 percent of Americans at some point in their lives, depending on their risk factors, the Framingham Heart Study recently reported.[28] Red flags for developing AF including the following:

Diabetes

Obesity and/or poor cardiovascular fitness

A resting heart rate above 84 beats per minute

Obstructive sleep apnea

High blood pressure

Chronic obstructive pulmonary disease (COPD)

Rheumatoid arthritis

Low levels of magnesium and/or potassium

Thyroid disorders

Kidney disease

A family history of AF

Use of alendronate (a medication for osteoporosis sold under such brand names as Fosamax and Binosto)

Having an ischemic (clot-caused) stroke, particularly if the cause was unclear

Advanced age (AF is most common in people sixty-five and older)

Given the many dangers of this disorder, and the widespread availability of a simple, inexpensive blood test to check for genetic risk, we think it makes sense to get tested, so you can act now to avoid atrial fibrillation and its devastating or even fatal complications if you're genetically susceptible. The same strategies that help keep your heart healthy can also reduce your risk for AF, such as exercising regularly, maintaining a healthy weight, avoiding all nicotine use or exposure, and managing high blood pressure. Reducing your systolic blood pressure (the top number) below 130 mm Hg has been shown to cut risk for AF by 30 percent, compared to a reading above 142 mm Hg.[29]

For people with particularly high risk for atrial fibrillation, medications may be advised, along with lifestyle modification. In a recent study of older adults, those with the highest levels of Omega-3 fatty acids in their blood had a 39 percent lower rate of AF, compared to people the same age with the lowest levels. Omega-3 fatty acids are found in oily fish (such as salmon, tuna, lake trout, sardines, and herring), nuts, flax seeds, vegetable oils, and leafy green vegetables.

If your levels of Omega-3 are low, ask your medical provider if a supplement is appropriate for you. In another recent study of adults fifty-five and older, those who followed a Mediterranean diet that included 50 grams (about 4 teaspoons) of extra-virgin olive oil daily had a 38 percent reduction in their rate of AF, compared to a control group.[30] Studies vary about the effects of drinking coffee, with most research finding that a daily intake of two to three cups is safe and either neutral or beneficial in protecting against AF and stroke.[31]

Haptoglobin Genotype: Predicts Cardiovascular Danger in Diabetics and Identifies People Who Can Benefit from a Gluten-Free Diet

This blood or saliva test, which can also be performed through a simple oral rinse, checks for variants of the haptoglobin (Hp) gene and provides valuable information if you have diabetes, which now ranks as the world's fastest-growing chronic disease. Not only can you find out if you have an Hp gene variant that quintuples the lifetime threat of CVD, but if you do have this high-risk genotype, one of our recent peer-reviewed publications and other new research suggests that the results can guide precision-medicine therapies that almost eliminate this risk.[32] These treatments include dietary changes and an inexpensive, over-the-counter supplement that most people should avoid. However, it can be lifesaving for diabetic patients with a certain Hp genotype.

If you don't have diabetes, you can still benefit from this test by finding out if you have a genotype linked to increased risk for intestinal, autoimmune, and inflammatory disorders and if you'd benefit from a gluten-free diet and probiotics to ward off these health threats. The Hp gene has two alleles, called Hp1 and Hp2. Since you inherit one allele from each of your parents, there are three possible combinations:

Hp 1-1 (low risk for heart disease)
Hp 2-1 (intermediate risk)
Hp 2-2 (high risk)

Seven independent long-term studies have demonstrated that the Hp 2-1 and 2-2 genotypes predict increased risk for coronary artery disease (CAD) in type 2 diabetes. If you are diabetic and have the Hp 2-2 genotype, your lifetime risk for CAD is triple that of a diabetic with the Hp 2-1 genotype and five times higher than that of a diabetic with the Hp 2-2 test.[33] About 16 percent of people carry the Hp 1-1 genotype, 48 percent carry the Hp 2-1 genotype, and 36 percent carry the Hp 2-2 genotype.

Finding out your Hp genotype is also extremely important for protecting your arterial wellness. The Hp gene regulates haptoglobin, a protein produced by the liver that binds to hemoglobin, a substance produced when red blood cells die.[34] If hemoglobin isn't bound quickly, it will release iron, which can harm your blood vessels. For example, the iron will oxidize LDL (bad) cholesterol, making it even more harmful to your arteries. When Hp binds to hemoglobin, white blood cells can quickly clear this damaging substance from your blood, neutralizing these dangers. In diabetics, iron can also bind to HDL (good) cholesterol, negating many of its usually heart-protective properties. Therefore, the Hp 2-2 genotype packs a double punch of bad news!

Our study, which was published in *Frontiers of Cardiovascular Medicine* in 2018, and other peer-reviewed research has revealed that type 2 diabetics can counteract almost all the increased risk for heart disease by taking 400 IU of vitamin E daily. While you might wonder if everyone with diabetes should take this inexpensive supplement—and skip the gene test—studies show that unless you have the Hp 2-2 genotype, taking vitamin E not only has no CV benefits, but it can be downright dangerous for your heart.

In most people, vitamin E supplementation raises the risk for heart attacks and early death. The only people who benefit from it are diabetics with the Hp 2-2 genotype. This actionable insight is why we recommend that all type 2 diabetics get this test. Before taking any dietary supplement, discuss the potential risks and benefits with your medical provider. We also recommend that all patients follow a diet based on their Apo E genotype, as described earlier in this chapter, whether they have diabetes or not.

It is also very important for diabetic patients with the Hp 2-1 and 2-2 genotypes to practice tight glycemic control, as we also recommend for those who carry the 9P21 gene. Talk to your medical provider about the best ways to manage your blood sugar. Many of our diabetic patients, including Neal, have benefitted from continuous glucose monitoring, using FDA-approved technologies like the Freestyle Libre sensor, which automatically measures blood sugar levels once a minute. Getting immediate feedback from the sensor helped Neal, who has the 2-1 genotype, better understand how his diet was impacting his sugar levels. For example, after switching to a gluten-free diet, he started including brown rice in his meals, only to discover via continuous glucose monitoring that it was causing his sugar to spike.

There is now strong scientific evidence that diabetic and nondiabetic patients with the Hp 1-2 and Hp 2-2 genotypes benefit from a gluten-free diet as part of their heart-attack-and-stroke-prevention plan, while there's no CV advantage for those with the Hp 1-1 genotype. Here's why: Recent studies have identified Hp2's precursor protein, zonulin, as "the biological door to inflammation, autoimmunity and cancer."[35] Zonulin has been linked to many chronic conditions, including autoimmune and inflammatory disorders.[36] As you learned in chapter eight, inflammation is also a key player in causing arterial disease. Once plaque has formed in the arteries, this fiery process can also ignite a heart attack or stroke. Think of plaque as kindling and inflammation as the match.

Since gluten activates the zonulin pathway with adverse effects on the intestines, the lining of blood vessels, and other parts of the body, increasing risk for chronic disease, including CAD, we recommend that people with the Hp 1-2 and Hp 2-2 genotypes limit or avoid gluten in their diet and consider taking a daily probiotic supplement to protect and enhance their gut health, after consulting with their medical provider to make sure a probiotic is appropriate for them.

Outsmarting Her Genes

Four years ago, Diane H. celebrated her fiftieth birthday, making her officially "old" by the standards of her maternal relatives. To mark this milestone, her friends took her on a surprise vacation at a hot springs resort with a five-star restaurant. "It was all about quality time and relaxation," she recalls. "I felt so special and got to reflect on all the blessings in my life." Now fifty-four, Diane H. had lost thirty pounds by following the DNA-based diet and exercise plan in this chapter. A carrier of the Hp 1-2 gene, she's gone gluten-free and reports that her energy level has dramatically improved. She's become an avid racewalker and has won several medals in this competitive sport.

"Every birthday is very emotional for me," she adds.

"Following the BaleDoneen Method has extended and enriched my life, and has helped my entire family become better keepers of our bodies," she says. "Without it, my husband, who is prediabetic, would probably be on insulin by now and my parents, whom I love dearly, might not be here at all. Getting the right preventive care has made an awesome difference and I'm eternally grateful for the life that has given us."

Action Step: Find Out If You Need Screening for Familial Hypercholesterolemia

Affecting about one in every 200 to 250 people, familial hyper-cholesterolemia (FH) is a genetic disorder that greatly increases the risk for developing arterial disease at a young age. It stems from an inherited abnormality in how the body recycles LDL cholesterol, leading to very high levels building up in the blood. Without treatment, people with this condition are twenty times more likely to develop coronary artery disease than those without it. If untreated, men with FH have a 50 percent risk of suffering a heart attack by fifty and untreated women have a 30 percent risk of having a heart attack by sixty, reports the CDC.[37]

However, if it's found and treated early, risk for CAD drops by 80 percent![38] Tragically, this potentially life-threatening condition often goes undiagnosed and untreated. Although it's estimated to affect about 1.3 million Americans, only about 10 percent of those with FH are aware they have it, leaving the other 90 percent in extreme vascular peril, according to the American Heart Association.[39] It's possible for people with this disorder to develop heart disease as early as their twenties.

The leading warning signs of FH are a total cholesterol level above 290 mg/dL or an LDL level above 190 mg/DL in an adult or total cholesterol above 260 mg/dL or LDL above 155 mg/dL in a child. Other clues that you could be at risk include a family history of early heart disease, high cholesterol levels, and/or FH.

To check for this disorder, most providers use a widely accepted diagnostic tool called Simon Broome criteria, which include an evaluation of the patient's cholesterol numbers, symptoms, family history, and, in some cases, genetic testing. Once it's diagnosed, FH is treatable with medications and lifestyle changes, helping people who have it avoid heart attacks, strokes, and other complications of arterial disease. In fact, early detection and treatment can be lifesaving!

CHAPTER 12

Three Smart Strategies to Protect Your Memory

"The size of your dreams must always exceed your current capacity to achieve them. If your dreams do not scare you, they're not big enough."

— ELLEN JOHNSON SIRLEAF, TWENTY-FOURTH
PRESIDENT OF LIBERIA AND AFRICA'S
FIRST WOMAN PRESIDENT

Robert and his wife, Kellee, the Texas couple you met in chapter ten, have both suffered the same tragedy: Each of them has lost a parent to dementia, which now affects 50 million people globally, with a new case occurring every three seconds.[1] Robert's mom, Jane Ann, a petite dynamo who loved to throw parties, dance the night away, and captivate a crowd with her witty anecdotes, began to show the first signs of memory loss at sixty-five. Robert's dad had to install locks on all the doors in the house to keep her from wandering away.

Formerly so agile that she could still do handstands and backflips in her early sixties, she became clumsy and disoriented in her own home. One night, she fell down a flight of stairs, breaking both arms. After that, her grace and charm disappeared and she grew increasingly confused, agitated, and paranoid. Many times, Robert recalls, "I'd get calls from my father asking me to explain to my mom who he was because she thought a stranger had broken into her home." Jane Ann spent her final years in a nursing home until her death at eighty.

Kellee's dad, Bruce, had a long battle with vascular dementia. "When I was growing up, I couldn't have asked for a better dad," she says. "He was a school superintendent and Sunday school teacher who loved reading so much that he'd go to the library every week, bring home a big stack of books and finish one almost every day. Ordained as a minister when he was young, he was also a brilliant orator and the smartest person I've ever known."

Shortly after turning seventy, Bruce began to have trouble remembering how to get to the library, and could no longer remember the content of a book he'd just read, adds Kellee. "It was so sad to see such a brilliant mind slowly erased by vascular dementia over the next ten years. It was heartbreaking to see this disease rob him of everything, especially in the last year and a half of his life when his eyes were blank and he no longer recognized us. After witnessing what happened to my father—and knowing what happened to Jane Ann—my husband and I pray that we don't have to go through that ourselves."

Compounding the couple's concern, Robert carries one copy of the Apo E4 gene you read about in chapter eleven, which multiplies risk for Alzheimer's disease, the most common form of dementia. Although Kellee, now fifty-nine, does not carry that gene, like many older adults, particularly those with a family history of dementia, she gets a flash of fear whenever she experiences even the slightest mental glitch. "Rather ironically, the other day, I blanked on what my mother-in-law's name was when I was talking about her fifteen-year battle with dementia. Whenever something like that happens or I forget where I put the car keys, there's always that nagging worry: *Is this normal or am I starting to lose it?*"

Are Alzheimer's Disease and Dementia Preventable?

Every sixty-five seconds, someone in the U.S. is diagnosed with Alzheimer's disease (AD). Dementia is a general term that includes several chronic diseases of the brain—including AD and vascular dementia—that cause progressive memory loss, personality changes, and impairments of reasoning and problem-solving severe enough to interfere with daily life. Later in this chapter, you'll find a three-part plan to help you avoid memory loss, as well as ten action steps to protect and preserve the wellness of your most important organ: your brain.

Dementia can have several causes, including damage to blood vessels that supply the brain. For example, vascular dementia is most common in people who have microvascular disease and have experienced symptomatic or silent strokes. Arterial disease and related conditions also play a key role in Alzheimer's disease, a factor that helps explain why we have long observed a remarkably low rate of dementia and AD in our older patients. Although much remains to be learned about AD, which has eluded effective treatment for decades, two specific brain abnormalities are now known to be hallmarks of the disease[2]:

The development of amyloid plaques: sticky clumps of proteins that form in the spaces between the brain's neurons (nerve cells), disrupting their communication.

Accumulation of neurofibrillary tangles: twisted fibers inside neurons that are mainly made of a protein called tau. This protein normally forms part of tiny tubes (microtubules) that ferry nutrients and other substances from one area of a brain cell to others. In AD, tau is abnormal and damages neurons, particularly those in brain regions involved in memory.

More than 6 million Americans are living with AD,[3] a

number that's projected to rise to 13.2 million by 2050, underscoring the urgent need for effective prevention strategies.[4] Currently, AD[5] affects one in ten people over sixty-five and one in three of those over eighty-five, and ranks as America's sixth leading cause of death.[6] While deaths from heart disease (the number one killer of U.S. men and women) dropped by 9 percent between 2000 and 2017, deaths from AD have soared by 145 percent.[7] Because this memory-robbing disorder has long eluded effective treatment, people who develop it, on average, die within four to eight years after their diagnosis.[8]

Although these are frightening statistics, there are now powerful reasons to be hopeful.

Until recently, the scientific consensus was that there was no known way to prevent AD and dementia. But is that really true? In 2017, the medical journal *The Lancet* commissioned a panel of twenty-eight of the world's leading experts on dementia to find out. Based on a rigorous review of the peer-reviewed evidence, the experts zeroed in on nine lifestyle factors and medical conditions (all of which are preventable and highly treatable) that contribute to the disease.[9] The key takeaway: Addressing these risks could prevent up to 35 percent of dementia cases.

The landmark discovery of these factors prompted the World Health Organization to conduct its own evidence review and issue the world's first guidelines for dementia and cognitive decline risk reduction in 2019, stating that for the first time, there is solid science to show that "prevention of dementia is possible [through] implementation of key interventions."[10] Since then, there has been an avalanche of exciting new peer-reviewed publications offering actionable, scientifically grounded insights on how to protect and preserve memory. In 2020, the *Lancet* team conducted a new analysis that identified three additional dementia risks. Their study concluded by addressing them and the nine they'd previously discovered. They learned that up to 40 percent of memory-loss cases could either be prevented or delayed.[11] Another 2020 paper reported that following an optimal lifestyle clobbered AD risk by 60 percent![12]

The Three Keys to Optimal Brain Health Throughout Your Life

One of the most important underlying messages from the hundreds of new publications on dementia prevention is simple: "Heart health equals brain health." For example, the landmark 2017 *Lancet* study and other groundbreaking new research has revealed that three interlocking strategies are central to slashing your risk for cognitive decline (the first stage of memory loss) and dementia, including AD. All three of the strategies summarized below are already part of our evidence-based AHA for Life plan and have helped many of our patients, including an octogenarian you'll meet in chapter fourteen, enjoy a health span that matches their life span.

1. Protect your brain from injury by optimizing your arterial wellness.

Healthy blood vessels are essential to your brain's well-being. Although your brain only accounts for about 2 percent, it is powered by 25 percent of your blood flow, which supplies it with about 20 percent of the oxygen you breathe and 25 percent of the calories you consume.[13] Each of the 100 billion neurons that comprise the wiring that the brain uses to communicate with the rest of your body has its own blood supply: tiny capillaries that both nourish the neurons and cleanse them of wastes.

So important are healthy blood vessels to brain function that several of the new recommendations for dementia prevention echo those for the prevention of CVD. One of the most important is avoiding nicotine use or exposure to secondhand smoke—factors that raise risk for memory loss by up to 214 percent.[14] Also crucial is getting your blood pressure, blood sugar, and cholesterol numbers into the healthy range, using the targets specified in our action steps.

2. Take action to avoid arterial and brain inflammation.

Chronic inflammation is more dangerous to your arteries than smoking. Inflammation and oxidative stress have also been linked to the buildup of brain deposits of beta-amyloid. Many scientists believe that accumulation of this sticky compound in the brain is the primary cause of Alzheimer's disease, with the buildup initially disrupting communication between neurons and ultimately killing them. According to this widely held theory, called the amyloid hypothesis, the development of the amyloid plaques that are the hallmark of AD activates immune cells, leading to inflammation that eventually destroys brain cells.[15]

As discussed more fully in chapter eight, this fiery condition has been linked to so many disorders that some scientists have called it "the root of all diseases." Proven strategies to combat inflammation include weight loss, aerobic exercise, eating anti-inflammatory foods and improving your oral health. Not only is inflammation a key characteristic of AD, but researchers are actively exploring therapies to extinguish fire in the brain as a potential new approach to treatment.

3. Boost your cognitive reserve.

Like your body, your mind needs exercise to stay fit. The *Lancet* paper and other studies show that highly educated people are less likely to suffer memory loss, possibly because keeping the brain active boosts its cognitive reserve, allowing it to work efficiently even if some of its neurons are damaged.[16] A wide range of activities provide healthy intellectual stimulation and help increase your cognitive reserve, including studying a foreign language, taking adult education classes, doing crossword and other puzzles, and brain training.

In a Harvard study of people in their fifties and sixties, those who were the most socially connected had half the rate of memory loss during the six-year study as those who were socially isolated.[17] Another new discovery: Several studies report that even mild hearing loss raises dementia risk, while more severe hearing loss doubles or triples the threat. Hearing may be important to protecting memory because of what the *Lancet* paper's lead author, Gill Livingston, calls the use it or lose it model. "We get a lot of intellectual stimulation through hearing," Dr. Livingston reports.[18]

Top Ten Action Steps to Help You Avoid Memory Loss

Shortly before writing this chapter, we conducted our own rigorous evidence review of the latest peer-reviewed findings about the best ways to prevent cognitive decline and dementia. Drawing on new and recent discoveries from the research front, here are ten proven steps that you can take—today—to safeguard and enhance your brain health at every age. They're easy, often enjoyable, and backed by the latest science.

Lifestyle matters!

Remember how we told you earlier in this chapter that an optimal lifestyle can clobber Alzheimer's risk by 60 percent? What, specifically, does that involve? The latest research suggests that one of your best bets is to follow a Mediterranean diet that is high in fruits, vegetables, fish, seeds, and nuts.[19] Healthy oils are also important, but as you learned in chapter eleven, the amount of fat in your diet should be guided by your Apo E genotype. Also stay hydrated and drink adequate water. In a healthy individual, research supports determining the daily amount based on weight, roughly half of body weight in ounces of water per day. If you weigh one hundred pounds, aim for fifty ounces per day, or if you are two hundred pounds, aim for one hundred ounces per day. Keeping your waistline trim (less than forty inches for men and less than thirty-five inches for women) also helps reduce dementia risk. If you're saddled with excess belly fat, check out the weight loss ideas in the next chapter. An excellent way to tone your muscles and rev up your brain is to get at least thirty minutes of cardiovascular exercise daily, plus resistance training twice a week. Fun ways to keep fit include Zumba, tai chi, yoga, brisk walking, biking, and dancing.

Make healthy brain activities a daily habit.

A systematic review of twelve randomized controlled trials concluded that meditation can offset age-related cognitive decline.[20] Other studies suggest that mindfulness may change the brain, by expanding areas involved in focused attention. We recommend fifteen minutes of mindful meditation daily, using a focus word or object or an app, such as Calm. Give your brain plenty of stimulation by listening to music, studying a new language, trying brain training games (such as Lumosity), volunteering, and social engagement. Great ways to connect with others include book clubs, current event discussions, online groups, and even chatting with friends. Laughter does your heart—and brain—good by improving blood pressure and increasing levels of nitric oxide, a naturally produced substance that acts as the best "food" for your arterial lining and protects its health.[21]

Get seven to eight hours of sound, refreshing sleep every night.

Skimping on slumber or not sleeping well contributes to beta-amyloid deposition, adversely affects blood pressure, and often causes weight gain, potentially leading to insulin resistance and diabetes, which in turn raises risk for developing dementia. A recent study found that even one night of sleep deprivation resulted in a significant increase in the brain's beta-amyloid burden.[22] There are many tools available to measure your sleep, including apps, wrist devices, certain beds, and the Ōura Ring. If you snore loudly or frequently experience unexplained daytime drowsiness, getting tested and, if necessary, treated for obstructive sleep apnea (OSA) can be lifesaving. A recent study of older adults found that those with untreated OSA had more than double the risk of developing AD within the next five years, as compared to people the same age without this sleep disease.[23]

The study also found that people whose OSA was treated reduced their risk for AD diagnosis and death by 77 percent, versus those who were untreated.

Get your vitamin D level checked.

In a study of Alzheimer's risk that included more than 378,000 participants sixty and older, those with high levels of vitamin D had a 38 percent lower risk for AD.[24] Why? The sunshine vitamin helps reduce oxidative stress, prevents neurons from dying, and aids the clearance of beta-amyloid plaques by activating macrophages (the Pac-Man-like immune cells that gobble up harmful substances). If you don't know your vitamin D level, ask your healthcare provider to check it. All that's involved is a simple, universally available blood test. The optimal level of the sunshine vitamin is 40–60 ng/mL. If yours is lower than that, you'll need a supplement. However, it's important to realize that vitamin D is a fat-soluble vitamin, so you can overdose. That's why it's important to get your level checked before taking a supplement and during treatment. If your level is low, taking 2,000 to 5,000 IU of vitamin D3 daily is usually effective.

Optimize your oral health.

The oral bacteria that cause periodontal (gum) disease can infect the brain and inflame your arteries. These oral pathogens have also been implicated in the development of AD. To tease out the associations between gum disease, the bacteria that cause it, and AD, a 2020 study by the National Institute of Aging analyzed the oral and cognitive health of more than eight thousand middle-aged and older adults. All participants received a baseline dental exam and blood tests for antibodies to nineteen species of causative bacteria, then were tracked for up to twenty-six years. Of the nineteen, *Porphyromonas gingivalis* (Pg) was the microbe most strongly linked to AD in older adults. Compared to people without antibodies to causative bacteria, those with Pg antibodies had a 36 percent higher risk for AD mortality.[25] Pg has also been found in the brains and spinal fluid of AD patients.[26] A key takeaway from the latest research: Your dental provider is a lifesaving member of your dementia prevention team! The findings also offer powerful motivation to follow the four-step oral health plan in chapter ten.

Get your cholesterol checked.

What cholesterol goal should you strive for to help prevent dementia? Studies show that if your total cholesterol is above 200 mg/dL, risk for AD rises by 23 percent, and if total cholesterol is above 250 mg/dL, risk is doubled.[27] Therefore, maintaining a cholesterol level below 200 mg/dL should be a top priority. Watch your total cholesterol-to-triglycerides ratio (your total cholesterol number divided by your triglycerides number), which should be below 3. Pay attention to your HDL level as well: this "good" cholesterol is brain food. In a recent study, people whose HDL level was below 40 mg/dL had a 53 percent higher risk for memory loss, compared to those with a level above 60 mg/dL.[28]

Maintain healthy blood pressure levels.

Your goal should be a blood pressure below 120/80 mm Hg. High blood pressure is the number one risk factor for stroke, which increases risk for vascular dementia. High blood pressure also increases the risk for AD and many chronic diseases, including heart failure, heart attacks, chronic kidney disease, aortic aneurysm, and vision loss.[29] A recent study of 4.28 million people thirty to ninety, who were tracked for seven years, found that the higher a person's blood pressure was, the greater the risk for

AD.[30] An even newer study linked having blood pressure above 120/80 at fifty-three to brain volume shrinkage and small vessel disease of the brain by seventy.[31] The best time to measure blood pressure is in the morning. Treatments for elevated blood pressure include exercise, laughter, mindfulness, proper sleep, a low-salt diet, staying hydrated, and, if necessary, medication, a topic that we will discuss more fully in chapter fourteen. In chapter fifteen, we'll take a closer look at new blood pressure guidelines, the best ways to check your blood pressure, and other key things to know about this and other important health metrics.

A healthy gut helps keep your brain healthy.

One of the latest discoveries is that an unhealthy gut microbiome (the trillions of bacteria and other microorganisms that live in your intestines) can activate your immune system, leading to systemic inflammation. This, in turn, can impair the blood–brain barrier, leading to neuroinflammation, nerve cell damage, and, ultimately, destruction, magnifying the threat of AD.[32] Ways to enhance gut health include eating prebiotic and probiotic foods such as fermented foods like sauerkraut, kombucha, kefir, and tempeh, and yogurt, asparagus, garlic, dandelion root, and apples. Epidemiological studies have shown that coffee intake can also be a healthy food for the gut because of its antioxidant, anti-inflammatory, and antiproliferative effects on the mucosa. Avoid saturated fats, artificial sweeteners, and all soft drinks.[33]

Know your blood sugar numbers.

Eighty percent of AD patients are either insulin resistant or diabetic. Insulin resistance (IR), as you learned in chapter nine, is the precursor to type 2 diabetes. It is an inflammatory condition of the arteries and whole body that, if untreated, can often progress silently for decades before someone is diagnosed with diabetes. For that entire time, the brain is suffering.[34] In short, the brain is on fire! The inflammatory effects of IR have been shown to drive the development of Alzheimer's disease, which is often called type 3 diabetes. That's because insulin signaling is important for many aspects of normal brain function and plays a key role in learning and memory. Levels of brain insulin are lower in AD because amyloid beta proteins render neurons insulin resistant.[35] This impairment is thought to be a central mechanism by which memory deficits develop in people with AD.[36]

Certain medications used to treat arterial disease may also protect against Alzheimer's.

In chapter fourteen, we'll take a deep dive into medications commonly used to treat heart disease. Recent studies suggest that some of them may also have an added benefit by supporting brain health and helping to preserve memory. For example, daily low-dose aspirin, which is frequently prescribed for heart attack and stroke prevention, has also been shown to decrease cognitive decline in women. However, this over-the-counter medication shouldn't be taken without a provider's supervision because it can have dangerous side effects, including increased risk for gastrointestinal bleeding. The signal from recent studies of statins, which are commonly prescribed to lower cholesterol, indicates that these medications may significantly lower risk for AD. That signal is so strong that the National Institutes of Health has started a $90 million clinical trial called PREVENTABLE to secure a definitive answer. ACE inhibitors, a class of blood pressure drugs, have been linked to slowing of cognitive decline and a 32 percent drop in stroke danger. *However, there's an important caveat: None of these drugs are approved solely for AD prevention. If your provider has prescribed them for the conditions listed above, or to treat arterial disease, you may also be getting a marvelous side effect: memory protection!*

A Dramatic Recovery

Seven years ago, Robert was so ill during his first visit to our center that he could barely walk. Despite meeting medical criteria for twenty-six different diseases and conditions, he had an excellent memory. During his initial evaluation, despite having severe chest pain and shortness of breath, he was still able to rattle off every detail of his complex medical history, including the exact dates of his two coronary artery stenting procedures and the names and dosages of the numerous medications he was then taking.

Now seventy-three, he is optimistic that our AHA for Life plan will be as effective at keeping him cognitively strong as it has been for reversing his arterial disease. Thanks to the therapies we advised—including changes in his medications, improved dental care, and a diet based on his DNA—he's achieved a remarkable health turnaround. He's overcome his myriad ailments, is taking fewer medications, at lower doses, than he used to, and recently told us that he's feeling better than he has for years. Because his arterial disease has been successfully halted and stabilized, he's avoided any additional trips to the OR for heart procedures. Instead, he and Kellee travel all over the country for fun and pleasure, without fear of heart attacks and strokes.

Robert is back to competing in his favorite cowboy sport: cutting horse shows, in which a horse and rider work together to "cut" at least two cattle from a herd within strict time limits. Along with literally being back in the saddle again, Robert continues to have a laser-sharp memory and remains firmly at the reins of his ranching, cattle, and trucking enterprises. He routinely makes—and recalls with perfect accuracy—complex business deals based solely on a handshake and can recite the entire pedigree of each of the thirty-six quarter horses in his stables. And he's looking forward to a bright future. "I love what I do and never want to retire," he told us recently.

Action Step: Learn Some New Dance Moves — and Teach Them to a Friend

If you love to dance, here's some delightful news from the research front: Moving to the beat boosts brain health and helps keep your memory sharp. One study examined the impact of eleven types of physical activities on older adults—including biking, exercise classes, golf, and swimming—and found that only one of them, dancing, decreased risk for memory loss.[37] Participants were tracked for about five years and those who danced frequently were 76 percent less likely to develop Alzheimer's disease or other forms of dementia, compared to those who danced rarely or never, even when a wide range of risk factors were taken into consideration.

In an intriguing paper published in *Scientific American*, Columbia University neurologist John Krakauer reports that synchronizing music and movement offers "a pleasure double play": Music lights up the brain's reward centers, while dance stimulates its sensory and motor circuitry.[38] Dr. Krakauer also reports that even watching others dance is intellectually stimulating because subconsciously you are choreographing their next moves, and if they execute them with expert skill, your brain's reward centers activate.

Moving to the beat improves mood, reduces stress, and helps the brain form new neural connections in regions involved in long-term memory, planning, and executive function according to a recent report from Harvard Medical School.[39] Busting some moves on the dance floor also provides an excellent cardiovascular workout, helps you maintain a healthy weight, and improves balance and coordination. Dancing also raises levels of the feel-good brain chemical serotonin. Ready to give it a try? Consider taking a Zumba, hip-hop, or jazz class or watching a YouTube video with some rock 'n' roll moves you've always wanted to learn. Then grab a partner and start shimmying. Or invite some friends over, put on your favorite tunes, and show them how to bust some moves!

CHAPTER 13

Lifestyle: the Ultimate Miracle Cure

"The only thing you can change about your life... is the future."

— Ross Dawson, motivational speaker

and futurist

During Jack's first visit to our center twenty years ago, he bantered with our staff and made us laugh when he suggested that we prescribe a tranquilizer—for ourselves. Predicting that we'd be shocked and horrified by his "wicked ways," he launched into a recital of his lifestyle sins. "I used to smoke like I was trying to start a fire—four packs a day—and drank like I was trying to put it out," the then fifty-six-year-old business owner from Post Falls, Idaho, said with a mischievous grin. Quickly adding that he quit both habits when he was in his late twenties, he then patted his ample belly and admitted that he'd spent most of his adult life "riding the double-cheeseburger-with-extra-large-fries-and-a-milkshake train."

Not surprisingly, his cholesterol levels shot up and his weight climbed to 190 on his five-foot-ten-inch frame, putting him in the borderline obese category. Starting when he was in his mid-thirties, he began to have occasional bouts of chest pain, sometimes accompanied by shortness of breath and a heavy feeling in his left arm. Each time, he consulted a doctor, received a tread-mill stress test, and was told that his results were normal or even "superb." With a note of pride, he reported that he'd passed his most recent treadmill test with flying colors and was told that his heart function was "optimal," all of which led him to believe that he'd escaped unscathed from what he acknowledged was a "horrible lifestyle."

Still, he added, a few years earlier, at the repeated urging of his family doctor, he'd attempted to improve his diet. "I started eating so much lettuce that the rabbits were picketing outside my house because there was nothing left for them, but nothing worked," he told us. "My weight stayed the same and my cholesterol actually went up." Then he gave us a sheepish grin, gripped the arms of his chair, and appeared to be bracing himself for a lecture about his lifestyle. We got the impression that he'd been scolded by many doctors, but we don't believe in shaming our patients. Instead, we see ourselves as coaches who help people take the necessary steps toward a healthier future.

We assured Jack that we'd develop a personalized treatment plan, but first we needed to find out if he had arterial plaque. Much to our surprise, Jack immediately perked up when we told him that we wanted to send him to a cardiologist for a then relatively new test: the coronary artery calcium score (CACS) test you read about in chapter seven. He immediately started regaling us with stories about how he'd beaten every heart test he'd ever had. "By the time I'm done running on the treadmill, it will be begging for mercy," he quipped. He looked a little crestfallen when we explained that CACS is an imaging test that doesn't involve any exercise. All he'd have to do was lie on an exam table while X-ray images were taken of his heart and its arteries to check for plaque. Still, he left our center in good spirits, firmly convinced that he'd get reassuring news from the scan.

A week later, the businessman looked pale and shaken when he returned to our center to discuss his CACS results. This time, he didn't stop to joke with our staff. Instead, he hurried into our office, shut the door, and said, "During the heart scan, when the cardiologist showed me on the screen what I looked like on the inside, I was so scared that I almost passed out. My coronary arteries were loaded with plaque and if things get any worse, the next stop will be the funeral home. I told my wife that she'd better start shopping online for a cheap casket." Jack grew even more despondent when he learned his other test results. Not only did he have high levels of small, dense LDL particles (the most dangerous kind), but he also had elevated levels of lipoprotein (a), the inherited cholesterol disorder that we call the mass murderer because it triples risk for heart attacks and strokes. What's more, his blood pressure was in the hypertensive range and he was prediabetic.

Slumping in his chair, he grimly remarked that, "It sounds like a race to see which fatal disease will get me first: a heart attack or stroke triggered by all the cholesterol bullets in my arteries, or diabetes, which killed my father at sixty-three." Then he added bleakly, "At this rate, I probably won't live long enough to worry about dementia, which killed my mom when she was eighty-nine." We quickly explained that Jack's CACS results were not nearly so dire as he thought—and that we've successfully treated patients with coronary artery calcium scores that were far worse than his, using our proven prevention plan, including the eight lifestyle moves we recommend in this chapter, to help them remain heart attack and stroke free.

A Healthier Future Is Just One Smart Decision Away

Looking as if he'd just gotten a reprieve from a death sentence, Jack immediately announced that he was ready—and eager—

to start taking his cardiovascular health seriously. "I'll get religion, I'll follow the straight and narrow, do whatever it takes, starting right now, and stick to the BaleDoneen Method lifestyle plan without any backsliding, but are you sure it's not too late to turn this around?" he asked anxiously. "Or have I screwed up my body beyond repair by doing everything wrong?" We've been asked similar questions many times, by patients with far worse lifestyles than Jack's, including people who weighed as much as four hundred pounds, those who had been smoking heavily for their entire adult lives, and men and women in such poor cardiovascular health that they had already suffered one or more heart attacks or strokes.

Our answer is that it's never too late — or too soon — to start reaping the miraculous benefits of adopting healthier habits. Numerous studies have come to the same conclusion: If optimal lifestyle was a medication, it would far outperform every drug on the market by preventing or treating dozens of dangerous disorders, including cardiovascular disease, diabetes, depression, obesity, high blood pressure, chronic inflammation, arthritis, and cancer.[1] It can also add years to your life and help keep your arteries young and healthy at every age.[2] In addition, two large studies have recently linked an optimal lifestyle to a 92 percent reduction in heart attack risk and a 60 percent drop in risk for Alzheimer's disease.[3] Therefore, Jack had every reason to be optimistic that he could overcome his maladies — and avoid the diseases that had killed his parents.

Even taking small steps toward a healthier future can make a surprisingly big difference. For example, a study of more than three thousand prediabetic patients found that a modest drop in body weight — as little as 3 percent — trimmed the risk of progressing to full-blown diabetes by 38 percent, and a drop of 10 percent slashed it by 85 percent.[4] What's more, the researchers reported that the effects of weight loss, attained through a healthy diet and exercise, were superior to those of medication for the prevention of type 2 diabetes and its many dangerous complications, such as heart attacks, strokes, and dementia.

Another study found that people who ate three hundred fewer calories a day—the equivalent of two chocolate chip cookies or a slice of pizza—not only lost an average of sixteen pounds over a two-year period, but also had significant improvements in their cholesterol, blood pressure, blood sugar, and other markers of cardiovascular and metabolic health.[5] In addition, simply by skipping a snack or two a day, the study participants also reduced their levels of C-reactive protein—an inflammatory marker linked to increased risk for CVD, cognitive decline, and cancer—and improved their mood, sleep, and energy levels. Compared to a control group of people who ate their usual diet, those who practiced calorie restriction also reduced their risk for insulin resistance (the root cause of 70 percent of heart attacks, many strokes, and a major contributor to memory loss).

Intriguingly, the study was both a success and a failure, in that its original goal was to investigate the effects of reducing daily calories by 25 percent—a goal that almost none of the participants were able to achieve. Instead, the calorie-cutting group, on average, only slashed their intake by 11.9 percent, or 297 calories. The study's lead author, Dr. William E. Kraus, a cardiologist and professor at Duke University School of Medicine, told the *New York Times* that the improvements in metabolic and cardiovascular health were much greater than would be expected from weight loss alone. "We weren't surprised that there were changes," he said. "But the magnitude was rather astounding. In a disease population, there aren't five drugs in combination that would cause this aggregate of an improvement."

Two studies have also shown that the simple act of using a pedometer or activity tracker on a watch or smartphone to count the number of steps walked per day leads to significant reductions in participants' weight, body mass index (BMI), blood pressure, and risk for cardiovascular events. In one of these studies, which included more than 2,700 people, tracking their physical activity motivated overweight, previously seden-tary participants to take 2,491 extra steps (a little over a mile) per day.[6] The study's lead author also reported that although the participants' blood pressure only dropped modestly, the improvement was enough to reduce their risk for fatal heart attacks and strokes by 10 percent. The other study, which included 7,454 people, had similar findings, leading the team to conclude that even slight improvements in physical activity can produce large changes in health.[7]

After we told Jack about a few of the thousands of other stud-ies showing that a wide range of easy-to-implement actions—including improving sleep quality, devoting a few minutes a day to mindful meditation, taking relaxation breaks, intermittent fasting, and for many patients, sipping a glass of wine—can powerfully improve cardiovascular wellness, he started to get excited about his prospects for a healthier future. "All I need to do is make one simple decision: to let my mind be the boss of my body, instead of letting my body lie around on the sofa eating ice cream bars," he said. "That's an easy decision since I want to live a long, fruitful life and not spend my final years slumped in a wheelchair, battling dementia, heart failure, or stroke-related disabilities."

We congratulated Jack for having already made a much harder lifestyle change that's been ranked as similar or even superior in power to the best available heart attack and stroke prevention medications: quitting smoking. In a recent study of 18,809 heart attack survivors, almost of all whom were treated with standard medications, those who also kicked the deadly nicotine habit reduced their risk for suffering a repeat heart attack by 43 percent, as compared to persistent smokers. Those who combined smoking cessation with an improved diet and increased physical activity *were nearly four times more likely to be alive six months later* than those who made none of these lifestyle upgrades after their heart attacks.[8]

As this and other recent studies suggest, for people who already have arterial disease, the combination of healthier behaviors and appropriate medications can have a synergistic effect that helps save lives, hearts, and brains. Although medications, which we'll discuss more fully in the next chapter, are also essential for the successful treatment of CVD, very often our patients find that after they lift their lifestyle to the next level, they are able to take fewer medications, at lower doses, and still enjoy excellent protection against cardiovascular events. In most cases, a combination of healthier habits and medication is also necessary to treat high blood pressure, high cholesterol, and diabetes.

Some of our other prescriptions for optimal cardiovascular wellness surprise and even delight our patients. These include laughter, hugs, making love with your significant other, taking frequent vacations, listening to your favorite music, getting a relaxing massage, and taking a daily "dose" of dark chocolate (in moderate amounts). As we like to tell our patients, "Not all heart medicines are hard to take!"

The Amazing Healing Power of an Optimal Lifestyle

What is the optimal lifestyle—and how do you achieve it? Is it about setting goals on your fitness tracker? Filling your fridge with fresh, vibrantly colored fruits and veggies? Trying intermittent fasting to slim down? Although many people assume that the key to arterial wellness is getting in better physical shape, we believe in a more holistic approach to heart-healthy living that goes beyond the numbers on the scale or even freedom from chronic illness. To us, an optimal lifestyle is one that supports and enhances all aspects of your physical, mental, and spiritual well-being, allowing you to flourish during your journey to a healthier and happier future.

All too often, healthcare providers and medical groups make the mistake of only telling patients *what* to do, while failing to adequately explain *how* to achieve an excellent lifestyle and *why* it's so important to attaining optimal heart health. For example, in 2010 the American Heart Association launched a public health campaign called "Life's Simple 7", which offers the following advice, "Stop Smoking. Eat Better. Get Active. Lose Weight. Manage Blood Pressure. Control Cholesterol. Reduce Blood Sugar."[9] The American Heart Association also advised healthcare providers to recommend these evidence-based lifestyle guidelines to their patients. Nearly a decade later, however, a 2019 study of more than thirteen thousand Americans found that fewer than 1 percent of them followed six or seven of these highly publicized directives.[10]

While it's easy for providers to conclude that many patients lack the will to get well, we find that the men and women we treat are excited—and eager—to upgrade their lifestyle after we explain the leading-edge science behind each of our recommendations. Instead of doling out one-size-fits-all advice, such as "eat less and move more," we work in partnership with our patients to develop a personalized lifestyle improvement plan that takes their genetics, medical conditions, and personal preferences into account. As a result, what we advise for one patient may be very different than the lifestyle guidance we give to another.

We also believe that providers and patients need to work in partnership to develop and implement realistic, achievable goals.

At the start of Neal's treatment, when he was in so much pain from his peripheral artery disease that he couldn't walk more than twenty-five steps, we suggested that he start improving his physical fitness by standing up during television commercials. When that became easy for him, we encouraged him to try marching slowly in place. Later, he progressed to short walks and then longer ones.

Jack, on the other hand, had already demonstrated an impressive level of cardiovascular fitness by his ability to "outrun" the treadmill during heart tests, despite rarely going to the gym. We suggested that he harness the competitive drive that motivated him to "beat" these tests by making a treadmill workout or brisk walk a daily habit. He set a goal of walking or jogging ten thousand steps a day. Other patients prefer taking Zumba or Pilates classes, dancing to their favorite music with their significant other, teaming up with an exercise buddy for a morning workout date, using a fitness app to challenge friends to an exercise duel to see who can log the most steps, or going for a nature hike or walking tour to explore new locales.

Along with helping our patients figure out enjoyable, sustainable ways to improve their physical, mental, and spiritual well-being, we also empower them with the knowledge they need to make informed choices and smart decisions that lead to arterial wellness. One of the latest scientific discoveries is that an optimal lifestyle has an effect comparable to hitting a grand slam in baseball because it protects and enhances arterial health on the cellular level in four different ways as follows:

Practicing healthy habits helps your arteries avoid forming cholesterol traps, by preventing the first step of the disease process: the creation of Velcro-like compounds that latch on to cholesterol particles that would otherwise flow harmlessly through the arterial walls. Essentially, safeguarding your cardiovascular wellness is all about avoiding arterial Velcro![11]

An optimal lifestyle helps keep the arterial lining (endothelium) from becoming inflamed. The cooler your arteries are, the lower your risk for a heart attack or stroke, since inflammation is what ignites these events in people who have plaque. Reducing inflammation also helps you avoid developing arterial disease in the first place, and lowers your risk for numerous other chronic diseases.[12]

Upgrading your lifestyle lowers your level of apolipoprotein B-100 (ApoB), the main component of all dangerous forms of cholesterol.[13]

Heart-healthy practices, including regular exercise, also help prevent blood clots that could otherwise block the flow of blood to your heart (causing a heart attack) or to your brain (causing a stroke).[14]

The Eight Best Ways to Boost Your Heart and Brain Health

Here's a look at eight easy actions that do your heart good—and what makes them so amazingly beneficial for all forms of prevention, from helping you avoid getting arterial plaque in the first place (primary prevention) to halting its progression if you already have it (secondary prevention) or heading off a repeat heart attack or stroke if you've already suffered one or more of these events (tertiary prevention). Following these easy and often enjoyable actions, all of which are backed by solid science, will help you score a grand slam in heart health.

Battle belly fat and keep chronic disease at bay with interval training, aerobics, and strength training.

If you saw an ad online for a pill that promised to protect your memory, aid weight loss, improve your sleep, reduce stress, anxiety, and depression, boost your sex drive, and prevent dozens of dangerous diseases, you'd rightfully dismiss it as an internet hoax. However, there is something that has been scientifically proven to do all these things and more: exercising regularly.[15] The benefits of physical activity start immediately and rapidly multiply over time: Even one exercise session improves cardiovascular health for several days.[16] In a twelve-week study, previously sedentary people who walked briskly for thirty minutes a day, five days a week, whittled their waists by about an inch, enjoyed a six-point drop in their systolic blood pressure (the top number), and reduced their hip measurement by an inch.[17]

At every age, keeping fit has numerous health perks. Regular exercise lowers your risk for thirteen types of cancer (including those of the breasts, colon, uterus, lungs, stomach, bladder, and kidneys) by up to 42 percent, halves it for heart attacks, and reduces it for diabetes by 70 percent.[18] A fifteen-year study that included nearly 140,000 older adults found that the more seniors walked, the longer they lived.[19] Another study found that on average, regular exercisers outlive their sedentary counterparts by seven years![20] Daily physical activity also enhances the brain's cognitive reserve and helps keep your memory sharp. In another recent study of seniors, those who kept fit were 31 percent less likely to develop dementia and 55 percent less likely to experience other brain-related disabilities or motor skills impairments.[21]

Along with helping to prevent chronic diseases, physical activity can also help treat these conditions. After a heart attack, physical activity has been shown to increase four-year survival.[22] Tai chi has been found to be a particularly effective option for such patients.[23] If you have insulin resistance (the root cause of type 2 diabetes and 70 percent of heart attacks) or metabolic syndrome (a cluster of heart attack risks that often includes too much belly fat), research shows that the most effective way to combat these problems is interval training, in which you alternate short bursts of more intense aerobic activity with intervals of lighter activity. In a recent study of people with metabolic syndrome, interval training increased insulin sensitivity and levels of heart-protective HDL cholesterol by 25 percent and reduced blood sugar levels and waist circumference. In a study of overweight and obese people, this type of exercise resulted in overall weight loss, a slimmer waist, improved lipid levels, and a 32.5 percent drop in risk for metabolic syndrome.[24]

The best way to keep your heart healthy is to combine aerobic exercise, such as walking, jogging, cycling, or swimming, with muscle strengthening activities, such as lifting weights or resistance training. Including weight lifting in your workout not only tones your muscles, but it can also help prevent age-related gain in waist size, according to a 2015 Harvard study.[25] That's because larger, stronger muscles help rev up metabolism, so you torch more calories even when you're at rest. To avoid injury, start with lighter weights and gradually build up to heavier ones as you gain strength. The American Heart Association and the BaleDoneen Method advise at least thirty minutes of moderate-intensity aerobic activity at least five days a week, plus moderate-to-high-intensity strength training twice a week. Both types of exercise help dieters avoid regaining belly fat after weight loss, suggesting that regular workouts are essential for maintaining a healthy weight and waistline.[26] Before starting a new exercise regimen, always check with your provider to make sure it's appropriate for you.

Intermittent fasting dials down inflammation, helps heal your gut, and burns fat.

Many diets focus on *what* to eat, but intermittent fasting is all about *when* to eat. There are a few variations of this popular eating plan, with the most common being the 16/8 approach, which involves fasting every day for about sixteen hours and limiting your daily eating to a window of eight hours, in which time you'll fit in two meals. Following this plan can be as easy as not eating anything after dinner and skipping breakfast the next morning. However, it's crucial to choose healthy foods, such as those we recommend later in this chapter, in moderate portions since you won't get any health benefits if you load up on high-fat or processed foods, sweet treats, and super-sized portions during the eating window.

Here's how the 16/8 plan works: If you finish your evening meal at eight p.m., you'd wait until noon the next day to eat again, thus completing a sixteen-hour fast. During the fasting window, it's important to stay hydrated by drinking plenty of water, which helps quell hunger pangs. It's also fine to drink coffee or tea during the fasting window as long as these beverages are unsweetened and don't contain anything with calories, such as milk or cream. *Before starting intermittent fasting, always check with your healthcare provider since this eating approach is not appropriate for everyone and may be harmful for people with certain medical conditions.*

Most people think of intermittent fasting (IF) as a weight-loss plan because it helps your body burn fat. That turned out to be the case for Catherine and Elaine, both of whom had tried numerous diets without success before we suggested they try IF. Each of them has lost more than thirty pounds with the 16/8 fasting plan and both report that they're feeling healthier than they have for years. However, intermittent fasting isn't just a way to get the pounds off. Even if you don't lose any weight with this eating plan, studies show that it's still the best anti-inflammatory diet around and can also help reverse insulin resistance, as Catherine, Elaine, and many of our other patients have discovered.

New and recent studies have shown that IF has a wide range of cardiovascular perks, including helping prevent the arterial Velcro that traps cholesterol and leads to plaque formation. People who follow this regimen also have reductions in endothelial inflammation, lower levels of small, dense LDL and ApoB particles, and decreased risk for blood clots, thus scoring a grand slam in protecting their arterial wellness.[27] In a 2021 clinical trial, participants who practiced IF for eight weeks had significant decreases in body fat, oxidative stress, and inflammatory markers, coupled with significant improvements in blood vessel function, food metabolism, and gut health, as compared to a control group who ate their normal diet without any fasting.

IF also helps keep your cells young and healthy by enhancing autophagy, the process cells use to clear out debris (such as broken-down cellular components) and recycle it as fuel.[28] Without this housekeeping process, which literally means "self-eating," cells would become overloaded with trash and die. Reduced autophagy has been linked to a range of diseases and is also thought to play a major role in aging. Exercise also acts as a fountain of youth for cells in another way, by helping to prevent premature senescence, an accelerated form of cellular aging that can be triggered by oxidative stress and chronic inflammation.

Soothe your spirit and defuse stress with mindful meditation or prayer.

Years ago, a large study conducted in fifty-two countries around the world found that psychological factors (including stress) nearly tripled the risk for a heart attack.[29] Until recently, however, scientists weren't sure *why* chronic stress was so toxic: A 2017 study revealed that activity in the amygdala—a brain area involved in stress—independently predicted risk for cardiovascular events, even when a wide range of other factors affecting arterial health were taken into account.[30]

The team also found activation of the amygdala due to fear and stress triggers a cascade of effects, including a rise in arterial inflammation. The research suggests that stress reduction doesn't just make people feel better psychologically—it may also enhance arterial wellness, potentially protecting against heart attacks and strokes. Other recent research offers a simple but remarkably effective way to tame tension: mindful meditation.

Mindfulness involves focusing on the present moment in an open, nonjudgmental way, while letting stressful thoughts about the past or future drift away. Try sitting quietly for ten minutes and paying attention to your breathing or a mantra (focus word) that you repeat silently as you allow distracting thoughts or worries to drift away like wisps of smoke. Some of our patients find that prayer fosters a similar sense of calm and inner peace, as well as fostering a spiritual connection with a higher power. A recent study found that daily prayer is highly effective at reducing stress and anxiety in patients with coronary artery disease—and instilling a sense of hope.[31]

To practice mindfulness, you may find it helpful to gaze at a meditation object, such as a smooth stone, during mindful meditation. There are many apps for meditation and stress reduction, such as Calm, Breethe, and Headspace. Many studies have reported health benefits from this mindful meditation, including:

Keeping your brain sharp throughout your life

In one of the most extensive studies to date, spanning seven years, researchers report that meditation may help prevent age-related mental decline.[32] Other studies suggest that mindfulness may change the brain, by expanding areas involved in focused attention.

Fighting inflammation and stress

In a small study, people who were highly stressed due to unemployment were randomly assigned to learn mindful meditation or a fake technique focused on relaxation.[33] While both groups felt less stressed after three days, follow-up tests found that only those who practiced mindfulness had reductions in inflammation. This group also had more communication in brain areas that process stress-related reactions and those related to focus and calm, suggesting that their brains may have undergone rewiring to manage tension more effectively.

Reducing chest pain and stress in heart patients

Significant decreases in frequency and severity of angina in women with heart disease were reported after eight weeks of mindfulness training in a recent study. Mindfulness also reduced the women's scores on tests measuring depression, anxiety, and perceived stress by 10 to 15 percent. No improvements in symptoms or mood were reported in a control group of patients who didn't get the training.

Lowering your blood pressure

A 2018 eight-week Harvard study found that people who meditated for fifteen minutes a day had striking changes in expression of genes that regulate inflammation, circadian rhythms, and glucose metabolism, leading to significant drops in their blood pressure.[34]

Combating or preventing depression

In an eight-week study published in *Annals of Family Medicine*, adults with mild depression were randomly assigned to either receive standard medical care or mindfulness training.[35] After twelve months, those who practiced mindfulness had a much lower rate of major depression than those who received standard care (10.8 versus 26.8 percent). That is an important CV benefit since major depression escalates the risk for arterial disease.

Weigh the pros and cons of moderate drinking to decide if it's right for you.

Does a drink a day keep the cardiologist away—or is there a cardiovascular downside to moderate drinking? Studies have contradictory findings. For example, a 2017 study of nearly 2 million initially healthy people who were tracked for up to 30 years reported that nondrinking elevated the threat of heart attack by 32 percent, fatal coronary artery disease by 56 percent, heart failure by 24 percent, peripheral artery disease by 22 percent, and stroke by 12 percent, as compared to moderate drinking, while heavy drinking was linked to *higher* risk for numerous blood vessel issues, including strokes, heart failure, and death from coronary artery disease.[36] Heavy alcohol intake also boosts the threat of dementia, according to a study of more than 31 million people.[37]

A 2018 study also found that moderate drinking was linked to longer survival in people with heart failure, as compared to abstinence.[38] The USDA's dietary guidelines for Americans define moderate drinking as a maximum of two alcoholic beverages a day for men and one for women.[39] A drink consists of twelve ounces of beer, five ounces of wine, or 1½ ounces of spirits, such as vodka, whiskey, or gin. According to the CDC, two-thirds of Americans exceed this amount at least once a month.[40] That's dangerous.

Over the years, many prospective studies have reported an association between moderate alcohol intake and a 25–40 percent lower risk for CVD. Some researchers have also reported reduced risk for heart attacks, strokes, type 2 diabetes, and high blood pressure, and improvements in levels of HDL (good) cholesterol and insulin sensitivity.[41] However, prospective studies are not designed to show a cause-and-effect relationship, so do not prove that alcohol is responsible for these effects, which could only be done with a randomized clinical trial.

Recent research suggests other possible explanations for the link between light drinking and reduced cardiovascular risk.[42] For example, the CDC reports that moderate drinkers are more likely to maintain a healthy weight, exercise regularly, and average the seven to eight hours of sleep a night that is optimal for heart health, compared to nondrinkers or heavy drinkers. A 2015 study found that after taking lifestyle and other factors into consideration, moderate alcohol intake provided little or no cardiovascular protection for most people.[43] The researchers analyzed health data from nearly twenty thousand men and women who were followed for about ten years.

It is also important to weigh the potential perils of moderate drinking. For example, in middle-aged women, even one drink a day is linked to increased risk for breast cancer, a factor that women with a family history of this disease should take into consideration.[44,45] Alcohol consumption has a wide range of short- and long-term risks that increase with the amount you drink, including high blood pressure, various cancers, injuries, and car crashes. In a 2017 study, quaffing more than one drink a day significantly increased the risk for atrial fibrillation, a dangerous type of irregular heart rhythm that is a major risk factor for strokes.[46]

What's the key takeaway from current research? If you don't currently drink, the CDC and the BaleDoneen Method recommend against starting. If you imbibe moderately, we advise discussing the risk and benefits with your healthcare provider. It's also important to take your genetics into account. If you are one of the 25 percent of Americans who carry the Apo E 3/4 or Apo E 4/4 genotypes, we strongly advise limiting or avoiding alcohol as part of your heart attack, stroke, dementia, and chronic disease prevention plan.

Eat an optimal diet based on your DNA to live long and well.

"Let food be thy medicine," wrote Hippocrates centuries ago. But which foods should you choose to protect the health of your heart, brain, and arteries—and which ones should you avoid? In chapter eleven, we discussed the cardiovascular benefits of an eating plan guided by your Apo E genotype—which provides insight into whether to follow a very low-fat diet, the conventional Mediterranean-style diet that is widely recommended to protect heart health, or a moderate-fat diet that includes heart-healthy oils—and your haptoglobin genotype, which helps you tell if you'd benefit from going gluten-free.

A 2017 analysis of American dietary patterns linked eating suboptimal amounts of ten specific foods and nutrients—too much of some and not enough of others—to nearly half of all deaths from cardiometabolic disease (CMD), such as heart disease, stroke, or type 2 diabetes.[47] Conversely, people who ate the recommended amounts of the ten foods had the lowest risk for CMD, according to the study, which was published in *Journal of the American Medical Association*.

Since then, however, new studies have yielded sometimes contradictory findings about these foods, leaving Americans confused about the best and worst dietary choices. Here's a look at the latest nutritional wisdom about these foods and how to optimize your diet for cardiometabolic wellness.

Eat More of These Foods

Nuts

People who eat nuts regularly have a lower risk for developing heart disease or experiencing cardiovascular events, such as heart attacks and strokes, compared to those who rarely or never eat nuts, according to a study of more than 210,000 men and women.[48] Although the tasty treats are high in calories, they can also help people avoid long-term weight gain or obesity, other research shows.[49] Moreover, eating almonds or hazelnuts may raise HDL (good) cholesterol, while pistachios help lower triglycerides. The BaleDoneen Method recommends eating a palmful of nuts daily, preferably tree nuts with skins, such as almonds, walnuts, hazelnuts, and pistachios.

Fish

The omega-3 fatty acids in seafood have a wide range of cardiovascular benefits, including helping prevent heart disease, strokes, heart failure, and sudden cardiac death; reducing triglycerides, blood pressure, and chronic inflammation; and improving insulin sensitivity.[50] The best sources of omega-3s are oily fish, such as salmon, herring, sardines, tuna, and lake trout. The American Heart Association recommends eating at least two 3½-ounce servings of non-fried fish per week.

Fresh vegetables

A diet high in these nutritional powerhouses could add years to your life. A study presented at Nutrition 2019, the annual meeting of the American Society for Nutrition, suggests that globally, low intake of vegetables is the culprit in more than 800,000 deaths from heart disease—and about 200,000 deaths from strokes—per year.[51] The USDA advises eating two to three cups of veggies daily. Yet only one in ten adults consumes the recommended amount. An easy way to meet your goal is to fill half of your plate with vegetables and fruit.

Fresh fruit

Do people who eat a lot of veggies get any extra cardiometabolic benefits from eating fresh fruit? A study of more than 510,000 adults in China, where fresh fruit intake is very low, found that those who ate it daily had 36 percent lower risk for heart attack and stroke than those who ate no fresh fruit.[52] Another recent study found that people who ate higher amounts of fresh fruit had a lower risk for diabetes.[53] Among those who were already diabetic, the study also reported reduced rates of diabetes-related deaths and complications in those who ate more fruit.

High-fiber foods

People who eat a diet high in fiber (found in most fruits and vegetables) were 56 to 59 percent less likely to die from CVD, infectious disease, or respiratory disorders, according to a study of nearly 400,000 older adults.[54] Another large study found that people who ate 25 to 29 grams of fiber daily received the greatest cardiovascular benefit.[55]

Dark chocolate

In a study of nearly twenty thousand people, those who ate an average of 7.5 grams of chocolate (about one small square) daily had a 27 percent lower risk for heart attack and 48 percent drop in stroke danger.[56] Ten grams of dark chocolate contains about fifty calories. The darker the chocolate, the lower the calories. Eating moderate amounts of the sweet treat also reduced participants' blood pressure.

Eat Less of These Foods

Salt

The American Heart Association recommends a limit of no more than 2,300 mg per day of sodium and an ideal limit of no more than 1,500 mg for most adults. Cut back on the "Salty Six": bread and rolls, pizza, sandwiches, cold cuts and cured meats, soup, and burritos and tacos, all of which typically contain high levels of sodium. Limiting or avoiding packaged, processed foods, which are typically high in salt, may lower your blood pressure or help you avoid hypertension in the first place, the American Heart Association reports.

Processed meats

People who eat the most processed meat—such as bacon, beef jerky, salami, and other deli meats—have a higher risk for CVD.[57] What's more, eating as little as one hot dog or a few strips of bacon daily raises colon cancer risk by 20 percent, according to a 2020 study published in *International Journal of Epidemiology*.[58] Processed meat has also been tied to increased risk for cancers of the breast, pancreas, and prostate.

Sugar-sweetened beverages

Consuming just one or two sugar-sweetened beverages daily— such as energy drinks, fruit drinks, soda, or coffee drinks— raises the risk for a heart attack or dying from CVD by 35 percent, diabetes risk by 26 percent, and stroke risk by 16 percent, according to a recent Harvard study.[59] Sweet drinks have been called liquid candy and rank as the top source of added sugar in the U.S. diet. Quench your thirst with plain or sparkling water flavored with a spritz of lemon or lime.

Red meat and plant meats

In the *IJE* study discussed above, eating 2½ ounces or more of red meat per day raised colon cancer risk by 20 percent. While plant-based veggie burgers and other "meatless meats" might sound like a healthier alternative, in reality these foods are ultra-processed and relatively high in saturated fat and sodium, delivering no cardiovascular benefits over animal-based meat, a 2020 study found.[60]

Saturated fat

For fifty years, saturated fats were demonized as the number one dietary culprit for arterial disease. However, the effect of cutting down on saturated fats depends on how you replace them. Swapping them with healthy fats (such as those found in oily fish, olive oil, most nuts, and avocados) or high-fiber carbs (such as whole grains) may benefit heart health, while replacing saturated fat with refined carbs (such as baked goods or sweets) is likely to do the opposite. In fact, sugar is worse for heart health than saturated fats.

If you smoke, keep trying to quit until you succeed!

A 2015 survey found that about 70 percent of current smokers want to quit, and 55 percent had attempted to kick the habit in the previous year. However, only 7 percent of them succeeded in remaining tobacco free for six to twelve months.[61] If you've made one or more unsuccessful quit attempts, don't get discouraged. We tell our patients that it can sometimes take ten or more attempts to break this deadly addiction that leads to 480,000 premature, preventable deaths each year.[62] The important thing is to look upon each of these efforts as a step forward—and learn from them.

"We know more about the science of quitting than ever before," U.S. Surgeon General Vice Admiral Jerome M. Adams reported in 2020.[63] Every year, nearly 3 million Americans succeed at kicking the nicotine habit—and with the right support and tactics, you can too! Here are some helpful insights from the research front.

Just quit.

You are much more likely to succeed if you quit cold turkey, instead of trying to gradually wean yourself off cigarettes, according to a 2016 randomized study of nearly 700 smokers.[64]

All the participants received nicotine patches and those who were trying to taper off cigarettes also received nicotine gums, lozenges or under-the-tongue tablets to help manage withdrawal symptoms. The study found that 22 percent of those who quit cold turkey were still smoke free six months after their quit date, versus only 15 percent of those who tried to taper off.

Replace a bad habit with a good one.

Researchers report smokers who try to stop thinking about cigarettes when they're trying to quit have a harder time doing so, and are more likely to backslide, even if the thoughts are about the negative consequences of their habit.[65] The key takeaway is that instead of just focusing on telling yourself not to smoke, it's much more effective to form healthy new habits to replace smoking. For example, when you get the urge to take a cigarette break, try replacing it with an exercise break (such as a short, brisk walk). Also try munching on healthy, crunchy foods, such as carrot or celery sticks and replacing the oral gratification of smoking with taking excellent care of your teeth (using the dental tips in chapter ten).

Get smoking cessation counseling and talk to your healthcare provider about nicotine replacement therapy.

A 2021 analysis of high-quality evidence from more than three hundred studies that included more than 250,000 people found that people who join stop-smoking support programs have a very high success rate, with up to 56 percent of them being smoke free six months later.[66] The surgeon general's 2020 report also endorses smoking cessation programs as being one of the most effective strategies to free yourself of the deadly nicotine addiction—and adds that using nicotine replacement therapy (such as patches, sprays, or gum) under medical supervision further enhances success rates.

Sexual activity is safe — and healthy — for most heart patients and an optimal lifestyle can heighten its pleasure.

It's very common for people with arterial disease, particularly those who have already suffered a heart attack or have undergone heart procedures, such as bypass surgery, to worry that engaging in sex might be dangerous. Because of such fears, many heart patients assume, mistakenly, that they must resign themselves to a celibate life. One reason why this misconception is so prevalent is that healthcare providers rarely discuss sexual matters with their patients, the American Heart Association reported in a 2012 scientific statement.[67]

In the statement, they reported that it's usually safe for patients with stable cardiovascular disease to have sex. However, people with severe heart disease that sparks symptoms, such as chest pain during light physical activity like walking short distances, or when they are at rest, should refrain from sexual activity until their symptoms have been successfully treated and stabilized. In the next chapter, you'll find a guide to commonly prescribed medications and supplements for heart disease and its major risk factors.

Contrary to urban legends, the risk of having a heart attack or going into cardiac arrest during sex is minuscule, even among people with known coronary artery disease (CAD), the American Heart Association emphasized in its statement. It also reported that drugs to treat erectile dysfunction (ED), such as Viagra, Levitra, and Cialis, are usually safe for men with CAD. However, men who take nitroglycerin for heart-related chest pain should not use these ED drugs due to the risk of harmful drug interactions.

Since the publication of the American Heart Association's scientific statement, new studies have shown that sex isn't just safe for people with heart disease — it can actually *enhance* their long-term survival, as well as their quality of life![68] A large study of older adults, sixty-five and older, who were tracked for fourteen years also found that seniors who remain sexually active had a 28 percent lower risk for death from any cause during the study period, compared to seniors who were celibate.[69]

A 2020 study identified some of the reasons why staying sexually active helped heart attack survivors live longer, including improved physical fitness, lower stress levels, reduced inflammation, and a stronger partner relationship that may enhance quality of life.[70] The study also found that resuming lovemaking after a heart attack may be an important indicator of recovery and thus reflect a mental ability to bounce back quickly from the shock of the event. Adding to the benefits of getting busy between the sheets, the researchers also reported that the more often people had sex after a heart attack, the lower their risk of dying in the next fourteen years was!

That's right — making love with your significant other can save your life! Other research has shown that men who have more than twenty-one orgasms a month have a 50 percent lower risk of prostate cancer, as compared to men who climax four to seven times a month.[71] Here's some extra motivation to follow the optimal lifestyle recommendations in this chapter: Staying physically fit has been shown to improve sexual performance, increase libido, and heighten sexual pleasure in both men and women.[72] Researchers have also linked a heart-healthy lifestyle to improved sexual function, increased sexual frequency, and having more fun in bed.

Laughter and a spirit of optimism do your heart good.

One of our favorite Bible verses starts, "A merry heart doeth good like medicine" (Proverbs 17:22). Numerous studies bear this out. For example, a 2020 study found that the more you laugh, the less likely you are to have a heart attack, stroke, or die from cardiovascular causes. The researchers tracked 17,152 patients for an average of 5.5 years and reported that laughing once or more a week slashed the risk for suffering a cardiovascular event by 40 percent and risk for death from heart-related causes by 50 percent, as compared to laughing less than once a month.[73]

We find this and other studies with similar findings so persuasive that we actually prescribe laughter to our patients. One wonderful way to include more humor in your life is laughter yoga, which combines self-triggered mirth with yogic breathing to draw oxygen deep into the body. Also try watching sitcoms on TV, taking your significant other to a comedy club on date night, reading funny books, or checking out hilarious internet videos of pets and children doing silly things. Ask your friends to tell their favorite jokes or get a joke-a-day calendar to help you start each day with a chuckle. All these actions contribute to better blood vessel function, reduce stress, and make life more fun.

We always enjoy a good laugh when Jack comes to our center for his quarterly checkups. Now seventy-five, he has a lot of reasons to rejoice: After following our AHA for Life plan for twenty years, his weight and cholesterol are in the ideal range. He's stopped cracking bleak jokes about shopping for a cheap casket because his plaque is completely stabilized and his arteries are no longer on fire. During a recent visit, he told us that he considers the improvement in all aspects of his health "miraculous," then added, "My wife smiles at how frisky her seventy-five-year-old husband is in the bedroom."

Jack also said, "Instead of worrying about cholesterol 'bullets' in my arteries, I'm completely bulletproof. I've stopped looking over my shoulder for the bogeyman and worrying about my health. I tell everyone that it's impossible for me to have a heart attack or stroke." Determined to get the most fun and joy out of each day, he recently went on a 1,500-mile motorcycle trip across the country with his twenty-six-year-old grandson. "We had a fantastic time, and if I felt any younger, I'd break out in pimples."

Action Step: Eat the Rainbow

Did you know that eating a variety of colorful fruits and vegetables can have amazing benefits, including lowering your risk for heart attacks, strokes, high blood pressure, diabetes, and several forms of cancer? What's more, eating certain vegetables may be linked to better memory and longer life, recent studies suggest. Yet fewer than one in ten adults eat the recommended amount of these nutritional powerhouses, according to the CDC.[74] One easy way to reach your goal: fill half your plate with fruits and vegetables at each meal. For a full spectrum of health benefits, include these colors in your daily diet:

Red

Lycopene is the pigment that gives some fruits, such as tomatoes, their ruby hue. Studies suggest that tomatoes, which are also high in disease-fighting antioxidants, vitamins A and C, folic acid, and beta carotene, have surprisingly powerful benefits for vascular health, including reducing levels of oxidized LDL cholesterol (the kind that can form plaque in the coronary arteries) and reducing blood sugar.[75] Eating tomatoes or tomato products is also linked to reductions in blood pressure and inflammation. A large study also found that high consumption of lycopene from tomatoes reduced stroke risk by 55 percent.[76]

Purple and blue

These colors result from pigments called anthocyanins that may enhance brain health. Indeed, blueberries are often called brain berries because studies link them to reduced risk for age-related memory loss. For example, the Nurses' Health Study reported that women who ate the most blueberries and strawberries had slower rates of cognitive decline and lower heart attack risk than those who ate the least.[77] A study of more than 500,000 people, published in The *New England Journal of Medicine*, found that people who ate fresh fruit daily had a 34 percent lower rate of coronary artery disease and were 25 percent less likely to suffer a stroke, compared to people who rarely or never ate fresh fruit.[78]

Green

A 2021 study that pooled data from more than 2 million people, who were tracked for up to thirty years, offered a delicious recipe for longevity: Those who ate five servings of produce daily (three of vegetables and two of fruit) had a 12 percent lower risk for dying from CVD and a 10 percent lower risk for cancer death than those who only ate two servings.[79] While all fresh produce boosts heart health, leafy green vegetables (such as spinach, Swiss chard, lettuce, and mustard greens) and cruciferous vegetables (such as broccoli, cabbage, and Brussels sprouts) are particularly beneficial.[80]

Yellow and orange

Citrus fruits, such as oranges, lemons, and grapefruit, also make important contributions to protecting against heart attacks and strokes.[81] These fruits contain citrus limonoids that have been shown to help fight cancers of the mouth, skin, lungs, stomach, and colon in lab tests and may help lower cholesterol.[82] A yellow fruit, the pineapple, contains bromelain, a mixture of enzymes that have been used for centuries to treat indigestion and fight inflammation. Although patients often worry that the natural sugar in fruit is fattening, the sweet truth is that most types of fruit have anti-obesity effects—and many health organizations recommend that dieters eat fresh fruit.[83]

CHAPTER 14

Are You Getting the Right Medications and Supplements, at the Right Dose?

"Medicine is anything which, in proper measure, moves us toward wholeness."

— MICHELE JENNAE, WRITER, ARTIST, AND HEALER

Like Diane H., whom you met earlier, Diane G. has a tragic family history. Her father had a fatal heart attack at forty-six — and three of her uncles suffered the same fate at relatively young ages. One of her brothers survived a heart attack at a relatively young age and her sister has suffered (and survived) two heart attacks. "It was a horrible thing, because during the first heart attack, she went to the hospital and was told nothing was wrong," says the retired teacher and hotel owner from Spokane, Washington. "They sent her home without any treatment and a few weeks later, during a diagnostic test, she had a second heart attack."

At fifty-five, Diane G. experienced similar medical neglect when she developed chest pain and shortness of breath. "I called my doctor and was told to take two aspirin," she recalls. That didn't help. Two days later, she says, "I had pain down my left arm like a piercing sword and demanded that my doctor order a coronary angiogram. It took five days before I was admitted to the hospital for the test and, even then, the doctor said, 'I'm doing this against my will because you are so healthy that you shouldn't have any heart problems.'"

During the imaging test, doctors inserted a thin tube into an artery in Diane G.'s leg and snaked it through her blood vessels up to her heart. Then a special dye was injected through the tube to map blood flow through her coronary arteries. "Almost immediately, I realized that something was terribly wrong, because on the computer screen, I saw that the dye had stopped in one area of my heart, like water pooling in a dam," she recalls. "Looking like a dog with his tail between his legs, my doctor said, 'You have a serious heart problem.' One of my coronary arteries was one hundred percent blocked and I was having a heart attack."

After treatment with balloon angioplasty to reopen the obstructed vessel, Diane G. was sent home a few days later with a couple of prescriptions. "Nobody explained what these medications were or why they'd help me," she says. Nor did the doctors recommend any lifestyle changes for Diane G., who was then about twenty-five pounds overweight. Fortunately, despite the long delay in diagnosing and treating her heart attack, she didn't suffer any permanent heart damage. Determined to avoid another event, she adds, "I took the pills as prescribed and tried to lead the right lifestyle, but it didn't work. Nine months later, my arteries got clogged again." This time, the obstructions were so severe that she needed emergency triple bypass surgery to avoid a second heart attack.

"After my open-heart surgery I wasn't given any new medications or lifestyle recommendations, so I started looking for a better doctor who could tell me what I needed to do."

"First, I went to a heart convention where several famous male cardiologists were speaking. All of them had totally different advice. One of them said I should eat bacon and red meat. That didn't sound right to me, but these doctors acted like they were gods—you weren't allowed to ask any questions. Their attitude was, 'Just follow my program, little lady, and you'll be fine.' I investigated further and found a specialist in women's heart health—Dr. Amy Doneen—who has a track record of success with heart attack prevention and was willing to explain *why* her method would help me."

Prescriptions for Better Heart Health

When we met Diane G. twenty-four years ago, she was terrified that she'd have a fatal heart attack, like the ones that had already killed her father and his three brothers. Then fifty-six, she was also understandably angry about the ineffective treatment she'd received after her heart attack—and was still in pain after having her chest split open less than a year later for emergency triple bypass surgery. During her initial evaluation, she posed a question that we've been asked many times by patients who have undergone multiple heart procedures that have failed to halt the seemingly relentless progression of their coronary artery disease (CAD): "How do I get off the express train to the OR?"

At the time, we'd just started using a new evidence-based treatment approach that has been shown in many excellent studies—including large, randomized clinical trials (the gold standard of scientific research)—to save lives by preventing heart attacks, strokes, and other devastating complications of CAD.[1] Called optimal medical therapy (OMT), it combines an optimal lifestyle with drug therapy to treat arterial disease *and* conditions that spark it, such as chronic inflammation, high cholesterol, and high blood pressure. OMT is sometimes confused with "aggressive treatment," which typically involves taking high doses of medication or several powerful drugs at once—an approach that's been shown in large studies to be ineffective, dangerous, or even fatal in some cases.

We define OMT as "individualized medical therapy," in which medications and, in some cases, supplements, are prescribed cautiously in situations when the benefits clearly outweigh the risks. It's also essential to identify and treat the root causes of the patient's disease. For example, along with genetic risk, Diane G. had two previously undiagnosed conditions. Similar to about one in three Americans—88 million adults—she had prediabetes.[2] It should have been obvious long before her heart attack that she needed to have her blood sugar checked, given that being overweight is the leading risk factor for prediabetes.

Yet prediabetes is so frequently missed by medical providers that 84 percent of people who have this highly treatable—and usually reversible—condition are unaware they have it, the CDC recently reported.[3] That's frightening, since prediabetes (which is also known as insulin resistance) is the root cause of about 70 percent of heart attacks, many strokes, and almost all cases of type 2 diabetes. It's also a major contributor to the arterial inflammation that causes plaque and can spark heart attacks and strokes in those who already have it.

In addition, we identified another culprit in Diane's arterial disease that had previously been overlooked by her medical providers: her long history of dental issues. "I've always had lots of cavities and other problems with my teeth," she told us. "When I was fourteen, my dentist said I'd need false teeth by twenty-one. Although that didn't happen, I have lots of crowns, bridges, and two implants." When we referred her to an excellent dental provider who is trained in our method, she turned out to have both gum disease and endodontic disease (tooth decay). Therefore, the treatment plan we recommended included optimal dental care, using the therapies discussed in chapter ten.

Diane G. was surprised—and excited—to hear that OMT is

just as effective at preventing cardiovascular events and early death from heart-related causes as the invasive, painful—and very expensive—procedures she'd already undergone to restore blood flow to clogged vessels, a type of treatment that is medically known as revascularization. She also wondered why none of the cardiologists she'd met at the heart conference had even mentioned that OMT was an option. Because we rapidly adapt the latest scientific findings into clinical practice, it's possible that these specialists were not yet aware of the value of this then novel approach to prevention.

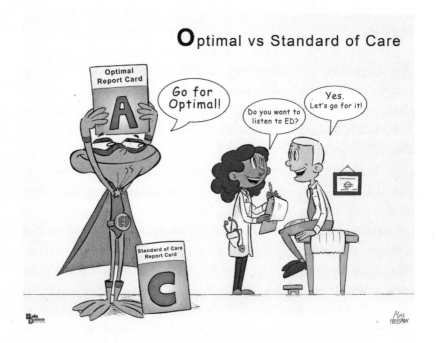

However, since then, numerous landmark studies have confirmed the lifesaving benefits of this inexpensive and extremely safe alternative to surgical interventions. Indeed, the scientific evidence supporting OMT is so overwhelming that in 2012, the four optimal medical therapies described later in this chapter, which we call the cornerstones of treating arterial disease, were formally endorsed clinical practice guidelines jointly issued by the American College of Physicians, the American Heart Association, the American College of Cardiology Foundation, the Preventive Cardiovascular Nurses Association, and other leading medical societies, based on a "scientifically valid, high-quality review of the evidence."[4]

Together, these cornerstones serve as the foundation of our AHA for Life plan for the prevention of heart attacks, strokes, and dementia in people with diseased arteries. In some cases, as we will explain in depth later in this chapter, these therapies can also be beneficial for people who *don't* have arterial disease but are at high risk for developing it due to such conditions as chronic inflammation, high blood pressure, high cholesterol, high blood sugar, or insulin resistance.

The Lifesaving Treatment Many Cardiologists Don't Prescribe

Even though OMT was endorsed in medical guidelines a decade ago, this excellent and easy-to-implement treatment remains underused, even as new studies continue to add to the mountain of proof supporting its powerful role in helping patients with arterial disease and major cardiovascular risk factors live long and well. In breaking news as we were writing this chapter, a major clinical trial called SYNTAX reported that OMT dramatically improved long-term survival in patients like Diane G.: those who have undergone revascularization procedures for severe CAD, such as triple bypass surgery.

In fact, the study found that those who received this guideline-recommended therapy, starting soon after their surgery, were 53 percent more likely to be alive ten years later than those who didn't get OMT![5] Conducted by an international team of cardiovascular specialists, the study included 1,472 patients who were tracked for up to ten years. In an interview with the medical press, one of the study's authors, Dr. Patrick Serruys, stated that the findings offered compelling data for providers to tell patients with CAD that OMT "is the best insurance for extended survival."

The study also found that people treated with this approach for five or more years significantly outlived those who were treated for shorter periods or didn't get this type of treatment at all. "The longer, the better," added Dr. Serruys. "OMT even outweighs the survival benefit from revascularization alone, so our patients should convince themselves of the value of rigorous adherence and compliance" to this type of treatment. Dr. Serruys and his team define OMT as receiving four types of heart medications: an antiplatelet drug, a statin, a renin-angiotensin system inhibitor, and a beta-blocker, all of which will be discussed in depth later in this chapter. People who received at least three OMT medications had a more than 50 percent drop in mortality risk, as compared to those who received two or fewer. That's an impressive improvement in survival from taking one additional medication!

So exciting and important did *The New England Journal of Medicine*, which published the SYNTAX findings, deem these results that it ran an accompanying editorial in which two leading experts made an impassioned plea for the widespread adoption of OMT in medical practice.[6] Calling the current rate of prescribing these treatments to high-risk patients—including those who have undergone heart procedures—"unacceptably low," the editorial's authors called upon providers to put patients with diseased arteries on OMT, calling it "the best warranty to blunt the progression of atherosclerosis and to reduce subsequent cardiac events." On the cellular level, OMT promotes biochemical changes that convert lipid-rich plaque (the most dangerous kind) into calcified plaque (the stable kind that does not cause heart attacks and strokes).

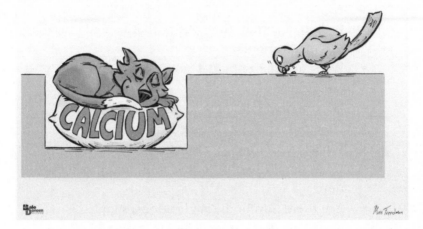

Questions to Ask Before You Take a Pill

If your healthcare provider advises you to take medication, ask the following questions to make sure you understand why the therapy is being prescribed and how it will help manage your coronary artery disease, treat coexisting conditions, or reduce your risk for a heart attack or stroke. Don't be shy about asking the provider to explain anything that is not clear. It's helpful to take notes to help you remember any important information about your treatment.

- Why do you recommend this medication and what does it treat?
- Could this medication interact with any of my other medications or supplements?
- How likely is this treatment to help me and how will I know if it's working?
- Should this medication be taken with food or on an empty stomach?

- Is there a certain time of day that I should take this medication?
- What are the potential side effects, and which are serious?
- What should I do if I have a side effect?
- How do I reach you in an emergency?
- What are my other treatment options?
- What should I do if I miss a dose of my medication?
- Are there any foods, medications, supplements, herbal products, or activities to avoid while I am taking this medication?
- When should I return for a follow-up appointment?
- Which tests will you do to see if this medication is helping or harming me?
- If this medication doesn't help me, what are the next steps?

The Four Cornerstones of Treating Arterial Disease

Discuss the risks and benefits of the treatments below with your healthcare provider and alert them if you are pregnant, breastfeeding or planning to conceive, or have any medication allergies or intolerances. Bring a complete list of all medications and supplements you are currently taking and ask your provider to review it before prescribing any new medications. Not only will that help you avoid dangerous drug interactions, but it's possible that your older prescriptions are no longer appropriate or the dosages need to be adjusted. Later in this chapter, we'll tell you about a new pharmacogenetic test that checks for genetic variants that affect your response to hundreds of commonly prescribed medications and supplements, helping you avoid treatments that don't work or are likely to cause harmful side effects.

Depending on which coexisting medical conditions you have, it may be necessary to layer additional medications on top of the four cornerstones of treatment for arterial disease discussed below. We suggest using the information in this chapter as a springboard to an informed discussion with your provider about the optimal medical therapy to help you avoid heart attacks, strokes, dementia, and other dangerous threats to your heart and brain health.

Cornerstone #1: Optimal Lifestyle

Whether your goal is to avoid getting arterial disease, to halt its progression and avoid devastating complications if you already have it, or to protect yourself from repeat events if you've suffered one or more heart attacks or strokes, an optimal lifestyle is the strongest cornerstone of your prevention plan. As discussed in chapter thirteen, an excellent lifestyle is the cardiovascular equivalent of hitting a grand slam in baseball, because it protects and enhances arterial health in four different ways. Studies have shown that taking optimal care of your heart through such simple steps as avoiding smoking, daily physical activity, getting adequate sleep, maintaining a healthy weight, and managing stress can reduce your risk for cardiovascular events by at least 80 percent.[7]

Diane G. has never smoked, but she needed help with other lifestyle factors. For example, she used to struggle with daytime drowsiness, despite averaging seven to eight hours of sleep a night. We ordered a sleep study, which revealed that she had obstructive sleep apnea, a disorder that's been found in several studies to double or even triple the risk for heart attacks and strokes.[8] The good news is that if it's treated, this excess risk can be eliminated, a recent study found. In Diane G.'s case, weight loss—achieved through increased exercise and following a heart-healthy diet based on her DNA—and the use of a CPAP machine successfully treated this disorder. She turned out to have a genotype that benefits from a Mediterranean diet and going gluten-free.

Along with helping Diane G. slim down, daily workouts that included a combination of cardio, strength training, and yoga had other important benefits for her. Like about 50 percent of Americans, she carries the 9P21 heart attack gene. Recent research suggests that keeping fit is particularly important for people who carry this or other high-risk genes—and can halve their risk for heart attacks, strokes, and other cardiovascular events.[9] In addition, increased physical activity dialed down Diane G.'s stress level, and when combined with a diet that was rich in anti-inflammatory foods and improved dental care, helped put out the fire in her arteries. She's also a firm believer in the healing power of prayer and a positive outlook on life.

Our optimal lifestyle plan for Diane G.—and for many of our other patients—also included taking certain supplements that have proven cardiovascular benefits. Here are a few of our favorites, all of which should be discussed with your provider before taking them to make sure they are appropriate for you:

Vitamin D

About 40 percent of the U.S. population is vitamin D deficient, raising their risk for many medical issues, including CVD, diabetes, Alzheimer's disease and other forms of dementia, autoimmune diseases, cancer, infections, and even severe complications of COVID-19 if they become infected with the virus that causes it.[10] A simple blood test can reveal if you are deficient in vitamin D (a level below 30 ng/dL).[11] If so, your provider will advise taking a daily vitamin D3 supplement so you reach a healthy level. Recent studies suggest that a level of 40–50 ng/dL may be optimal for heart health and chronic disease prevention.[12] Benefits of getting enough vitamin D are reduced inflammation, decreased risk for side effects in statin users, improved insulin sensitivity, and protection against developing type 2 diabetes—even if you are prediabetic. For example, a six-month study found that only 3 percent of prediabetic patients treated with vitamin D supplements progressed to full-blown diabetes, as compared to 28 percent of those who received a placebo.[13] However, it's possible to get too much of a good thing: Taking ultra-high doses of vitamin D can be toxic, so if you need a supplement, stick to the dosage advised by your healthcare provider.

Vitamin C

An extensive 2018 analysis of earlier publications linked higher intake of vitamin C (a powerful antioxidant found in many foods, particularly fresh fruit and vegetables) to many cardiovascular health perks, including improvements in blood pressure, blood sugar, lipids, arterial stiffness, and endothelial function.[14] The analysis also found that vitamin C supplements were particularly beneficial to older adults, obese people, people with low levels of vitamin C, and those with cardiovascular risk factors. Another important finding: Unlike other antioxidants, vitamin C showed *no* adverse effects in any of the subgroups the researchers looked at.

Omega-3 fatty acids

Found in foods—including oily fish (such as rainbow trout, salmon, mackerel, tuna, sardines, and herring), caviar, oysters, and nuts—as well as supplements, omega-3 fatty acids offer a delicious recipe for better heart health and longer life. In a 2020 study of 427,678 initially healthy men and women forty to sixty-nine, those who took fish oil supplements were 20 percent less likely to suffer fatal heart attacks and also reduced the threat of other fatal and nonfatal CV events.[15] An even newer analysis of 40 studies that included 135,267 people linked taking omega-3 supplements to a 41 percent drop in rates of CV events, leading the researchers to conclude, "Supplementation with [omega-3] is an effective lifestyle strategy for CVD prevention, and the protection likely increases with dosage."[16] We use the patient's Apo E genotype to guide the dosing. For example, we prescribe a lower dose for people with the Apo E 3-4 or 4-4 genotypes, who benefit from a very low-fat diet, than the dose we recommend for people with other genotypes.

Coenzyme Q10 (CoQ10)

If you take statin medication, this supplement can improve muscle-related side effects, according to 2018 analysis of twelve clinical trials in which participants were randomly assigned to take CoQ10 or a placebo.[17] Compared to the placebo group, the CoQ10 group had reductions of 60 percent or more in muscle pain, weakness, cramps, and fatigue. There are two forms of CoQ10: ubiquinol and ubiquinone. We recommend the use of ubiquinol, the active form of CoQ10.

Berberine

Berberine is a natural compound found in several plants, including goldenseal, tree turmeric, Oregon grape, and barberry. Used in traditional Chinese and Ayurvedic medicine for centuries, this botanical supplement has anti-inflammatory effects. It can also improve gut health, lower cholesterol, reduce fat in the liver, and aid weight loss.[18] It is also helpful for people with diabetes and prediabetes because it reduces glucose production in the liver and lowers blood sugar.

Cinnamon

This tasty spice helps reduce blood sugar and lipid levels in people with type 2 diabetes, according to an extensive literature review and pooled analysis of studies.[19] In a 2020 randomized clinical trial, cinnamon was also shown to improve glucose tolerance significantly in prediabetic patients, as compared to a placebo.[20]

Cornerstone #2: Low-Dose Aspirin

Aspirin is the world's most widely used drug—and one of the most controversial. Its medicinal use dates to circa 1500 BCE, when extracts of willow bark (which contain salicylate, the active ingredient in aspirin) were described in an ancient Egyptian papyrus as a remedy for pain and fever.[21] Also known as acetylsalicylic acid (ASA), aspirin has proven anti-clotting effects, thus helping to prevent heart attacks and strokes, which occur when a clot blocks flow of blood to the heart or brain. However, ASA can also be dangerous due to a significant risk for internal bleeding.[22]

In 2018, findings from three large randomized clinical trial (RCT) studies were published that highlighted the challenges of deciding if the benefits of low-dose aspirin therapy (taking one 81 mg tablet daily) outweigh the potential harms. You may have seen media headlines like these: "Daily Aspirin Could Be Harmful for Older Adults," "Daily Aspirin: Risks Outweigh Benefits, According to New Research," and "Does Daily Aspirin Therapy Work?" Here is a look at some of the latest scientific findings, including those from these three trials, with key takeaways about how to decide, in consultation with your healthcare provider, if daily low-dose ASA is right for you.

The effectiveness of low-dose ASA for people who have already suffered one or more heart attacks or strokes remains undisputed. The standard of care calls this use of daily aspirin secondary prevention, while primary prevention is defined as aspirin therapy to prevent cardiovascular disease (CVD) in people who have not yet had a heart attack or stroke. For secondary prevention, more than two hundred studies have shown that ASA significantly reduces rates of repeat heart attacks and strokes, with this potentially lifesaving benefit clearly outweighing the low, but serious risk for bleeding associated with this drug.[23]

As an added benefit, taking daily low-dose aspirin has been shown to reduce risk for colon cancer, and there is some evidence that it may also help protect against prostate, gastroesophageal, and breast cancer.[24] In addition, a 2021 pooled analysis of studies that included more than 100,000 people linked the use of low-dose aspirin to a 25 percent reduction in risk for developing dementia or major cognitive impairment, compared to nonusers of ASA. The researchers also reported that ASA users had a 46 percent lower risk for Alzheimer's disease.[25] Several RCTs have evaluated the effects of treating pregnant women at high risk for preeclampsia (a dangerous pregnancy complication marked by high blood pressure, swelling of the legs, and signs of damage to the liver, kidneys, or other organs) with aspirin. A recent comprehensive review of evidence from these trials found that low-dose ASA use reduced rates of preeclampsia by 24 percent and preterm birth by 14 percent, with no harms to the mom or baby identified.[26]

Current guidelines from the U.S. Preventive Services Task Force (USPSTF) base the decision on use of low-dose ASA for primary prevention of CVD and colon cancer on the patient's risk for developing CVD, using the Framingham Risk Score

(FRS).[27] The USPSTF only recommends the drug for people who are fifty to sixty-nine, have a 10 percent or higher ten-year risk for CVD, and are at no increased risk for bleeding. The USPSTF considers the evidence insufficient to recommend low-dose ASA for people under fifty or over sixty-nine, regardless of the magnitude of their risk.

This is where the standard of care and the BaleDoneen Method differ. As discussed more fully in chapter three, risk-factor profiling has been shown to be a highly inaccurate predictor of heart attack and stroke danger. Indeed, a 2017 systematic review of randomized clinical trials of widely used risk-factor scoring systems, including FRS, found no evidence that these tools save lives or reduce rates of CV events.[28] Instead, unsuspecting patients like Diane G., Melinda, Nikki, Camille, and J.P. are left in deadly peril because they didn't have the specific risk factors that these scoring systems checked for. As a result, they were deemed too "healthy" to qualify for low-dose ASA—a drug that costs a few cents a day—even though it might have prevented their heart attacks and strokes! Conversely, some people with lots of risk factors never suffer heart attacks or strokes because they don't have disease in their arteries. Taking aspirin daily would put these patients at needless risk for bleeding or other side effects, with no cardiovascular benefit.

Despite thirty years of randomized controlled trials—the gold standard of scientific research—the role of ASA in primary prevention has remained controversial. Five RCTs conducted between 1988 and 2003 linked aspirin use to a 32 percent reduction in first-time heart attacks.[29] Since then, additional RCTs have been published with inconsistent findings, leading to inconsistent guidelines, with some medical societies and government agencies in the U.S. and Europe recommending low-dose aspirin for primary prevention and others recommending *against* it. Here are key findings from the three latest RCTs (the ones that made headlines in 2018):

ASPREE (studied aspirin and the elderly)

Nearly twenty thousand older adults of diverse ethnicities were randomly assigned to either take 100 mg of aspirin daily or a placebo.[30] During nearly five years of follow-up, rates of CV events were 11 percent lower in the ASA group, but the researchers didn't consider the difference to be statistically significant. No testing was done to find out if the participants had arterial plaque. The authors concluded that "The use of low-dose aspirin as a primary prevention strategy in older adults resulted in a significantly higher risk of major hemorrhage and did not result in a significantly lower risk of CVD than placebo."

ASCENT (studied aspirin in people with diabetes)

More than fifteen thousand adults with type 2 diabetes, but no evident CVD, were randomly assigned to take ASA at a dose of 100 mg or a placebo, then were tracked for a mean of 7.4 years. The authors concluded that "Aspirin use prevented serious vascular events in persons who had diabetes and no evident cardiovascular disease at trial entry, but it also caused major bleeding events. The absolute benefits were largely counterbalanced by the bleeding hazard."

ARRIVE (studied aspirin for people at moderate risk for CVD)

In this multicenter trial conducted in seven countries, 12,546 patients were randomly assigned to either receive 100 mg aspirin tablets daily or a placebo, then were tracked for a median of five years. Eligible patients were fifty-five or older for men and sixty-five or older for women, deemed to have a 20 to 30 percent ten-year risk for CVD, based on various U.S. and European risk calculators. The authors concluded that "The event rate was much lower than expected, which is probably reflective of contemporary risk management strategies, making the study more representative of a low-risk population. The role of aspirin in primary prevention among patients at moderate risk could therefore not be addressed."

Given the conflicting findings of thirty years of research on the role of low-dose ASA in primary prevention, and recent RCTs raising questions as to whether the benefits outweigh the harms, what should patients and medical providers conclude? Our takeaway is that the decision about low-dose aspirin use is about proper patient selection. While the standard of care divides patients into two groups based on whether they have experienced a CV event, we advocate a precision-medicine, three-tiered approach, in which the decision about which patients would benefit from ASA is based on the presence or absence of disease (plaque):

Primary prevention

In the absence of arterial disease, the risk for a heart attack or stroke is so low that the benefits of ASA would be overshadowed by its potential harms. Instead, these patients should receive personalized therapies to reduce any potential risks they may have for future development of CVD, including genetic risks.

Secondary prevention

We propose the use of this term for patients who have arterial plaque but have not yet experienced a CV event. Given the presence of plaque, especially in patients who also have chronic inflammation, the risk for a heart attack or stroke outweighs the potential harms of low-dose ASA.

Tertiary prevention

We propose this term to describe what the standard of care currently calls secondary prevention, i.e., patients who have already experienced one or more CV events. The benefits of aspirin for this group are thoroughly documented in numerous studies.

We strongly recommend that patients who are being treated with low-dose ASA for prevention of CV events be screened for aspirin resistance, using a simple, inexpensive, and widely available urine test, such as AspirinWorks. This testing, which we typically perform one month after starting a patient on low-dose aspirin, checks levels of a biomarker called thromboxane, the compound that makes platelets sticky. High levels of thromboxane indicate that your dosage of aspirin is not effective, in which case, your healthcare provider may increase your dose to full-strength aspirin (325 mg) or switch you to a different anti-platelet medication, such as Plavix. In addition, if your levels of thromboxane are high, this result will alert your provider to check you for coexisting conditions that can cause aspirin resistance, such as insulin resistance, high blood pressure, heart failure, and inflammatory disorders.[31]

Here's another reason why it's important to find out if you are aspirin resistant. In a meta-analysis of 1,813 patients with CVD from twelve prospective studies, the average prevalence of aspirin resistance was 28 percent.[32] Aspirin-resistant patients were also found to have nearly quadruple the rate of CV events, compared to aspirin-responsive patients. Despite the dangers of aspirin resistance, many providers neglect to tell patients about this simple test, which only needs to be done once in a lifetime and costs about twenty dollars. If you are on aspirin therapy and your provider hasn't ordered this test, ask for it! Finding out if you have this common condition—and if so, having your treatment adjusted accordingly—could save your life.

Cornerstone #3: Statin Therapy

Remember how Juli quit taking the statin medication her doctors had prescribed after her second heart attack? Because her providers hadn't explained *why* this drug was advised, the thirty-seven-year-old mom—who had previously been told that her cholesterol levels were "beautiful, like a teenager's"—mistakenly thought she was being treated for a problem she didn't have. Actually, Juli made a very dangerous error when she halted statin therapy without seeking medical advice.

Like most patients and some providers, Juli didn't know that statin medications—sold under such brand names as Lipitor, Crestor, and Zocor, among others—can be potentially lifesaving after a heart attack or stroke, even in people with optimal cholesterol levels. In a randomized clinical trial with 4,295 heart patients, most of whom already had very low levels of LDL (bad) cholesterol, statin therapy reduced their risk of dying in the next two years by 35 percent, as compared to a control group.[33] In addition, a number of RCTs have reported sizable reductions in heart attack and stroke rates in at-risk patients with average or even superb lipid numbers.[34]

There is also an excellent reason why the BaleDoneen Method advises statin therapy for *all* patients with arterial disease, regardless of their cholesterol numbers: These medications deliver a cardiovascular grand slam by protecting and enhancing arterial health in several ways.

Statins, which block a liver enzyme involved in cholesterol production, are best known for their ability to drive down cholesterol. On average, people who take these drugs will see their LDL (bad) cholesterol numbers plummet by 40 to 60 percent, according to an analysis of 164 RCTs, published in *British Medical Journal*.[35] The researchers, who only examined short-term trials, also linked statin use to a 60 percent drop in heart attacks

and a 17 percent reduction in strokes, compared to study participants who received a placebo.

However, it's not just people with an LDL problem who get
extra protection against CV events if they take a statin. Many
excellent studies have shown that these medications also have
powerful anti-inflammatory effects.[36] In fact, there is overwhelming proof that statins are the best firefighting medications we have. Here are a few of the more significant discoveries:

Statins do a superb job of reducing two biomarkers that
warn of arterial peril: high-sensitivity C-reactive protein (hs-CRP),
which rises when the endothelium (tennis court) becomes
inflamed, and Lp-PLA2, which can signal that arterial plaque is
hot and growing. Having high levels of Lp-PLA2 doubles heart
attack risk in people with diseased arteries.[37] In a recent statin
trial, participants who achieved the greatest drop in their initial
Lp-PLA2 levels over the next twelve months had a 27 percent
lower rate of heart attacks and other major coronary events.[38]
The researchers reported that the majority of the risk reduction
from the statin was due to its lowering of Lp-PLA2, as opposed
to its lowering of LDL.

Statins also have immediate antiplatelet and antioxidant
effects that start to kick in within two hours of the first dose and
progressively increase during the first week of treatment, a study
published in *Circulation* reported.[39] Earlier research suggests
that these medications also help prevent the creation of the
arterial Velcro that snares cholesterol, decrease the amount of
cholesterol in plaque, and strengthen the fibrous cap that keeps
the cat in the gutter safely caged. These factors help protect
against the formation of a clot that could stop the flow of blood
to your heart.[40]

A small but intriguing twelve-week 2012 study found that
statin therapy reduced periodontal inflammation by 57 percent
in people with gum disease. The researchers also reported that

improvements in periodontal inflammation correlated to similar improvements in carotid artery inflammation. In other words, statin therapy appears to quell oral-systemic fire.[41] Another dental study reported that statins protect smiles as well as arteries: People who take these drugs have a 30 percent lower risk for tooth loss.[42]

In a five-year study of 1,674 older adults (sixty or older), those who were taking statins had 48 percent lower risk for dementia, even after the researchers took a variety of risk factors, including genes and history of strokes or diabetes, into account.[43] A much larger 2016 study of more than 405,000 Medicare patients linked statin use to a 20 to 25 decrease in Alzheimer's incidence.[44]

Does it matter which statin you take? Combined results of the large statin trials indicate that these medications are highly effective at reducing cardiovascular risk and vascular inflammation, but when you look at some of the newer trials individually, important differences emerge. It appears that one statin, Lipitor (atorvastatin), may not be the best choice for women or people with insulin resistance (IR), including those with type 2 diabetes or metabolic syndrome. In fact, in one RCT, taking atorvastatin *increased* IR by up to 45 percent and *raised* blood sugar, as compared with a placebo.[45]

Several randomized, placebo-controlled trials have looked at the effects of atorvastatin on women with high cardiovascular risk. In the large ASCOT trial, which included both men and women, women in the Lipitor group had a 10 percent *higher* rate of CV events of atorvastatin (including heart attacks and strokes) than women in the placebo group, while this medication reduced rates of these events by 42 percent in male study participants.[46] In a women-only RCT called CASHMERE, which included about four hundred participants who were postmenopausal with arterial plaque, the statin-treated women had no improvement whatsoever in their carotid intima-media thickness, suggesting that atorvastatin had failed to halt or regress their disease.

Based on these findings and other research with similar results, we avoid prescribing Lipitor to our female patients, such as Diane G., and those with IR/prediabetes, diabetes, or metabolic syndrome. For women with arterial disease, Crestor (rosuvastatin) can be an excellent option. In a recent gender-specific analysis of outcomes in the very large JUPITER primary prevention trial, which included more than 6,800 women, this statin reduced CV events in women at a rate similar to that in men.[47] Specifically, Crestor-treated women's rates of these events fell by 46 percent, compared to a 42 percent drop in men.

Along with taking your gender and coexisting conditions into account when considering which statin to prescribe, your provider should also be guided by your genetics. As discussed more fully in chapter eleven, Lipitor or Pravachol (pravastatin) only provide cardiovascular protection to the 60 percent of Americans who carry the KIF6 variant. Three large randomized clinical trials found that these drugs *do not* reduce the risk for heart attacks, strokes, and death from cardiovascular causes in the 40 percent of Americans who are noncarriers of the KIF6 variant, such as Juli, Diane H., Jack, Melinda, and Catherine.[48] We advise noncarriers of the KIF6 variant to discuss other treatment options with their providers.

We also prescribe statins to certain patients who *don't* have a cat in the gutter, such as those with elevated LDL or ApoB cholesterol and people with vascular inflammation. Until recently, the mainstays of cholesterol management were lifestyle modification and statins. If these treatments are not effective enough, current guidelines from the American Heart Association and American College of Cardiology also advise the use of non-statin drugs, such as ezetimibe and PCSK9 inhibitors, for two categories of patients: those who can't achieve the guideline-recommended cholesterol targets even on the maximum tolerated dosage of statin therapy and those with the inherited cholesterol disorder familial hypercholesterolemia.[49]

For example, Diane G. was not able to achieve her cholesterol goal with a statin alone, so we also prescribed a PCSK9 inhibitor. With this additional medication, her LDL numbers quickly fell to the optimal range. Currently, there are two FDA-approved PCSK9 inhibitors: alirocumab (Praluent) and evolocumab (Repatha). Recent studies suggest that these drugs can help prevent heart attacks and strokes, but they are much more expensive than other cholesterol drugs. Several trials have shown that PCSK9 inhibitors reduce cardiovascular risk in patients with stable CVD or a history of recent CV events who are already on moderate- or high-intensity statin therapy.[50]

Side effects of statins can include muscle pain and weakness or, in rare cases, muscle breakdown. Frequently, statin-related myopathy (muscle pain) is driven by vitamin D deficiency, low level of CoQ10, or even obstructive sleep apnea (OSA). In these cases, myopathy can be mitigated through using a statin at a very low dose, along with supplements to boost vitamin D or CoQ10, or treating the OSA. In a 2019 scientific statement, the American Heart Association recommended against the use of statins during pregnancy or breastfeeding.[51] Although statins have been rumored to potentially increase risk for dementia, in reality, the signal from the latest studies suggest that the opposite may be true. In fact, the National Institutes of Health (NIH) has sponsored a $90 million, seven-year study to explore the possibility that these medications may help *prevent* dementia.[52]

Cornerstone #4: Renin-Angiotensin Aldosterone System Inhibitors

The renin-angiotensin aldosterone system (RAAS) regulates blood pressure and the body's fluid balance. RAAS inhibitors reduce the effects of angiotensin II, a hormone that constricts arteries and boosts blood pressure. By causing blood vessels to relax and widen, these drugs lower blood pressure. Since angiotensin II also promotes blood clotting and can contribute to arterial wall inflammation and oxidative stress, it's not surprising that medications that decrease the effects of this hormone have been shown in many studies over the past two decades to lower heart attack and stroke risk.[53]

Indeed, the scientific evidence is so overwhelming that in 2004, the American College of Physicians issued a recommendation that all patients with coronary artery disease be treated with an angiotensin-blocking medication.[54] We strongly support that recommendation; however, we go one step further and prescribe RAAS inhibitors for patients with plaque in *any* of their arteries, not just those that supply the heart. To us, it doesn't make sense to focus only on heart attack prevention (by treating patients with CAD) and ignore patients with plaque in their neck arteries that could trigger a devastating ischemic stroke.

RAAS inhibitors relax the wall of the artery, resulting in lower blood pressure. That's an important benefit, since high blood pressure is a leading cause of stroke (and a major risk factor for heart attack, dementia, and many other chronic diseases). In the 2015 SPRINT trial, which looked at the effects of reducing blood pressure to a level below 120/80, achieving this goal reduced rates of heart attacks and strokes by 33 percent, and also decreased fatalities by as much as 25 percent.[55] However, just as statins are beneficial for patients with arterial disease—even if they have normal or optimal cholesterol levels—RAAS inhibitors have been shown to shrink cardiovascular risk in patients with blood pressure as low as 110/70 mm Hg (a superb level). RAAS inhibitors also help promote nitrous oxide to the artery wall, making it stronger and more resistant to plaque rupture.

There are two main types of RAAS inhibitors, both of which

target the same process that constricts blood vessels. Each type inhibits or blocks a different step of the process.

Angiotensin-converting enzyme inhibitors

Also known as ACE inhibitors, these medications prevent an enzyme called renin from producing angiotensin. We love the medical slang for these drugs, because we like having this ace up our sleeve! The ACEs are the oldest medications in the RAAS inhibitor category and have a wealth of data showing significant reductions in heart attacks, strokes, heart failure, and kidney failure.[56] Among the RAAS inhibitors, the ACEs have the best outcome data for preventing both cardiovascular events and fatalities.

There are many different ACEs, but we feel that the one called ramipril has superior data, with the very large HOPE trial reporting a 32 percent drop in the risk for stroke, 20 percent for heart attack, 26 percent for cardiovascular fatalities, *and* a 34 percent decrease in new-onset cases of diabetes.[57] No other ACE has been shown to be nearly as effective for preventing diabetes. That's a very important benefit for our patients with arterial disease and/or high blood pressure, since many of them are also on the road to type 2 diabetes, as Diane G. was at the start of her treatment. For people who are already diabetic, ACEs are superior to other types of RAAS inhibitors for reducing CV risk.[58] A 2018 study found that in patients with Alzheimer's disease, ACEs may slow cognitive decline, independent of their effect on blood pressure.[59]

However, ACEs do have some drawbacks. The most common side effect, occurring in about 5 percent of those who take this type of medication, is a dry, hacking cough. While nitrous oxide is marvelous for the blood vessel lining, it can irritate the airway lining, leading to coughing. If this occurs, we switch patients to a different type of RAAS inhibitor, such as angiotensin receptor blockers (ARBs). The most serious side effect of the

ACEs—affecting about one in 1,000 users—is sudden swelling of the mouth and back of the throat that demands immediate treatment in an emergency room. Like many drugs, ACEs are not safe during pregnancy.

Angiotensin receptor blockers

Many healthcare providers prefer to prescribe angiotensin receptor blockers (ARBs) instead of ACEs, because the ARBs don't cause coughing. Commonly prescribed ARBs include Benecar (olmesartan) and Diovan (valsartan). As the name suggests, ARBs block the action of angiotensin by preventing it from binding to receptors in blood vessels and other tissues, much as filling the lock on your front door with cement would render your house key useless. In effect, an ARB tells the body, "Make all the angiotensin you want. It doesn't matter, because I am going to stop its actions."

How effective are ARBs for heart attack and stroke prevention? In a review of thirty-seven RCTs that included about 150,000 patients who were tracked for at least one year, ARBs significantly reduced stroke danger (by about 10 percent), but had almost no impact on heart attack risk.[60]

They are effective at preventing and treating heart and kidney failure, with very few side effects. They also help prevent type 2 diabetes, but not as effectively as the ACEs.[61] Taking an ARB trims the threat of new-onset diabetes by about 14 percent, compared to the 34 percent risk reduction associated with ACE use. For people who already have diabetes, ACEs are superior to ARBs for cutting the threat of cardiovascular events and fatalities.[62]

We warn patients who are being treated with RAAS inhibitors not to take an antibiotic sulfamethoxazole-trimethoprim, sold under such trade names as Septra and Bactrim. Combining these drugs can cause your potassium level to become dangerously or even fatally high.[63] This antibiotic is frequently ordered for bladder, kidney, or middle-ear infections.

Other antibiotics are not associated with this danger. Make sure any healthcare provider who treats you checks for potential drug interactions with your current therapies whenever any new medication is prescribed. Also keep a list of your medications (including dosages) in your wallet or stored on your mobile device, so it's handy for medical appointments or an emergency.

Two Additional Cornerstones for Cardiovascular Protection

For patients who need tertiary prevention to avoid repeat cardiovascular events, such as Diane G., Juli, Camille, and Melinda, and those with certain medical conditions, we layer two additional types of medication on top of the four cornerstones discussed earlier in this chapter. Think of these two additional cornerstones as building an extra-strong foundation on your house to protect it from being damaged by earthquakes and other disasters. Decades of excellent research have shown that these two medication types can be extremely beneficial—and often lifesaving—when prescribed for appropriate patients:

Beta blockers

Sold under such brand names as Corgard (nadolol), Bystolic (nebivolol), Coreg (carvedilol), and Torol (metoprolol), beta blockers lower your blood pressure and reduce stress on your heart. They work by blocking the effects of certain hormones, such as adrenaline, the fight-or-flight chemical that revs up the body for exertion to escape danger. In one of the newest studies, published in 2020, the use of beta blockers after a heart attack reduced risk for suffering additional CV events in the next year by 20 percent and decreased mortality risk by 31 percent.[64] When beta blockers were prescribed in combination with RAAS inhibitors, one-year risk for CV events dropped by 30 percent and mortality risk by 45 percent. The study included more than fifteen thousand heart attack survivors.

Dual anti-platelet therapy (DAPT)

This type of treatment involves combining low-dose daily aspirin therapy with an additional medication that also helps prevent clots, such as Plavix (clopidogrel), Effient (prasugrel), or Brilinta (ticagrelor). DAPT is most commonly prescribed to patients who have experienced a stroke or transient ischemic attack (TIA or mini-stroke), have been treated with stents, or have peripheral artery disease. In a 2019 study of 5,590 stroke and TIA patients, those started on DAPT within twenty-four hours of their events had a 26 percent lower rate of subsequent strokes, as opposed to patients who only received aspirin.[65]

Treatment for Insulin Resistance and Type 2 Diabetes

Since insulin resistance—the culprit in 70 percent of heart attacks—is the leading cause of both atherosclerosis and high blood pressure, it's essential to treat this prediabetic condition. Research shows that people with prediabetes can substantially reduce their risk for progressing to full-blown type 2 disease through losing 5 to 10 percent of their body weight and exercising moderately thirty minutes a day, at least five days a week.

In some cases, diet and exercise aren't enough to halt further loss of insulin-producing beta cells in the pancreas and further damage to blood vessels. In this situation, we sometimes prescribe Actos (pioglitazone), a drug that improves insulin sensitivity, thereby reducing blood sugar. Like optimal lifestyle and statin therapy, Actos delivers a wealth of arterial benefits: It reduces inflammation, reduces the trapping of ApoB cholesterol in the wall of the artery, supports endothelial health, slows or halts the progression of CVD in both prediabetic and diabetic patients, and has antiplatelet effects, recent studies have revealed.[66] It also helps prevent new-onset diabetes.[67]

How do pioglitazone's cardiovascular perks compare to those other anti-diabetes medications? In a head-to-head 2018 study comparing patients treated with Actos versus those who were treated with alternative anti-diabetes drugs, pioglitazone slashed rates of CV mortality by 42 percent during 2.5 years of follow-up.[68] In another recent trial comparing pioglitazone to a placebo in nondiabetic stroke survivors, the group that received this drug had 24 percent lower rate of stroke and 31 percent decrease in risk for fatal and nonfatal heart attacks.[69] A 2019 paper published in *JAMA Neurology* suggested that pioglitazone's benefits for secondary stroke prevention may also encompass dementia prevention, since stroke, in particularly, is a strong predictor of risk for memory loss. However, further research is needed to explore this exciting possibility.

Some diabetic patients may need additional medications to optimize their blood sugar control. There are many options available, including newer drugs, some of which also have CV benefits. If you are diabetic or prediabetic, talk to your health-care provider about which therapies are best for you. Also inquire about continuous glucose monitors, such as the Free-Style Libre, which Diane G. and many of our other diabetic and prediabetic patients use to get immediate feedback on how their diet and activities are affecting their blood sugar. For example, like Neal, Diane G. discovered that her blood sugar spiked after consuming rice or products containing rice flour, so she now limits or avoids these items.

Celebrating a Marvelous Milestone

During the quarter century that Diane G. has been our patient, she has been treated with *all* the medications and supplements discussed in this chapter. How has twenty-four years of optimal medical therapy worked out for her? All her plaque is completely stabilized and she's had no further trips to the OR for heart procedures. In addition, she has avoided progressing to type 2 diabetes and all her health metrics—including blood pressure, weight, and lipid levels—are completely normal. Earlier this year, she turned eighty and calls the four cornerstones of our prevention plan "the secret of my longevity." The octogenarian celebrated her milestone birthday surrounded by her extended family, including her ninety-year-old husband, their four children, five grandkids, and a great grandchild.

In a recent visit to our center, Diane G. told us, "It's hard to believe that I'm feeling so good at my age. I still drive, exercise every day, and love to travel. I recently went to Mexico, where I had a great time walking on the beach, drinking margaritas, and going on a walking tour. I believe that God has many more things for me to do on this earth and I'm living like a fifty-year-old, thanks to the BaleDoneen Method."

Action Step: Find Out If You Are Getting the Most Effective Medications and Supplements at the Right Dose

If you're one of the 226 million Americans who take prescription drugs to treat arterial disease or other conditions, a new pharmacogenetic test can help your healthcare provider personalize your care, so you get the safest and most effective medications at the right dose. Called MyPGt, it checks for genetic variants that affect your response to hundreds of commonly prescribed medications and supplements.

Not only can your results help you avoid drugs that don't work, or are likely to cause side effects, but this one-time saliva test can also offer guidance on medications that may be prescribed in the future, thus enabling your provider to fine-tune your medical care throughout your life, based on your unique DNA.

Your healthcare provider collects a sample of your DNA, using a simple oral rinse method, and sends it to the MyGenetx laboratory for analysis. You will also be asked for a list of your current medications, so a personalized report can be sent to your provider. The test covers many genes that determine how your body processes a wide range of common medications, including those often prescribed for heart disease, high blood pressure, chronic pain, depression, and other disorders.

Here's an example of how this testing can be valuable. When Robert came to our center, he was suffering from twenty-six different conditions (including arterial plaque) and had a wide range of debilitating symptoms, despite being on numerous medications. When we ordered the MyPGt test, it revealed that the beta blocker he was on was completely ineffective for his genotype, so he was getting no cardiovascular protection from this medication. Therefore, we switched him to a different beta blocker that did work for people with his genotype.

In addition, when we reviewed the other medications he was on, we found that many of his symptoms were actually drug side effects that could be eliminated by other changes in his medication. Instead of reevaluating him every time a new medication had been prescribed, using the results of MyPGt testing, the doctors who were previously treating him had prescribed additional drugs to manage the side effects caused by his other therapies, leading to new side effects and worse health for Robert.

Simply by switching him to medications that were appropriate for his genotype and taking him off the drugs that were causing him harm, we were able to dramatically and rapidly improve Robert's health, while still treating his various medical conditions effectively with evidence-based therapies, such as the four cornerstones of treatment of arterial disease discussed in this chapter, and the two additional cornerstones for tertiary prevention of cardiovascular events and complications.

Here is another example of how this testing can be helpful: Let's say you need a statin to lower your cholesterol or as one of the cornerstones of treating arterial disease. The traditional approach is to prescribe a low dose and gradually adjust it up or down, trying to find the sweet spot. However, you might have a gene variant that makes that statin ineffective for you or increases the risk for side effects, such as severe muscle pain. Without this test, it could take weeks or even months of trial and error, and many medical visits, to find the right statin and the most appropriate dose.

Moreover, some patients have genes that cause them to metabolize certain drugs faster than average, so they need a higher dose, while others process those drugs more slowly and need a lower dose to avoid adverse reactions. Results from MyPGt or other pharmacogenetic tests take the guesswork out of choosing the right prescription drugs and dosages for each individual, leading to faster, safer, and more effective medical care to protect and enhance your arterial health. Also, if you are under the care of multiple providers, each them can use your pharmacogenetic results to avoid prescribing drugs or supplements that would interact in a harmful way with therapies prescribed by your other providers.

CHAPTER 15

Achieving Optimal Arterial Wellness

"When you reach the top, keep climbing."

— Zen proverb

When Joe arrived at our center for his initial evaluation, he had such severe chest pain that he was unable to walk across the exam room without stopping to take nitroglycerin to temporarily quell the angina. Looking pale and shaky, he said that he was terrified that he was on the same tragic trajectory as his father, who had died at sixty-two, five years after undergoing quadruple bypass surgery to treat severe coronary artery disease (CAD).

Getting a little choked up as he continued his story, Joe added that his own battle with CAD had started two years earlier, when he developed chest pain during exercise. He was rushed to the OR, where he underwent open-heart surgery and a quadruple bypass. Then fifty-seven, Joe was almost the same age his dad had been when the older man had had these procedures decades earlier. After Joe's bypass surgery, he spent six weeks in cardiac rehabilitation. These programs are customized with exercise, nutritional counseling, and education to teach patients healthy lifestyle habits and help them recover after a heart attack or cardiac surgery. Determined to avoid his father's fate, he quit smoking, began working out regularly, and dramatically improved his diet.

"During cardiac rehab, I told the nurse that I knew this treatment would help slow down my disease, and I might live a little longer, but I thought my heart would get me in the end," says the retired real estate broker from Granbury, Texas. "She said that physicians used to think that all they could do was keep patients from getting worse, but there were two doctors in Spokane who had success in halting and reversing this disease. She also told me that she was planning to send her own mother to these specialists because the standard treatments weren't helping her."

Initially, however, lifestyle improvements seemed to do the trick. Before long, Joe, an avid nature photographer, felt well enough to resume his favorite activities: hiking, kayaking, and training his three German short-haired pointers for bird-dog competitions—physically challenging events that required following the fast-moving dogs through rough terrain on horseback to find hidden birds.

However, the seemingly miraculous improvement only lasted eighteen months. Not only did the angina return, but it became so severe that despite treatment with nitroglycerin and several other medications, even the slightest exertion—such as walking from his house to his car—left him in agony. His cardiologist ordered heart tests. "He told me that I had new blockages, which I kind of knew, and sent me to the hospital for an angiogram," says Joe, who still gets choked up remembering what happened next.

"When the cardiologist came into my hospital room with the results, my two sons and their wives were with me," recalls the divorced dad. "I was told that two of the vein grafts in my bypasses had totally failed. Then the cardiologist—with a heart doctor standing next to him—said that if they tried stenting or putting in new grafts, it could cause a heart attack. He said that I might not even survive the surgery and they felt I needed to consider a heart transplant. That really shook me and my family started crying."

After pausing to blink back tears, Joe adds, "I told my sons, 'Maybe this is what it boils down to, but I want a second option and a lot more answers first.' I felt that the cardiologist wasn't looking at why I'd gone downhill so fast after the quadruple bypass. Even on medication, my blood pressure was staying at 150/90 and I'd done enough research to know that was not normal. But when I asked him about that, he'd say, 'For your age, that's a decent number: You can live with that.' I felt I was just being herded along, like sheep in a pen, from one surgery to another. Basically, I was being told, 'You've drawn a bad hand of cards in life and all we can do is put in a new heart.'"

Joe's face brightened a little when he shared what the nurse at the cardiac rehab program had said about us. He'd attended one of our lectures and hoped that we could help him feel better. However, he still had a fatalistic attitude about his long-term prospects for survival and worried that it might be too late to turn his disease around. We assured him that we'd successfully treated patients who were even sicker than he was with the optimal medical therapy discussed in the last chapter. First, however, we needed to do some detective work and testing to uncover the root causes of his severe CAD and persistently highly blood pressure to identify the best personalized therapies. At the end of the visit, Joe said he'd give our method a shot, but we could see that he remained skeptical that it would save his life.

Stopping a Silent Killer

Contrary to what Joe had been told, high blood pressure is *not* a problem that people can live with. Also called hypertension, this condition kills nearly 500,000 Americans annually.[1] What's more, rates of hypertension-related fatalities have skyrocketed by 66 percent since 2003, according to an alarming report from the National Center for Health Statistics.[2]

Nearly half of all U.S. adults—108 million people—have hypertension under recently updated guidelines from the American Heart Association (AHA) and the American College of Cardiology (ACC).[3]

Issued in December 2017 by the AHA/ACC and endorsed by many other medical groups, the new guidelines set a lower threshold for a disorder often called the silent killer because hypertension typically causes few or no symptoms as it wreaks slow mayhem on your blood vessels and vital organs such as your heart, brain, and kidneys, if untreated.[4] Under the old guidelines, only one in three Americans were deemed to have high blood pressure, which was defined as a reading of 140/90 mm Hg or higher. The new guidelines define hypertension as 130/80 mm Hg or higher, putting an additional 30 million Americans in the danger zone.

The new guidelines eliminate the category of prehypertension (previously defined as systolic pressure between 120 and 139 or diastolic pressure between 80 and 89). Until recently, the 67 million Americans with blood pressure in this range were often told that their pressure was "a little high, but nothing to worry about." Actually, studies show that having prehypertension doubles the risk for cardiovascular events, such as heart attacks and strokes. Recognizing that serious or fatal complications of high blood pressure can occur at lower numbers, and to encourage earlier treatment, the guidelines create the following new blood pressure categories:

Normal: Less than 120/80 mm Hg.

Elevated: Systolic blood pressure (the top number) between 120–129 and diastolic pressure (the bottom number) less than 80.

Stage 1 hypertension: Systolic between 130–139 or diastolic between 80–89.

Stage 2 hypertension: Systolic at least 140 or diastolic at least 90 mm Hg.

Under the new guidelines, 46 percent of U.S. adults meet criteria for hypertension. Only one in four of them, however, have their condition under control, the CDC reported in 2019.[5] Yet research has found that most people with uncontrolled high blood pressure have health insurance and visit a healthcare provider at least twice a year but remain undiagnosed and untreated. In our practice, we frequently see patients who don't know what their blood pressure is but tell us they have always been assured that it's in the "healthy range." Very often, however, their numbers fall into the danger zone.

We also see many patients who know they have high blood pressure—including Joe, Neal, and Catherine—and are on medications or other therapies for it, but still don't have the problem under control. That's alarming because if untreated, high blood pressure is the leading risk factor for strokes and a major contributor to heart disease, chronic kidney disease, heart failure, vision impairment or loss, and many other debilitating conditions. For example, a 2019 study in which people born in 1946 were tracked for decades found that those who had hypertension at fifty-three were at much higher risk for developing dementia or Alzheimer's disease later in life, compared to their peers with normal blood pressure.[6] Those with high blood pressure in midlife were also more likely than their healthy counterparts to show signs of brain shrinkage at seventy and had higher rates of cerebral small-vessel disease, further undermining their brain health.

The Dangerous Problem of "Therapeutic Inertia"

Since the AHA/ACC guidelines and numerous public health campaigns strongly emphasize the importance of treating hypertension, why does it remain the most common uncontrolled chronic condition in the U.S.? In a 2010 paper we wrote about this issue, published in *Journal of the National Medical Association*, we pointed to the problem of therapeutic inertia, a provider's failure to increase therapy or try different treatments when blood pressure targets are not met.[7]

For example, one of the studies we examined found that medication adjustments were only made for 13 percent of patients with uncontrolled hypertension. Yet just reducing therapeutic inertia by as little as 20 percent would have improved blood pressure control for 46 to 66 percent of the patients studied, the researchers calculated, underscoring the need for healthcare providers to work harder on fine-tuning treatment, rather than giving up in despair if the first medication they try doesn't work. Joe appeared to have fallen victim to this scenario since the blood pressure medication he was on was not helping him at all—and he'd been told that he'd just have to live with high blood pressure and ineffective treatment.

A major reason why providers often find hypertension tricky to treat, even if they *are* willing to prescribe additional therapies, is that all too often, doctors don't look for the root cause of high blood pressure. Just as many heart attack and stroke survivors are told that their event was a medical mystery that was impossible to predict or prevent, people with high blood pressure are often led to believe that their condition defies medical explanation. Actually, high blood pressure is frequently triggered by the same disorder that causes 70 percent of heart attacks: insulin resistance.

When we reviewed Joe's medical records, we found a glaring red flag: the results of a blood sugar test performed several years earlier. "How long have you been prediabetic?" we asked. Joe looked bewildered and then angry that none of his doctors had told him that his blood sugar was too high. Like 84 percent of the 88 million Americans with prediabetes, he was walking around undiagnosed and untreated while this highly treatable and often reversible disease silently damaged his blood vessels.[8] To improve his insulin sensitivity, we added the diabetes drug pioglitazone to his treatment plan, which also included the four cornerstones and other therapies discussed in the previous chapter.

As discussed earlier, previously undiagnosed obstructive sleep apnea (OSA) is another common cause of hard-to-control blood pressure. The frequent, sudden drops in blood oxygen levels that result from this condition strain the cardiovascular system, raising the risk for elevated blood pressure. And the more severe OSA is, the higher the threat of developing hypertension and other cardiovascular complications. Sleep apnea boosts risk for strokes, irregular heartbeats (atrial fibrillation), congestive heart failure, and sudden cardiac death.

Several years ago, we had a patient whose blood pressure numbers remained horrible after an entire year of treatment with four different medications and other therapies. Since he had normal blood sugar levels (as measured with the highly accurate two-hour oral glucose tolerance test discussed in chapter nine), we questioned the patient about OSA symptoms, such as loud snoring, waking up at night for no apparent reason, persistent daytime drowsiness despite adequate rest, and morning headache or sore throat. He denied having any of these symptoms, so we also questioned his wife.

People with OSA are often unaware of their loud snoring—the leading warning sign of this frequently undiagnosed disorder. His wife was equally adamant that OSA couldn't possibly be the problem. Nevertheless, we persuaded the patient to go, very reluctantly, to a lab near his home for an overnight sleep study. The next morning, we received an urgent call from the sleep specialist who conducted the test, telling us that our patient had the worst case of OSA that the physician had ever seen in his many years of clinical practice. Joe, Catherine, and Neal also turned out to have this disorder (though not as severely). In all four cases, once our patients' OSA was treated, using CPAP (continuous positive airway pressure) machines, which blow pressured air into a patient's nose and mouth during sleep, we were able to get their high blood pressure under control.

Four Important Things to Know About High Blood Pressure

A common misconception is that hypertension is mainly a problem for middle-aged and older adults. In reality, it's relatively common in younger people, affecting about 26 percent of those twenty to forty-four.[9] That's why the American Heart Association advises having your blood pressure checked regularly, starting at twenty.[10] If your blood pressure is below 120/80 (normal), the AHA advises being screened for hypertension at least once every two years (since risk rises with age). If your blood pressure is higher, have your provider check it more frequently and discuss treatment, which is likely to include lifestyle changes and, in many cases, medication. Here are four other things to know about high blood pressure, particularly your systolic blood pressure (the top number in a blood pressure reading):

Your morning blood pressure may be the best predictor of heart attack and stroke risk.

A recent study of nearly twenty-two thousand people with hypertension found that morning measurements (when blood pressure tends to be the highest) were more accurate for predicting heart attack and stroke risk than readings taken at home in the evening or those taken by clinicians in medical settings.[11] The study found a significantly higher rate of CV events in people whose morning systolic blood pressure was 145 or higher, versus those with a reading below 125.

The new AHA/ACC guidelines encourage home blood pressure monitoring as an important way for people with hypertension to track their health.

However, it's essential to know the right technique: When using a wrist blood-pressure cuff, the reading will be inaccurate unless the device is positioned at heart level.[12] A good way to tell if the device is correctly positioned is to hold the arm with the cuff across your chest as you would if the national anthem were playing.

Elevated systolic blood pressure is more dangerous than smoking or obesity!

A 2017 study that examined data from 8.69 million people from 154 countries found that systolic blood pressure (SBP) of 110 or higher is one of the leading risks for health problems, including coronary artery disease, stroke, and chronic kidney disease. The researchers also reported that 30 percent of the disease burden fell on those with SBP of 110 to 135. While SBP of 110 to 119 is *not* cause for concern, you may want to discuss natural ways to maintain healthy blood pressure with your medical provider. These include mindful meditation to reduce stress (an important contributor to elevated blood pressure), beet juice (which has been shown to reduce SPB 4 to 5 points within hours of drinking it), eating foods that are rich in magnesium (which helps regulate blood pressure), such as dark green leafy vegetables, unrefined grains, and legumes, and getting seven to eight hours of sleep a night (skimping on slumber boosts risk for hypertension).

Lowering systolic blood pressure from 140 to 120 saves lives!

Until recently, a commonly recommended treatment target for systolic blood pressure was 140. The landmark SPRINT clinical trial compared outcomes in people treated to this goal (with an average of two medications) to those who received a more intensive therapy to lower SBP to 120. The researchers found that the more intensive therapy (using an average of three medications) lowered rates of cardiovascular events, such as heart attacks, strokes, and heart failure, by nearly one-third, and fatalities by 25 percent. The study included about 9,300 people fifty and older of diverse ethnicities with high blood pressure and at least one other risk factor for heart disease.

What's the Optimal Goal for Blood Pressure?

We are often asked what the optimal blood pressure numbers are. Like all the other optimal goals listed in the appendix for the tests advised in this book, your blood pressure target needs to be personalized according to your overall health and other medical conditions. The heart muscle is nourished mainly by diastolic pressure (the lower number) pushing nutrients and oxygen through the coronary arteries. Therefore, some patients with very narrowed channels in their coronary arteries need a higher diastolic pressure to squeeze the blood through.

If a patient with obstructive CAD, such as Joe, sets a goal to reduce the pressure to 75 mm Hg or less, they may not be able to adequately perfuse the heart muscle with blood, which might lead to a heart attack. In addition, patients like Joe may need a higher goal for systolic pressure, which is what perfuses the brain with oxygenated blood. If systolic pressure is reduced excessively in such patients, they may find themselves feeling confused or foggy-headed. Based on these considerations, we set an initial blood pressure target of 130 for his SBP and 70 to 88 for his diastolic pressure.

Similarly, some people with significant chronic kidney disease, which can result in narrowing of the arteries feeding the kidney, may also be in trouble if their pressure is lowered too much. For certain patients with heart failure, a 2018 study linked SBP levels below 120 to a 36 percent higher risk of death within the ensuing year and a 17 percent jump in risk mortality within six years.[13] The key takeaway from this research is that each patient needs to be followed closely when they are receiving BP treatment and appropriate lab tests should be followed to make sure the pressure is not reduced too much.

In a healthy population, scientific data would suggest that we'd be better off with a blood pressure just above the point where we might pass out. Some trials, however, have set very low blood-pressure goals for people who are not healthy, such as diabetics. Tragically, some participants in the "aggressive" treatment arm of these studies did very poorly and some even died. In this type of study, everyone in a certain arm of the study is treated the same. However, no two people are exactly alike. Excellent outcomes require personalizing care — not standardizing the same care for everyone!

Is Your Heart Happy?

Most people have pondered the question of how "happy" their heart is from the emotional standpoint—and a positive answer is beneficial for their psychological well-being. But most patients don't know that it can also be important to find out if their heart is happy from the physical standpoint as well. That's right— there is a simple, widely available blood test that can quantify how "happy" your heart is.

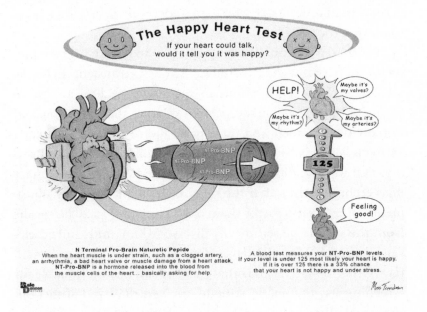

N Terminal Pro-Brain Naturetic Pepide
When the heart muscle is under strain, such as a clogged artery, an arrhythmia, a bad heart valve or muscle damage from a heart attack, **NT-Pro-BNP** is a hormone released into the blood from the muscle cells of the heart... basically asking for help.

A blood test measures your **NT-Pro-BNP** levels. If your level is under 125 most likely your heart is happy. If it is over 125 there is a 33% chance that your heart is not happy and under stress.

When the heart muscle is under stress or struggling to function properly—due to such conditions as a clogged artery, an arrhythmia, muscle damage from a heart attack, heart failure, or issues with a heart valve—it produces extra amounts of a hormone called B-type naturetic peptide (BNP). Essentially SOS messages that the heart is in distress, naturetic peptides cause the body to excrete more fluid, decreasing the amount the heart has to pump each time it beats. These peptides also cause arteries to dilate, lessening the force the heart must generate to circulate blood. Both effects reduce a struggling heart's workload.

B-type naturetic peptide is easy to measure with a rapid, inexpensive blood test known as NT-proBNP. We call it the happy heart test, because when the level of this cardiac distress marker is below 125 pg/mL, there is a 98 percent probability your heart is very happy![14] Any test in medicine that can give you those odds is phenomenal. We recommend this test for everyone over fifty and younger people who have hypertension, arterial disease, or a history of heart attacks, strokes, and other cardiovascular events, or who have undergone heart procedures to prevent these events.

Elevated NT-proBNP has been shown to be a significant predictor of risk for heart attacks, strokes, transient ischemic attacks, and other CV events in seemingly healthy, symptom-free people. In fact, in a recent study of more than five thousand initially healthy men and women who were tracked for nearly thirteen years, NT-proBNP was the *only* biomarker test, of several that were studied, that accurately predicted both coronary *and* cerebral danger after the researchers made rigorous adjustments for every risk factor they could think of.[15] In 2020, results from the very large, ethnically diverse MESA study linked elevated levels of NT-proBNP to a 55 percent rise in risk for dementia.[16] Other research shows that this test can be also valuable for screening asymptomatic patients for ventricular dysfunction: abnormal stiffness in the heart's lower chambers (the ventricles), which pump blood out of the heart.

How worried should you be if your NT-proBNP level is 125 ng/dL or higher? If that's the case, there is a 33 percent chance that your heart is not totally happy and is experiencing dysfunction.[17] While there is still a decent chance that you are okay even if this biomarker is elevated, the odds that there may be a problem are high enough that your provider may order additional tests to further evaluate your heart health, such as an electrocardiogram (EKG) or an echocardiogram.

In Joe's case, this test revealed that his heart was extremely unhappy in the physical sense since his level of NT-proBNT was extremely high. In addition, his heart was also very unhappy in the emotional sense since the divorced dad was convinced that he was doomed to a short, lonely, and celibate life. During the initial visit, he told us, in a wistful tone, "People are meant to share their lives with others, but I don't allow myself to even attempt a romantic relationship because I'm not healthy enough for *any* sustained physical activity, including sex or even going on a date."

A Lifesaving Treatment Strategy

At the start of his treatment fourteen years ago, Joe, then fifty-nine, told us that he needed to take nitroglycerin so frequently for his chronic chest pain that he had to ration the hundred nitroglycerin pills that his health plan allowed him to have each month so he didn't run out. And even though he was on several other medications his cardiologists had prescribed, he was still unable to walk even one block. He was also rather overweight, carrying 215 pounds on his five-foot-eleven-inch frame, and had all five of the disorders that define metabolic syndrome: a large waistline, high blood pressure, high blood sugar, low levels of HDL (good) cholesterol, and high triglycerides.

Although Joe needed several changes in his medications, transitioning him to more effective treatments was a gradual process. In this scenario, we only make one medication change at a time, then follow up in four to six weeks with lab or other testing to see how well the new medication is working. Managing Joe's blood pressure proved challenging since we had to try three different drugs to find one that was effective for him.

Ultimately, ramipril helped him achieve—and then exceed—the blood pressure target we'd set for him. During his first year of treatment his blood pressure gradually dropped from 150/90 to 120/70. That's a blood pressure he really can live with!

We also helped him improve his lifestyle. Like Neal, Joe had to start improving his fitness with very small steps, such as standing up during TV commercials, then marching in place and taking short walks. He also followed a gluten-free, Mediterranean diet based on his DNA and started taking some of the supplements discussed in chapter thirteen. Little by little, his health began to improve. During the second year of his treatment, after we'd finished switching him to the cornerstones of optimal medical therapy, he reported that he no longer had to ration his nitroglycerin pills, because he hardly ever needed to take them. By year three, his health metrics, including his weight, were in the normal range and he was able to resume his favorite hobbies.

Now seventy-three, Joe says that his heart is very happy. "I can go on hikes and ride horses all day in bird-dog trials without any chest pain," says the Texan. "If I hadn't found these treatments and the BaleDoneen Method, I doubt I'd still be alive today." Not only has he far outlived his father, but his heart has healed in other ways, too. Now that he's healthy again, he's rediscovered the joys of romance and sex. "I have a significant other and feel extremely thankful and fulfilled to be sharing my life with someone I care about deeply."

Making Heart-Smart Choices

While Joe's journey toward cardiovascular wellness progressed smoothly, with steady improvement year after year, Catherine, who became our patient around the same time that Joe did, encountered many challenges and faced some very difficult decisions. Initially, her numbers started to improve, but she continued her relentless schedule as a nurse-midwife and was unable to prioritize her health. "I knew I was supposed to exercise, get more sleep, improve my diet, and reduce my stress level, but babies are born at all hours and I continued to work very long shifts."

Because Catherine wasn't achieving any of the lifestyle goals we'd agreed upon, we needed to intensify her treatment to keep her safe from cardiovascular events. To protect her heart and brain, we added more medications to her treatment, and raised the dosages of some of those she was already taking. From a cardiovascular viewpoint, her treatment was working: Her arteries were cool and her plaque was starting to stabilize. However, her weight, blood pressure, and blood sugar remained too high.

"After seeing my lab results, I realized that I was making a dying, not a living—and had to stop what I was doing," she adds. "I rested for nine months—the length of a pregnancy—and thought about other ways to follow my passion for helping people." She switched to working as a midwifery instructor, but that job also proved grueling. "I was traveling from city to city observing student midwives in their clinical practice, showing them how to catch babies, and was on the computer all day long."

Once again, Catherine's weight, blood pressure, and blood sugar failed to improve. At that time, she was sixty-one and realized that her health metrics did not support her goal of a long and healthy life. A hard decision had to be made: Should she continue to dedicate every waking hour to her patients and students, when her own health was suffering, or make major lifestyle changes? Soon after that, she decided to retire and focus on her emotional, spiritual, and physical well-being. "I had an amazing work life, but it almost ended my life," she says. "I was so exhausted and stressed out that I wasn't even excited to see my patients and their babies anymore—and I used to love that."

Instead of grabbing meals on the go out of hospital vending

machines, and only working out on her rare days off, she became diligent about following a diet and exercise plan based on her DNA, including aerobic workouts, strength training, and yoga. She also dramatically changed her eating habits. "I have the gluten gene and as soon as I stopped eating foods with gluten—such as cakes, muffins, and bagels—and picked up my exercise to thirty or more minutes a day, I noticed a rapid impact," she reports. "My 'wheat belly' disappeared and my weight decreased. One day I realized that instead of being soft, weak, and chronically tired, I was actually slim and strong!"

Catherine subsequently moved to the country, got married, and became a part-time yoga instructor. She loves to take long walks in the woods and practices mindfulness every day. "I carry the heart attack gene, but at seventy, I'm healthier than I've ever been. As a nurse midwife, my purpose was to provide a safe, quiet, and sacred environment where the mother's preferences and needs were honored. Now I do the same thing for myself with a sense of optimism, gratitude, and purpose. I have an amazing husband and family and I don't want to leave them early by being too stubborn to take good care of myself."

Reimagining the Future

As we were writing this chapter, Neal came to our center for a checkup, accompanied by his wife, Anne. Two years earlier, he'd turned to us for help for the much same reasons that Joe had: Neal had also been told that his only hope for staying alive was a heart transplant and was in such excruciating pain from peripheral artery disease that he was unable to walk more than twenty-five steps. During Neal's initial evaluation, Anne was so terrified that she'd lose the love of her life—and the father of their three teenaged children—that she spent most of the visit crying.

During the checkup, Anne again wept when she reminded

us how sick Neal used to be. "After his quadruple bypass surgery, he had eleven heart catheterization procedures and every time they had to put a couple more stents into his coronary arteries," she recalls. "After one of these procedures, Neal suddenly went pale, his eyes rolled back into his head, his blood pressure dropped, and every monitor he was hooked up to started blaring. The nurse ran in and screamed, 'We're losing him!'"

After a long pause to wipe away the tears that were pouring down her face, Anne added, "After seeing the doctors working frantically to resuscitate him, I was terrified that the next time he had to go to the hospital for an invasive procedure—which happened at least once a year—he'd never come home again." Again stopping to blot her tears, Anne eventually added that she and Neal used to avoid talking about the future. "We didn't even make vacation plans and never discussed what we'd do after retirement, since we both thought I'd spend my sunset years alone, sitting on the porch with one rocking chair."

Seeing that his wife was too distraught to say anything else, Neal jumped in to talk about the astonishing progress he'd made under our care. "Not only is the heart transplant off the table, but this summer, we bought a used trailer and I'm feeling so good that I'm able to work four to six hours a day fixing it up for family vacations. It's very hot in Spokane during the summer, and for the first time in years, I was able to set up our aboveground pool so Anne and I can splash around with the kids and cool down."

Adds Anne, "Neal has so much more stamina now that he can walk a mile, with only one thirty-second pause to rest, and even took our daughter, Olivia, to the school's father-daughter dance. Previously, all he could have done was sit in a chair and watch her dance with someone else, but this time, he was able to twirl her around on the dance floor and was very proud to be doing that. He also helped our two sons earn their Boy Scout

Eagle Awards—the highest honor in scouting—which involved many physically demanding activities that would have previously been impossible for him."

Our testing confirmed that Neal's heart was extremely happy and his other health metrics have improved dramatically. His blood pressure has dropped from 145/90 to 130/70 (an excellent value for someone with obstructive CAD), he's lost twenty-five pounds, and his diabetes, OSA, and metabolic syndrome are all under optimal control. Vascular imaging revealed that his arterial plaque is now stable and lab testing revealed that his arteries are no longer on fire. Giving her husband an affectionate hug, Anne told us that Neal, who used to struggle with erectile dysfunction, also has increased stamina in the bedroom. "The other day, we were talking about how he almost has too much stamina, because he sometimes wants to make love two or three times a day, when all he could manage previously was attempting sex maybe twice a week and was often unable to maintain an erection for very long."

The couple has also regained their lust for life in other ways as well, Anne reported. "Very recently, we've started talking about *our* retirement ten to fifteen years from now. Instead of picturing myself as a lonely widow in a solitary rocking chair, we envision ourselves as a duo, holding hands as we stroll down a Caribbean beach together. Or maybe we'll travel around the U.S. in our trailer, camping out in beautiful national parks and seeing spectacular natural wonders, as we celebrate our sunset years as two soul mates who love each other so much."

Neal and Anne's story—and those of the men and women you've met in this book—are what inspires us. Their journey toward optimal health—and seeing a brighter future dawn—is ongoing. We are profoundly grateful for the opportunity to make a real difference in their health and help them live well, without constant fear of a heart attack, stroke, or dementia. Seeing these outcomes is what fuels our passion for prevention.

Anne calls Neal's improvement "miraculous" and we couldn't agree more.

Even after more than two decades of practicing the Bale-Doneen Method, we continue to marvel at the heart's amazing ability to heal and regain happiness, even in the most challenging scenarios, when it's provided with optimal medical therapy, an excellent lifestyle and genetically guided care. As you strive to improve your arterial wellness, we urge you to follow the sage advice of Martin Luther King, Jr.: "Take the first step in faith. You don't have to see the whole staircase, just take the first step."

Afterword:
Letter to the Reader

We hope that you enjoyed our book. We also hope that it has empowered you to protect and enhance your heart and brain health. Consequently, the wellness of the sixty thousand miles of blood vessels nourishing every organ and muscle in your body will be improved. If you have any questions or comments to share about the Bale-Doneen Method, the AHA for Life plan, or are interested in becoming a patient, contact us via our websites: baledoneen.com and theheartattackandstrokeprevention center.com.

Although we cannot offer specific medical advice about your case, we encourage you to be proactive about your health. Please use the recommendations in this book in conjunction with your medical and dental providers' recommendations. Work in partnership with your healthcare providers to receive the optimal personalized care that every patient deserves. The tests we recommend are available at laboratories around the country. If your provider does not suggest them, ask for them!

You and your providers can interact with us through other avenues. We speak to the public and healthcare providers around the U.S. and internationally. You can find a schedule of our upcoming events on our websites. We offer an accredited course for all clinicians in all specialties. The category 1 CME/CE (Continuing Medical Education/Continuing Education) program covers the essentials of the BaleDoneen Method and the latest peer-reviewed science on cardiovascular care and chronic disease prevention. We would love to have the opportunity to influence the care your healthcare team delivers. We encourage your providers to visit the BaleDoneen website to access many educational resources, including monthly scientific updates and recent publications.

As new research offers additional insights into the best ways to maintain cardiovascular wellness, our evidence-based prevention plan will continue to evolve. We suggest visiting our websites, signing up for our free newsletter and reading our blog, Facebook, Twitter, and Instagram pages for the latest news, study findings, and recommendations about how to protect your cardiovascular system. Our goal is to help you live a long and full life by achieving optimal arterial health.

—Bradley Bale, MD, Gallatin, Tennessee, and
Amy Doneen, DNP, Spokane, Washington

Acknowledgments

"Great things in business are never done by one person; they're done by a team of people."

— STEVE JOBS

This sagacious quote is accurate for any accomplishment. It is our pleasure to acknowledge the marvelous colleagues, friends, and patients who were instrumental in the creation of this book.

First of all, we thank our superb agent, Jessica Papin, who encouraged us to consider writing another book about cardiovascular prevention. Jessica secured the nation's oldest and most revered publisher for our book: Little, Brown. As a result, we have wonderful editors Marisa Vigilante and Fanta Diallo, who have been instrumental in getting our book to production.

Fortunately, we were able to engage Lisa Collier Cool again as our writer. She is one of the nation's most renowned health writers. She can take complicated science and make it palatable to a general audience. That ability requires a thorough understanding of the science coupled with incredible communication skills. Lisa holds a scholarly understanding of the medical literature. We thank Lisa for protecting our patients' vulnerability while writing each of their stories with honesty and integrity. It is a privilege to write this book with her.

Thanks to our patients—Babs, Camille, Casey, Catherine, Courtney, Diane G., Diane H., Dwayne, Elaine, J.P., Jack, Joe, Juli, Kellee, Melinda, Neal, Nikki, Paul, and Robert—for so generously sharing their stories in our book. We would also like to thank our patients for their trust and partnership in health over the past two decades. Their trust in us has allowed the Bale-Doneen Method to evolve.

ACKNOWLEDGMENTS

Thanks to the thousands of medical and dental providers who have participated in our CME/CE courses. Many of these clinicians are engaged with our BaleDoneen Method Academy, which supports incorporating our method into practice. These providers support our mission to enhance and save lives by offering a cure for arterial disease. We are humbled by their testimonials about the BaleDoneen Method.

Thanks to the pioneering cardiologist Dr. Paul Shields, who was one of the first cardiologists in Spokane, Washington. Decades ago, Paul's wisdom alerted us to the value of identifying asymptomatic arterial disease with imaging and taught us that inflammation was causal of atherosclerosis. These two pieces of knowledge are at the core of our method. We also want to thank one of Paul's protégés, Dr. Pierre Leimgruber, who is one of the most respected cardiologists in the country. Pierre's support over the many years boosted our courage to forge ahead. We are honored to have him now practicing prevention, utilizing the BaleDoneen Method. Thanks to the numerous scientists who have published the evidence we use in our method. They are our true heroes and mentors.

A huge thanks to our BaleDoneen COO and business partner, Randy Kembel, who is committed to enlightening everyone about our cure for arterial disease. He has enthusiastically supported our efforts and dedication to the creation of this book. We also thank our BaleDoneen clinical coach, Dr. David Wright, who provides critical aid in our academy, allowing our method to be translated into practice. Dr. Dave Vigerust provides in-depth scientific insight on numerous topics. He is a coauthor of many of our peer-reviewed manuscripts. These individuals comprise a powerful team maintaining the BaleDoneen Method at peak performance.

Brad's personal acknowledgment:
A tremendous thank-you to my daughter and nurse, Brittany Bale Woodcock, RN, BSN, who has comprehensive expertise in

our method. She is instrumental in the clinical care of my patients. Her dedication and impeccable reliability are stellar. She also periodically creates educational material for providers and patients of the method in general. My wife, Pam, was instrumental in my migration into preventative care and does a fabulous job as the administrator of my practice.

To Amy Doneen: Her collaboration and dedication for more than two decades are phenomenal. Her wisdom is only surpassed by her love and caring for others. If there is a secret to her fantastic clinical success, it rests in a quote from Theodore Roosevelt: "Nobody cares how much you know, until they know how much you care." Her birth was a precious gift to humanity. I cherish her partnership as one of my life's greatest treasures.

Amy's personal acknowledgment:
My team at the Heart Attack & Stroke Prevention Center (The HASPC) are key members of the BaleDoneen community. The dedication and care of our patients is demonstrated daily and I am so grateful to work with such amazing individuals—Karen Dominguez, Cathy Thornton, Dawn Korlock, Marin Wright, RN, BSN, Josie Shultes, Kayla Ring and Patty Neilsen. Each of you treat our patients with respect, integrity, and kindness, and I am thankful for the culture we have created. I thank Dr. Pierre Leimgruber for trusting and joining me at my center. Pierre's expertise and passion for prevention meld with his thirty-two years of traditional cardiology, creating a level of care for our patients that is exceptional.

To my business partner, collaborator, mentor, and dear friend, Bradley Bale, I cherish the twenty years we have spent together. Your love of humanity, as demonstrated through your care of patients, and passion for science, through your love of teaching others, continue to inspire me. You exemplify Kahlil Gibran's definition of work: "Work is love made visible."

About the Authors

Dr. Bradley Bale and Dr. Amy Doneen are international leaders in the prevention of heart attacks, strokes, type 2 diabetes, and chronic disease such as dementia and heart failure. They Co-founded the BaleDoneen Method in 1999, which has shown in peer-reviewed studies to effectively identify, stabilize, and reverse arterial disease. Drs. Bale and Doneen have been called "disease detectives" because their method uses leading-edge laboratory and imaging tests to check for hidden signs of arterial disease and inflammation. Using a genetic, precision-based approach, the BaleDoneen Method treats each patient as a unique and special individual. Both share academic appointments at Texas Tech Health Sciences, University of Kentucky College of Dentistry, and Washington State University College of Medicine. Dr. Doneen owns the Heart Attack & Stroke Prevention Center in Spokane Washington, seeing patients and training providers in the BaleDoneen Method.

Lisa Collier Cool is a bestselling author, blogger, and winner of twenty journalism awards. Her previous books include *Beat the Heart Attack Gene,* coauthored with Bradley Bale, MD, and Amy Doneen, DNP; and *Deliver Us From Evil: A NYC Cop Investigates the Supernatural,* coauthored with Ralph Sarchie. She has written hundreds of articles for *Good Housekeeping, Oprah Magazine, Parade, Prevention, Reader's Digest, the Wall Street Journal,* WebMD and many others.

APPENDIX

Optimal Goals And Health Metrics Chart

In the chart below, you'll find the optimal goals we recommend for the tests and cardiovascular health metrics discussed in this book, based on the latest scientific evidence from peer-reviewed research. However, no two people are exactly alike. Therefore, to achieve excellent cardiovascular outcomes, healthcare requires personalization—not standardizing the same care for everyone. It's essential to discuss your prevention and treatment goals with your provider, individualize them according to your genes, overall health, and any medical or dental conditions you may have, and then be carefully monitored with periodic follow-up visits and testing as you strive to optimize your arterial wellness.

Test	Chapter	Purpose	Optimal Range
Highly sensitive Troponin T (hsTnT)	Chapter 2	Detects if heart muscle cells are being stressed or dying.	Less than or equal to 14 ng/L
Body Mass Index	Chapter 3	Being overweight or obese increases risk for many chronic diseases, including cardiovascular disease, cancer, and joint disorders. Can cause arterial inflammation; also associated with dementia. However, it's important to know that BMI is not an accurate way to check for obesity in highly muscular or athletic individuals.	18–25

Test	Chapter	Purpose	Optimal Range
Basic lipid panel	Chapter 4	Measures levels of cholesterol, a blood fat that is the main ingredient of new plaque; also associated with dementia risk if levels are high.	Optimal levels of total cholesterol, triglycerides, HDL, and LDL as below.
Total Cholesterol	Chapter 4	Combined measurement of certain cholesterol components.	Less than 200 mg/dL
Triglycerides	Chapter 4	Measures levels of triglycerides, a type of fat, in your blood. Elevated levels can be a signal for insulin resistance and increased risk for heart attacks and strokes.	Less than 100 mg/dL
High-Density Lipoprotein (HDL)	Chapter 4	Measures levels of HDL (good) cholesterol; if levels are low, may signal insulin resistance.	Men, less than 50 mg/dL; women, less than 60 mg/dL
Low-Density Lipoprotein (LDL)	Chapter 4	Measures levels of LDL (bad) cholesterol.	Less than 70 mg/dL
Apolipoprotein B-100 (ApoB)	Chapter 4	Measures levels of ApoB, a major component of all four types of cholesterol that are most harmful to your arteries. This blood test is not included in the standard cholesterol test but can be performed at the same time. Big studies show that a strong predictor of heart attack and stroke risk is your ApoB level plus your triglyceride level.	Less than 80 mg/dL
Lipoprotein (a) Lp(a)	Chapter 4	Checks for inherited disorder marked by elevated levels of this dangerous cholesterol, which is not included in the standard cholesterol test. Elevated levels, if untreated, greatly increased heart attack and stroke risk, often at a relatively young age.	Less than 75 nmol/L

APPENDIX

Test	Chapter	Purpose	Optimal Range
Total Cholesterol/HDL Ratio (TC/HDL)	Chapter 4	Most predictive calculation for predicting risk of heart attack and stroke; calculated by dividing total cholesterol number by HDL (good) cholesterol number.	Less than 3 mg/dL
Imaging	Chapter 6	Checks for arterial disease.	No plaque (diseas)
Chart review of radiology reports, e.g., X-rays and mammograms	Chapter 6	Checks for calcified plaque. Calcium seen in any arteries proves presence of arterial disease.	No calcium reported in any arteries
Carotid Intima-Media Thickness Test (cIMT)	Chapter 6	Checks for plaque in the neck arteries (carotid) and arterial age.	No plaque; chronological to arterial age disparity < 5 years
Femoral Intimal-Media Thickness Test (fIMT)	Chapter 6	Checks for plaque in the groin arteries (femoral).	No plaque
Coronary Artery Calcium Scan (CACS)	Chapter 6	Checks for calcium in the heart arteries (coronary).	No calcium = Score of 0
Abdominal Aortic Aneurysm Scan	Chapter 6	Checks for a weak, ballooning area (aneurysm) in the main artery that carries blood away from the heart to the rest of the body (the aorta) and plaque (disease) in that artery.	Less than 3 cm in diameter and no plaque noted
Inflammatory Testing	Chapter 8	Checks for elevated levels of inflammatory biomarkers linked to increased risk for developing arterial disease or having a heart attack or stroke; elevated levels also linked to increased dementia risk.	No evidence of arterial inflammation
F2-Isoprotane/Creatinine Ratio	Chapter 8	Checks for amount of oxidative stress in the body and provides insight into the effects of patient's lifestyle.	Less than 0.86 ng/mg

APPENDIX

Test	Chapter	Purpose	Optimal Range
Microalbumin/ Creatinine Urine Ratio (MACR)	Chapter 8	Checks the wellness of the blood vessel lining, also called the endothelium (tennis court).	Men, less than 4 mg/L; women, less than 7.5 mg/L
Highly Sensitive C-Reactive Protein (hsCRP)	Chapter 8	Checks for inflammation in the body; is not specific for the endothelium, but when optimal, suggests that the tennis court is not inflamed.	Less than 0.5 mg/L
Fibrinogen	Chapter 8	Checks for inflammation in the body; is not specific for the endothelium, but when optimal, suggests that the tennis court is not inflamed. [match more streamlined language from cell above]	Less than 350 mg/dL
Lipoprotein Associated Phospholipase A-2 (Lp-PLA2)	Chapter 8	Checks for inflammation inside the artery where the plaque resides.	Less than 123 nmol/min/mL
Myeloperoxidase (MPO)	Chapter 8	Checks for very dangerous inflammation of the artery and imminent risk of a heart attack or stroke.	Less than 420 pmol/L
Insulin Resistance	Chapter 9	Check for the root cause of type 2 diabetes: insulin resistance (IR), a prediabetic condition that causes arterial inflammation. IR raises risk for heart attack, stroke, dementia, and hypertension.	Sensitive to insulin
Fasting Glucose	Chapter 9	If elevated, signals insulin resistance. Test also checks for prediabetes and diabetes.	Less than 100 mg/dL
One-hour 75 gm Oral Glucose Tolerance Test (OGTT)	Chapter 9	If elevated, signals insulin resistance and prediabetes.	Less than 125 mg/dL
Two-hour 75 gm Oral Glucose Tolerance Test	Chapter 9	Considered the gold standard for checking for diabetes, prediabetes, and insulin resistance.	Less than 120 mg/dL

Test	Chapter	Purpose	Optimal Range
Hemoglobin A1C test	Chapter 9	Measures 3-month average glucose level and may identify prediabetes or diabetes. (Less accurate than OGTT test above.)	Less than 5.7%
Triglyceride/HDL Ratio	Chapter 9	If elevated, strong signal for insulin resistance and prediabetes.	Less than 3.5 (white); Less than 3.0 (Hispanic); less than 2.0 (Black)
Oral Health Evaluation	Chapter 10	Evaluates overall oral health; checks for tooth and gum infections linked to arterial inflammation and increased dementia and prediabetes risk.	No periodontal or endodontic disease
Periodontal Chart Pocket Depth (PD); Bleeding of gums (BOP); Clinical attachment level of teeth (CAL)	Chapter 10	Three elements of periodontal exam used to identify patients with signs of periodontal disease, including loose teeth, pockets of infection, and gum bleeding.	PD less than 4 mm BOP 0 CAL less than 1 mm
Oral Pathogen Testing	Chapter 10		Absence of high-risk oral pathogens
Imaging with X-ray or computed tomography with 3D cone beam	Chapter 10	Identifies infected teeth, abscess formation at base of teeth, and may detect calcified plaque in the carotid artery.	No endodontic (tooth) infection; No calcification in the carotid artery
Genetic panel	Chapter 11	Personalize healthcare and lifestyle.	Optimal genotypes for the 5 genes below
9P21	Chapter 11	Identifies carriers of "the heart attack gene" and guides lifestyle, medication, and supplement advice to protect heart health.	Noncarrier of 9P21

Test	Chapter	Purpose	Optimal Range
Apo E	Chapter 11	Identifies Apo E genotype and people at increased genetic risk for cardiovascular disease and dementia, as well as the best lifestyle strategies to avoid these threats.	Apo E 3/3 genotype
Haptoglobin	Chapter 11	Identifies haptoglobin genotype, offering critical knowledge for type 2 diabetics to guide lifestyle advice; establish goals for glucose control and potential need for vitamin E. Also provides guidance on value of a gluten-free diet for nondiabetic patients.	Haptoglobin 1-1 genotype
KIF6	Chapter 11	Checks for presence or absence of KIF6 genetic variant. Evaluates lifetime risk of developing cardiovascular disease and provides insight into statin response.	Noncarrier of the arginine variant
4Q25	Chapter 11	Identifies inherited risk for atrial fibrillation.	Noncarrier of the 4Q25 gene
Sleep study to check for obstructive sleep apnea (OSA) and other sleep disturbances	Chapter 12	Checks for episodes of interrupted breathing (apnea) during sleep. OSA can be a root cause of high blood pressure, and can cause arterial inflammation; also associated with insulin resistance and risk for dementia.	Apnea Hypopnea Index (AHI) fewer than five events per hour. Sleep six to eight hours nightly on average without interruptions
Mental Health Screening	Chapter 13	Screens for psychological factors, including for depression, anxiety, substance abuse disorders, posttraumatic stress disorder (PTSD), and high stress levels, associated with increased risk for arterial disease, chronic inflammation, and dementia.	Good mental health and effective stress management. If screening demonstrates concern, a referral to a mental health specialist for

Test	Chapter	Purpose	Optimal Range
		Stress is defined as "being in an environment where you feel a lack of control." Your provider should also assess your use of tools for stress management techniques, such as mindfulness meditation.	formal evaluation and counseling is essential.
Waist Circumference	Chapter 13	Checks for abdominal obesity. A large waistline can be a common warning sign of insulin resistance, prediabetes, and metabolic syndrome. Too much belly fat is also linked to increased risk for arterial disease, dementia, cancer, and other chronic diseases.	Men, less than 40 inches; women, less than 35 inches
Vitamin D Blood Test	Chapter 14	When low, it can cause arterial inflammation; also associated with insulin resistance and increased risk for heart disease, dementia, certain cancers, and other chronic conditions.	Less than 30 ng/mL
Blood Pressure	Chapter 15	Measures levels of systolic and diastolic blood pressure. If elevated, can cause arterial inflammation; also associated with dementia, heart attack, and many chronic diseases. High blood pressure is the number one risk factor for stroke.	Less than 120/80 mm Hg in healthy individuals
Pharmacogenetic Panel	Chapter 15	Identifies which medications and supplements are genetically best for patients and offers insight into most effective dosages.	Genotype and allele for metabolism
N-terminal Pro Brain Naturetic Peptide (NT-ProBNP)	Chapter 15	"Happy heart" test to evaluate health of the heart; if abnormal, may signal inadequate blood flow to heart, faulty heart valves, arrhythmia, or heart failure.	Less than 125 pg/mL

NOTES

Introduction

1. Centers for Disease Control and Prevention, "Heart Disease Facts," https://www.cdc.gov/heartdisease/facts.htm.
2. A. Doneen, "The Relationship between Electron Beam Computed Tomography Calcium Scores and Established Clinical and Serologic Risk Factors for Coronary Artery Disease," University Press (2003), Gonzaga University.

Chapter 1: A Plan That Is Guaranteed to Prevent Heart Attacks and Strokes

1. U.S. Department of Health and Human Services, Centers for Disease Control and Prevention, "Heart Disease Facts," https://www.cdc.gov/heartdisease/facts.htm.
2. Centers for Disease Control and Prevention, "Stroke Facts," https://www.cdc.gov/stroke/facts.htm.
3. M. Sanz et al., "Scientific Evidence on the Links Between Periodontal Diseases and Diabetes: Consensus Report and Guidelines of the Joint Workshop On Periodontal Diseases and Diabetes by the International Diabetes Federation and the European Federation of Periodontology," *Diabetes Research and Clinical Practice* 137 (2018): 231–41; Y. Zadik et al., "Erectile Dysfunction Might Be Associated with Chronic Periodontal Disease: Two Ends of the Cardiovascular Spectrum," *The Journal of Sexual Medicine*, 6, no. 4 (2009): 1111–16.
4. Yao-Tung Lee et al., "Periodontitis as a Modifiable Risk Factor for Dementia: A Nationwide Population-Based Cohort Study," *Journal of the American Geriatrics Society* 65, no. 2 (February 2017): 301–5; James M. Noble, Nikolaos Scarmeas, and Panos N. Papapanou, "Poor Oral Health as a Chronic, Potentially Modifiable Dementia Risk Factor: Review of the Literature," *Current Neurology and Neuroscience Reports,* no. 13 (August 2013): 384; S. L. Arvikar et al., "Clinical Correlations with Porphyromonas gingivalis Antibody Responses in Patients with Early Rheumatoid

Arthritis," *Arthritis Research & Therapy* 15, no. 5 (2013): R109; J. L. Freudenheim et al., "Periodontal Disease and Breast Cancer: Prospective Cohort Study of Postmenopausal Women," *Cancer, Epidemiology, Biomarkers & Prevention* 25, no. 1 (2016): 43–50; Y. W. Han, "Fusobacterium nucleatum: A Commensal-Turned Pathogen," *Current Opinion in Microbiology* 23 (2015): 141–47; J. Koziel et al., "The Link between Periodontal Disease and Rheumatoid Arthritis: An Updated Review," *Current Rheumatology Reports*, 16, no. 3 (2014): 1; D. S. Michaud et al., "A Prospective Study of Periodontal Disease and Pancreatic Cancer in US Male Health Professionals," *Journal of the National Cancer Institute* 99, no. 2 (2007): 171–75; B. A. Peters et al., "Oral Microbiome Composition Reflects Prospective Risk for Esophageal Cancers," *Cancer Research* 77, no. 23 (2017): 6777–87; E. L. Vander Haar et al., "Fusobacterium Nucleatum and Adverse Pregnancy Outcomes: Epidemiological and Mechanistic Evidence," *Anaerobe* 50 (2018): 55–59.

5. G. Livingston et al., "Dementia Prevention, Intervention, and Care: 2020 Report of the *Lancet* Commission," *The Lancet* 396, no. 10248 (2020): 413–46; World Health Organization, "Risk Reduction of Cognitive Decline and Dementia," *WHO Guidelines* (2019), https://www.who.int/mental_health/neurology/dementia/guidelines_risk_reduction/en/.

6. H. G. Cheng et al., "Effect of Comprehensive Cardiovascular Disease Risk Management on Longitudinal Changes in Carotid Artery Intima-Media Thickness in a Community-Based Prevention Clinic," *Archives of Medical Science* 4, no. 4 (2016): 728–35.

7. Du Feng et al., "8-Year Outcomes of a Program for Early Prevention of Cardiovascular Events: A Growth-Curve Analysis," *Journal of Cardiovascular Nursing* 30, no. 4 (July–August 2014): 281–91.

8. Y. B. Pride et al., "Prevalence, Consequences, and Implications for Clinical Trials of Unrecognized Myocardial Infarction," *The American Journal of Cardiology* 111, no. 6 (2013): 914–18; W. T. Qureshi et al., "Silent Myocardial Infarction and Long-Term Risk of Heart Failure: The ARIC Study," *Journal of the American College of Cardiology* 71, no. 1 (2018): 1–8; J. P. Fanning et al., "Emerging Spectra of Silent Brain Infarction." *Stroke* 45 (2014): 3461–71; A. E. Merkler et al., "Association between Unrecognized Myocardial Infarction and Cerebral Infarction on Magnetic Resonance Imaging," *JAMA Neurology* 76, no. 8 (2019): 956; T. Acharya et al., "Association of Unrecognized Myocardial Infarction with Long-Term Outcomes in Community-Dwelling Older Adults," *JAMA Cardiology* 3, no. 11 (2018): 1101.

9. American Heart Association, "Living Longer Is Important, but Those Years Need to Be Healthy Ones," January 29, 2020, https://newsroom.heart.org/news/living-longer-is-important-but-those-years-need-to-be-healthy-ones.

10. Cheryl D. Fryar, Teng-Ching Chen, and Xiafen Li, "Prevalence of Uncontrolled Risk Factors for Cardiovascular Disease: United States, 1999–2010," *NCHS Data Brief*, no. 103 (August 2012), https://pubmed.ncbi.nlm.nih.gov/23101933/.

Chapter 2: Arterial Health Assurance (AHA) for Life Program

1. Center for Disease Control and Prevention, "Peripheral Arterial Disease (PAD)," https://www.cdc.gov/heartdisease /PAD.htm; Salim S. Virani et al., "Heart Disease and Stroke Statistics—2020 Update: A Report from the American Heart Association," *Circulation* 141, no. 9 (March 2020): e139–e596.

2. Betsy McKay, "Heart Attack at 49—America's Biggest Killer Makes a Deadly Comeback," *The Wall Street Journal*, June 21, 2019; Sadiya S. Kahn et al., "Association of Body Mass Index with Lifetime Risk of Cardiovascular Disease and Compression of Morbidity," *Cardiology* 3, no. 4 (April 2018): 280–87.

3. Samuel S. Gidding and Jennifer Robinson, "It Is Now Time to Focus on Risk before Age 40," *Journal of the American College of Cardiology* 74, no. 3 (July 2019): 342–45.

4. Robert H. Eckel and Michael J. Blaha, "Cardiometabolic Medicine: A Call for a New Subspecialty Training Track in Internal Medicine," *The American Journal of Medicine* 132, no. 7 (July 2019): 788–90.

5. Ibid.

6. Ibid.

7. Matthew D. Ritchey et al., "US Trends in Premature Heart Disease Mortality over the Past 50 Years: Where Do We Go from Here?," *Trends in Cardiovascular Medicine* 30, no. 6 (August 2020): 364–74.

8. Craig M. Hales et al., "Prevalence of Obesity and Severe Obesity among Adults: United States, 2017–2018," *NCHS Data Brief*, no. 360 (February 2020): 1–8.

9. Pilar Garrido et al., "Proposal for the Creation of a National Strategy for Precision Medicine in Cancer: A Position Statement of SEOM, SEAP, and SEFH," *Clinical and Translational Oncology* 20, no. 4 (April 2018): 443–47.

10. Marcus A. DeWood et al., "Coronary Arteriographic Findings Soon after Non-Q-Wave Myocardial Infarction," *New England Journal of Medicine* 315, no. 7, (August 1986): 417–23.

11. Michael J. Davies, "The Pathophysiology of Acute Coronary Syndromes," *Heart* 83, no. 3 (March 2000): 361–66; Miranda C. A. Kramer et al., "Relationship of Thrombus Healing to Underlying Plaque Morphology in Sudden Coronary Death," *Journal of the American College of Cardiology* 55, no. 2 (January 2010): 122–32.

12. Erling Falk, Prediman K. Shah, and Valentin Fuster, "Coronary Plaque Disruption," *Circulation* 92, no. 3 (August 1995): 657–71; Renu Virmani et al., "Lessons from Sudden Coronary Death: A Comprehensive Morphological Classification Scheme for Atherosclerotic Lesions," *Arteriosclerosis Thrombosis, and Vascular Biology* 20, no. 5 (May 2000): 1262–75; Annachiara Aldrovandi et al., "Computed Tomography Coronary Angiography in Patients with

Acute Myocardial Infarction with Significant Coronary Stenosis," *Circulation* 126, no. 25 (December 2012): 3000–3007.

13. Alexander E. Merkler et al., "Association between Unrecognized Myocardial Infarction and Cerebral Infarction on Magnetic Resonance Imaging," *Neurology* 76, no. 8 (August 2019): 956–61; Tushar Acharya et al., "Association of Unrecognized Myocardial Infarction with Long-Term Outcomes in Community-Dwelling Older Adults," *Cardiology* 3, no. 11 (November 2018): 1101–6; Yuri B. Pride, Bryan J. Piccirillo, and C. Michael Gibson, "Prevalence, Consequences, and Implications for Clinical Trials of Unrecognized Myocardial Infarction," *The American Journal of Cardiology* 111, no. 6 (March 2013): 914–18; Waqas T. Qureshi et al., "Silent Myocardial Infarction and Long-Term Risk of Heart Failure: The ARIC Study," *Journal of the American College of Cardiology* 71, no. 1 (January 2018): 1–8; Juha H. Vähätalo et al., "Association of Silent Myocardial Infarction and Sudden Cardiac Death," *Cardiology* 4, no. 8 (August 2019): 796–802.

14. Eric E. Smith et al., "Prevention of Stroke in Patients with Silent Cerebrovascular Disease: A Scientific Statement for Healthcare Professionals from the American Heart Association/American Stroke Association," *Stroke* 48, no. 2 (February 2017): e44–71.

15. B. M. Everett et al., "High Sensitivity Cardiac Troponin I and B-Type Natriuretic Peptide as Predictors of Vascular Events in Primary Prevention: Impact of Statin Therapy, *Circulation* 131, no. 2 (2015): 1851–60.

16. D. Tsounis et al., "High Sensitivity Troponin in Cardiovascular Disease: Is There More Than a Marker of Myocardial Death?" *Current Topics in Medicinal Chemistry* 13, no. 2 (2013): 201–15.

17. Alan S. Go et al., "Heart Disease and Stroke Statistics—2014 Update: A Report from the American Heart Association," *Circulation* 129, no. 3 (January 2014): e28–292.

18. Damiano Baldassarre et al., "Measurements of Carotid Intima-Media Thickness and of Interadventitia Common Carotid Diameter Improve Prediction of Cardiovascular Events: Results of the IMPROVE (Carotid Intima Media Thickness [IMT] and IMT-Progression as Predictors of Vascular Events in a High Risk European Population) Study," *Journal of the American College of Cardiology* 60, no. 16 (October 2012): 1489–99; Joseph F. Polak et al., "Carotid-Wall Intima-Media Thickness and Cardiovascular Events," *New England Journal of Medicine* 365, no. 3 (July 2011): 213–21; Arie Steinvil et al., "Impact of Carotid Atherosclerosis on the Risk of Adverse Cardiac Events in Patients with and without Coronary Disease," *Stroke* 45, no. 8 (August 2014): 2311–17; Jae Hoon Moon et al., "Carotid Intima-Media Thickness Is Associated with the Progression of Cognitive Impairment in Older Adults," *Stroke* 46, no. 4 (April 2015): 1024–30; Pavla Cermakova et al., "Carotid Intima–Media Thickness and Markers of Brain Health in a Biracial Middle-Aged Cohort: CARDIA Brain MRI Sub-study," *The Journals of Gerontology: Series A* 75 (February 2019): 380–86.

19. Wanda Y. Wu et al., "Recent Trends in Acute Myocardial Infarction among the Young," *Current Opinion in Cardiology* 35, no. 5 (September 2020): 524–30.

20. Mary G. George, Xin Tong, and Barbara A. Bowman, "Prevalence of Cardiovascular Risk Factors and Strokes in Younger Adults," *Neurology* 7, no. 6 (June 2017): 695–703.

21. Robert S. Rosenson and Christine C. Tangney, "Antiatherothrombotic Properties of Statins: Implications for Cardiovascular Event Reduction," *Journal of the American Medical Association* 279, no. 20 (May 1998): 1643–50; David J. Maron, Sergio Fazio, and MacRae F. Linton, "Current Perspectives on Statins," *Circulation* 101, no. 2 (January 2000): 207–13; Peter S. Sever et al., "Prevention of Coronary and Stroke Events with Atorvastatin in Hypertensive Patients Who Have Average or Lower-Than-Average Cholesterol Concentrations, in the Anglo-Scandinavian Cardiac Outcomes Trial-Lipid Lowering Arm (ASCOT-LLA): A Multicentre Randomised Controlled Trial," *The Lancet* 361, no. 9364 (April 2003): 1149–58; Nicholas J. Leeper et al., "Statin Use in Patients with Extremely Low Low-Density Lipoprotein Levels Is Associated with Improved Survival," *Circulation* 116, no. 6 (August 2007): 613–18; Paul M. Ridker et al., "Rosuvastatin to Prevent Vascular Events in Men and Women with Elevated C-Reactive Protein," *New England Journal of Medicine* 359, no. 21 (November 2008): 2195–207; Pasquale Pignatelli et al., "Immediate Antioxidant and Antiplatelet Effect of Atorvastatin Via Inhibition of Nox2," *Circulation* 126, no. 1 (July 2012): 92–103; Harvey D. White et al., "Changes in Lipoprotein-Associated Phospholipase A2 Activity Predict Coronary Events and Partly Account for the Treatment Effect of Pravastatin: Results from the Long-Term Intervention with Pravastatin in Ischemic Disease Study," *Journal of the American Heart Association* 2, no. 5 (September 2013): e000360; Parmanand Singh et al., "Coronary Plaque Morphology and the Anti-Inflammatory Impact of Atorvastatin: A Multicenter 18F-Fluorodeoxyglucose Positron Emission Tomographic/Computed Tomographic Study," *Circulation: Cardiovascular Imaging* 9, no. 12 (December 2016): e004195; Diego F. Gualtero et al., "Rosuvastatin Inhibits Interleukin (IL)-8 and IL-6 Production in Human Coronary Artery Endothelial Cells Stimulated with Aggregatibacter actinomycetemcomitans Serotype b," *Journal of Periodontology* 88, no. 2 (February 2017): 225–35.

22. Paul M. Ridker et al., "Anti-inflammatory Therapy with Canakinumab for Atherosclerotic Disease," *New England Journal of Medicine* 377, no. 12 (September 2017): 1119–31.

23. Bradley F. Bale, Amy L. Doneen, and David J. Vigerust, "High-Risk Periodontal Pathogens Contribute to the Pathogenesis of Atherosclerosis," *Postgrad Medical Journal* 93, no. 1098 (April 2017): 215–20.

24. Carl J. Lavie, John H. Lee, and Richard V. Milani, "Vitamin D and Cardiovascular Disease: Will It Live Up to Its Hype?" *Journal of the American College of Cardiology* 58, no. 15 (October 2011): 1547–56;

Samantha M. Kimball et al., "Retrospective Analysis of Cardiovascular Disease Risk Parameters in Participants of a Preventive Health and Wellness Program," *Integrative Medicine: A Clinicians Journal* 18, no. 3 (June 2019): 78–95; Banaz Al-Khalidi et al., "Standardized Serum 25-Hydroxyvitamin D Concentrations Are Inversely Associated with Cardiometabolic Disease in U.S. Adults: A Cross-Sectional Analysis of NHANES, 2001–2010," *Nutrition Journal* 16, no. 1 (February 2017): 16; Thomas J. Littlejohns et al., "Vitamin D and the Risk of Dementia and Alzheimer Disease," *Neurology* 83, no. 10 (September 2014): 920–28.

25. Edward Giovannucci et al., "25-Hydroxyvitamin D and Risk of Myocardial Infarction in Men: A Prospective Study," *Archives of Internal Medicine* 168, no. 11 (June 2008): 1174–80; Peter Brøndum-Jacobsen et al., "25-Hydroxyvitamin D Levels and Risk of Ischemic Heart Disease, Myocardial Infarction, and Early Death," *Arteriosclerosis, Thrombosis, and Vascular Biology* 32, no. 11 (November 2012): 2794–802.

26. Olivier Milleron et al., "Benefits of Obstructive Sleep Apnoea Treatment in Coronary Artery Disease: A Long-Term Follow-Up Study," *European Heart Journal* 25, no. 9 (May 2004): 728–34; Francisco Campos-Rodriguez et al., "Cardiovascular Mortality in Women with Obstructive Sleep Apnea with or without Continuous Positive Airway Pressure Treatment: A Cohort Study," *Annals of Internal Medicine* 156 no. 2 (January 2012): 115–22; Yosuke Nishihata et al., "Continuous Positive Airway Pressure Treatment Improves Cardiovascular Outcomes in Elderly Patients with Cardiovascular Disease and Obstructive Sleep Apnea," *Heart Vessels* 30, no. 1 (January 2015): 61–69; Christina Parsons et al., "The Efficacy of Continuous Positive Airway Pressure Therapy in Reducing Cardiovascular Events in Obstructive Sleep Apnea: A Systematic Review," *Future Cardiology* 13, no. 4 (July 2017): 397–412; Minna Myllylä et al., "Nonfatal and Fatal Cardiovascular Disease Events in CPAP Compliant Obstructive Sleep Apnea Patients," *Sleep Breath* 23, no. 4 (December 2019): 1209–17; Kazuo Chin et al., "Falls in Blood Pressure in Patients with Obstructive Sleep Apnoea after Long-Term Nasal Continuous Positive Airway Pressure Treatment," *Journal of Hypertension* 24, no. 10 (October 2006): 2091–99; Kensaku Aihara et al., "Long-Term Nasal Continuous Positive Airway Pressure Treatment Lowers Blood Pressure in Patients with Obstructive Sleep Apnea Regardless of Age," *Hypertension Research* 33, no. 10 (July 2010): 1025–31.

Chapter 3: The New Red Flags for Heart Attack, Stroke, and Dementia Risk

1. Erica C. Leifheit-Limson et al., "Sex Differences in Cardiac Risk Factors, Perceived Risk, and Health Care Provider Discussion of Risk and Risk Modification among Young Patients with Acute Myocardial Infarction: The VIRGO Study," *Journal of the American College of Cardiology* 66, no. 18 (November 2015): 1949–57.

2. "AHA News: High Blood Pressure Top Risk Factor for Stroke in Young Adults," *U.S. News,* February 5, 2019, https://www.usnews.com/news /health-news/articles/2019-02-05/aha-news-high-blood-pressure-top -risk-factor-for-stroke-in-young-adults.

3. Mark J. Pletcher et al., "Young Adult Exposure to Cardiovascular Risk Factors and Risk of Events Later in Life: The Framingham Offspring Study," *Plos One* 11, no. 5 (May 2016): e0154288.

4. Véronique L. Roger et al., "Heart Disease and Stroke Statistics—2012 Update: A Report from the American Heart Association," *Circulation* 125, no. 1 (January 2012): e2–220; Society of Nuclear Medicine, "Many Die of Heart Attacks without Prior History or Symptoms: PET Imaging Can Offer Early Warning," *ScienceDaily* (June 2008), https://www .sciencedaily.com/releases/2008/06/080616124938.htm; American Heart Association, "Common Myths about Heart Disease," Go Red for Women, https://www.goredforwomen.org/en/about-heart-disease-in-women /facts/common-myths-about-heart-disease.

5. Judith H. Lichtman et al., "Sex Differences in the Presentation and Perception of Symptoms among Young Patients with MI: VIRGO Study," *Circulation* 137, no. 8 (February 2018): 781–90.

6. Jean C. McSweeney et al., "Women's Early Warning Symptoms of Acute Myocardial Infarction," *Circulation* 108, no. 21 (November 2003): 2619–23.

7. Ann Smith Barnes, "The Epidemic of Obesity and Diabetes: Trends and Treatments," *Texas Heart Institute Journal* 38, no. 2 (2011): 142–44.

8. Maren T. Scheuner et al., "Expanding the Definition of a Positive Family History for Early-Onset Coronary Heart Disease," *Genetics in Medicine* 8 (August 2006): 491–501; Justin M. Bachmann et al., "Association between Family History and Coronary Heart Disease Death across Long-Term Follow-Up in Men: The Cooper Center Longitudinal Study," *Circulation* 125, no. 25 (June 2012): 3092–98; Donald M. Lloyd-Jones et al., "Parental Cardiovascular Disease as a Risk Factor for Cardiovascular Disease in Middle-Aged Adults: A Prospective Study of Parents and Offspring," *Journal of the American Medical Association* 291, no. 18 (May 2004): 2204–11.

9. Martin Reriani et al., "Microvascular Endothelial Dysfunction Predicts the Development of Erectile Dysfunction in Men with Coronary Atherosclerosis without Critical Stenoses," *Coronary Artery Disease* 25, no. 7 (November 2014): 552–57; S. M. Iftekhar Uddin et al., "Erectile Dysfunction as an Independent Predictor of Future Cardiovascular Events: The Multi-Ethnic Study of Atherosclerosis," *Circulation* 138, no. 5 (July 2018): 540–42.

10. Binghao Zhao et al., "Erectile Dysfunction Predicts Cardiovascular Events as an Independent Risk Factor: A Systematic Review and Meta-Analysis," *The Journal of Sexual Medicine* 16, no. 7 (July 2019): 1005–17.

11. Ann I. Scher and Lenore J. Launer, "Migraine with Aura Increases the Risk of Stroke," *Nature Reviews Neurology* 6, no. 3 (March 2010): 128–29.

12. Tobias Kurth et al., "Migraine, Vascular Risk, and Cardiovascular Events in Women: Prospective Cohort Study," *British Medical Journal* 337 (August 2008): a636.

13. Bradley F. Bale, Amy L. Doneen, and David J. Vigerust, "High-Risk Periodontal Pathogens Contribute to the Pathogenesis of Atherosclerosis," *Postgraduate Medical Journal* 93 (April 2017): 215–20.

14. Chang-Kai Chen, Yung-Tsan Wu, & Yu-Chao Chang, "Association between Chronic Periodontitis and the Risk of Alzheimer's Disease: A Retrospective, Population-Based, Matched-Cohort Study," *Alzheimer's Research & Therapy* 9, no. 56 (August 2017); Mark Ide et al., "Periodontitis and Cognitive Decline in Alzheimer's Disease," *PLoS One* 11, no. 3 (March 2016): e0151081.

15. Mara Roxana Rubinstein et al., "Fusobacterium Nucleatum Promotes Colorectal Carcinogenesis by Modulating E-cadherin/β-catenin Signaling Via Its FadA Adhesin," *Cell Host Microbe* 14, no. 2 (August 2013): 195–206; S. Kaur, S. White, and P. M. Bartold, "Periodontal Disease and Rheumatoid Arthritis: A Systematic Review," *Journal of Dental Research* 92, no. 5 (March 2013): 399–408; Manoj Kumar et al., "Diabetes and Gum Disease: The Diabolic Duo," *Diabetes and Metabolic Syndrome* 8, no. 4 (October 2014): 255–58.

16. Nadya Marouf et al., "Association between Periodontitis and Severity of COVID-19 Infection: A Case-Control Study," *Journal of Clinical Periodontology* 48, no. 4 (April 2021): 483–91.

17. Joel M. Gelfand et al., "Risk of Myocardial Infarction in Patients with Psoriasis," *Journal of the American Medical Association* 296, no. 14 (October 2006): 1735–41; Julia Shlyankevich et al., "Accumulating Evidence for the Association and Shared Pathogenic Mechanisms between Psoriasis and Cardiovascular-Related Comorbidities," *The American Journal of Medicine* 127, no. 12 (December 2014): 1148–53.

18. Alex Dregan et al., "Chronic Inflammatory Disorders and Risk of Type 2 Diabetes Mellitus, Coronary Heart Disease, and Stroke," *Circulation* 130, no. 10 (September 2014): 837–44.

19. Philip M. Carlucci et al., "Neutrophil Subsets and Their Gene Signature Associate with Vascular Inflammation and Coronary Atherosclerosis in Lupus," *Journal of Clinical Investigation Insight* 3, no. 8 (April 2018): e99276.

20. José L. Peñalvo et al., "Association between a Social-Business Eating Pattern and Early Asymptomatic Atherosclerosis," *Journal of the American College of Cardiology* 68, no. 8 (August 2016): 805–14.

21. Wei-Shih Huang et al., "Association of Gout with CAD and Effect of Antigout Therapy on CVD Risk among Gout Patients," *Journal of Investigative Medicine* 68, no. 5 (June 2020): 972–79.

22. Neha J. Pagidipati et al., "Association of Gout with Long-Term Cardiovascular Outcomes among Patients with Obstructive Coronary Artery Disease," *Journal of the American Heart Association* 7, no. 16 (August 2018): e009328.

23. Lorna E. Clarson et al., "Increased Risk of Vascular Disease Associated with Gout: A Retrospective, Matched Cohort Study in the UK Clinical

Practice Research Datalink," *Annals of the Rheumatic Diseases* 74, no. 4 (August 2014): 642–47.

24. Wei-Shih Huang et al., "Association of Gout with CAD and Effect of Antigout Therapy on CVD Risk among Gout Patients," *Journal of Investigative Medicine* 68, no. 5 (June 2020): 972–79.

25. M. Kivimaki et al., "Long Working Hours and Risk of Coronary Heart Disease and Stroke: A Systematic Review and Meta-Analysis of Published and Unpublished Data for 603,838 Individuals," *The Lancet* 386 (2015): 1739–46.

26. M. Shields, "Long Working Hours and Health," *Health Reports* 11, no. 2 (Autumn 1999): 33–48.

27. Duk Won Bang et al., "Asthma Status and Risk of Incident Myocardial Infarction: A Population-Based Case-Control Study," *The Journal of Allergy and Clinical Immunology in Practice* 4, no. 5 (September–October 2016): 917–23.

28. Matthew C. Tattersall et al., "Asthma Predicts Cardiovascular Disease Events: The Multi-Ethnic Study of Atherosclerosis," *Arteriosclerosis, Thrombosis, and Vascular Biology* 35, no. 6 (June 2015): 1520–25.

29. Augusto A. Litonjua et al., "Parental History and the Risk for Childhood Asthma: Does Mother Confer More Risk Than Father? *American Journal of Respiratory Critical Care Medicine* 158, no. 1 (July 1998): 176–81.

30. Daniel H. Solomon et al., "Cardiovascular Morbidity and Mortality in Women Diagnosed with Rheumatoid Arthritis," *Circulation* 107, no. 9 (March 2003): 13037; Lewis H. Kuller et al., "Inflammatory and Coagulation Biomarkers and Mortality in Patients with HIV Infection," *PLoS Medicine* 5, no. 10 (October 2008): 1496–1508

31. Matthew E. Dupre et al., "Association between Divorce and Risks for Acute Myocardial Infarction," *Circulation: Cardiovascular Quality and Outcomes* 8, no. 3 (May 2015): 244–51.

32. Alan Rozanski et al., "Association of Optimism with Cardiovascular Events and All-Cause Mortality: A Systematic Review and Meta-Analysis," *JAMA Network Open* 2, no. 9 (September 2019): e1912200.

33. Ersilia Lucenteforte et al., "Ear Lobe Crease as a Marker of Coronary Artery Disease: A Meta-Analysis," *International Journal of Cardiology* 175, no. 1 (April 2014): 171–75.

34. S. T. Frank, "Aural Sign of Coronary-Artery Disease," *New England Journal of Medicine* 289, no. 6 (August 1973): 327–28.

35. J. S. Christiansen et al., "Diagonal Ear-Lobe Crease in Coronary Heart Disease," *New England Journal of Medicine* 293, no. 6 (August 1975): 3089; Y. Shoenfeld et al., "Diagonal Ear Lobe Crease and Coronary Risk Factors," *Journal of the American Geriatric Society* 28, no. 4 (April 1980): 184–87; Harun Evrengül et al., "Bilateral Diagonal Earlobe Crease and Coronary Artery Disease: A Significant Association," *Dermatology* 209, no. 4 (November 2004): 271–75; Y. Kobayashi et al., "The Evaluation of the Diagonal Ear Lobe Crease (ELC) as a Atherosclerotic Sign," *Nihon Ronen Igakkai Zasshi* 24, no. 6 (November 1987): 525–31; Aris P. Agouridis et al.,

"Ear Lobe Crease: A Marker of Coronary Artery Disease?" *Archives of Medical Science* 11, no. 6 (December 2015): 1145–55.

36. Mette Christoffersen et al., "Visible Age-Related Signs and Risk of Ischemic Heart Disease in the General Population: A Prospective Cohort Study," *Circulation* 129, no. 9 (March 2014): 990–98.

37. Ragip Ertas et al., "Androgenetic Alopecia as an Indicator of Metabolic Syndrome and Cardiovascular Risk," *Blood Pressure* 25, no. 3 (June 2016): 141–48.

38. Jane H. Lock, Carolyn A. Ross, and Maree Flaherty, "Corneal Arcus as the Presenting Sign of Familial Hypercholesterolemia," *Journal of American Association for Pediatric Ophthalmology and Strabismus* 22, no. 6 (December 2018): 467–68.

39. "Familial Hypercholesterolemia," National Organization for Rare Diseases, https://rarediseases.org/rare-diseases/familial-hypercholes terolemia/

40. Mette Christoffersen et al., "Xanthelasmata, Arcus Corneae, and Ischaemic Vascular Disease and Death in General Population: Prospective Cohort Study," *British Medical Journal* 343 (September 2011): db497.

Chapter 4: How Faulty Medical Guidelines Harm "Healthy" Patients

1. Damiano Baldassarre et al., "Measurement of Carotid Intima-Media Thickness in Dyslipidemic Patients Increases the Power of Traditional Risk Factors to Predict Cardiovascular Events," *Atherosclerosis* 191, no. 2 (April 2007): 403–38; Mario De Michele, Daniel J. Zaccaro, and Gene Bond, "Assessment of Carotid Intima-Media Thickness in Subjects with Ischemic Cerebrovascular Events Undergoing Endarterectomy," *Nutrition, Metabolism, Cardiovascular Diseases* 16, no. 8 (April 2006): 536–42.

2. Alexander C. Fanaroff et al., "Levels of Evidence Supporting American College of Cardiology/American Heart Association and European Society of Cardiology Guidelines, 2008–2018," *Journal of the American Medical Association* 321, no. 11 (March 2019): 1069–80; Donna K. Arnett et al., "2019 ACC/AHA Guideline on the Primary Prevention of Cardiovascular Disease: A Report of the American College of Cardiology/American Heart Association Task Force on Clinical Practice Guidelines," *Circulation* 140, no. 11 (March 2019): e596–646; Kevin M. Johnson and David A. Dowe, "The Detection of Any Coronary Calcium Outperforms Framingham Risk Score as a First Step in Screening for Coronary Atherosclerosis," *American Journal of Roentgenology* 194, no. 5 (May 2010): 1235–43; Khurram Nasir et al., "Comprehensive Coronary Risk Determination in Primary Prevention: An Imaging and Clinical Based Definition Combining Computed Tomographic Coronary Artery Calcium Score and National Cholesterol Education Program Risk Score," *International Journal of Cardiology* 110, no. 2 (June 2006): 129–36.

3. Naveen Garg et al., "Comparison of Different Cardiovascular Risk Score Calculators for Cardiovascular Risk Prediction and Guideline Recommended Statin Uses," *Indian Heart Journal* 69, no. 4 (July–August 2017): 458–63.

4. Matthew C. Tattersall et al., "Women Up, Men Down: The Clinical Impact of Replacing the Framingham Risk Score with the Reynolds Risk Score in the United States Population," *PLoS One* 7, no. 9 (September 2012): e44347.

5. Michael R. Langlois and Joris R. Delanghe, "Biological and Clinical Significance of Haptoglobin Polymorphism in Humans," *Clinical Chemistry* 41, no. 10 (October 1996): 1589–1600.

6. Scott M. Grundy et al., "AHA/ACC/AACVPR/AAPA/ABC/ACPM/ ADA/AGS/APhA/ASPC/NLA/PCNA Guideline on the Management of Blood Cholesterol: A Report of the American College of Cardiology/ American Heart Association Task Force on Clinical Practice Guidelines," *Circulation* 139, no. 25 (June 2019): e1082–1143.

7. Allan D. Sniderman et al., "Apolipoprotein B Particles and Cardiovascular Disease: A Narrative Review," *Cardiology* 4, no 12 (December 2019): 1287–95.

8. Wei-Qi Wei et al., "LAP Variants Are Associated with Residual Cardiovascular Risk in Patients Receiving Statins," *Circulation* 138, no. 17 (April 2018): 1839–49.

9. Byambaa Enkhmaa et al., "Lipoprotein(a): Genotype-Phenotype Relationship and Impact on Atherogenic Risk," *Metabolic Syndrome and Related Disorders* 9, no. 6 (July 2011): 411–18.

10. Anahad O'Connor, "A Heart Risk Factor Even Doctors Know Little About," *New York Times,* January 9, 2018.

11. Karim El Harchaoui et al., "Value of Low-Density Lipoprotein Particle Number and Size as Predictors of Coronary Artery Disease in Apparently Healthy Men and Women: The EPIC-Norfolk Prospective Population Study," *Journal of the American College of Cardiology* 49, no. 5 (February 2007): 547–53; Samia Mora et al., "Atherogenic Lipoprotein Subfractions Determined by Ion Mobility and First Cardiovascular Events after Random Allocation to High-Intensity Statin or Placebo: The JUPITER Trial," *Circulation* 132, no. 23 (December 2015): 2220–29.

12. John T. Wilkins et al., "Discordance between Apolipoprotein B and LDL-Cholesterol in Young Adults Predicts Coronary Artery Calcification: The CARDIA Study," *Journal of the American College of Cardiology* 67, no. 2 (January 2016): 193–201.

13. Samia Mora et al., "On-Treatment Non-High-Density Lipoprotein Cholesterol, Apolipoprotein B, Triglycerides, and Lipid Ratios in Relation to Residual Vascular Risk after Treatment with Potent Statin Therapy: JUPITER (Justification for the Use of Statins in Prevention: An Intervention Trial Evaluating Rosuvastatin)," *Journal of the American College of Cardiology* 59, no. 17 (April 2012): 1521–28.

14. A. Tirosh et al., "Changes in Triglyceride Levels over Time and Risk of Type 2 Diabetes in Young Men," *Diabetes Care* 31, no. 110 (October 2008): 2032–37.
15. A. Khan et al., "Cinnamon Improves Glucose and Lipids of People with Type 2 Diabetes," *Diabetes Care* 26, no. 12 (December 2003): 3215–18.
16. R. Akilen et al., "Glycated Haemoglobin and Blood Pressure-Lowering Effect of Cinnamon in Multi-Ethnic Type 2 Diabetic Patients in the UK: A Randomized, Placebo-Controlled, Double-Blind Clinical Trial," *Diabetic Medicine* 27, no. 10 (October 2010): 1159–67.
17. Mohammadreza Vafa et al., "Effects of cinnamon consumption on glycemic status, lipid profile and body composition in type 2 diabetic patients," *International Journal of Preventive Medicine* 3, no. 8 (2012): 531–36.
18. "Calculator: Cardiovascular Risk Assessment (10-Year, Men: Patient Education)," https://www.uptodate.com/contents/calculator-cardio vascular-risk-assessment-10-year-men-patient-education.
19. G. Belcaro et al., "Carotid and Femoral Ultrasound Morphology Screening and Cardiovascular Events in Low Risk Subjects: A 10-Year Follow-Up Study (The CAFES-CAVE Study[1])," *Atherosclerosis* 156, no. 2 (June 2001): 379–87.
20. Amy L. Doneen et al., "Cardiovascular Prevention: Migrating from a Binary to a Ternary Classification," *Frontiers in Cardiovascular Medicine* 7, no. 92 (May 2020).

Chapter 5: The Truth About Women and Heart Disease

1. Jonathan G. Zaroff et al., "Association of Azithromycin Use with Cardiovascular Mortality," *JAMA Network Open* 3, no. 6 (June 2020): e208199.
2. Gowtham A. Rao et al., "Azithromycin and Levofloxacin Use and Increased Risk of Cardiac Arrhythmia and Death," *Annals of Family Medicine* 12, no. 2 (March 2014): 121–27; Hsu-Chen Chou et al., "Risks of Cardiac Arrhythmia and Mortality among Patients Using New-Generation Macrolides, Fluoroquinolones, and β-lactam/β-lactamase Inhibitors: A Taiwanese Nationwide Study," *Clinical Infectious Diseases* 60, no. 4 (February 2015): 566–77; Eric M. Mortensen et al., "Association of Azithromycin with Mortality and Cardiovascular Events among Older Patients Hospitalized with Pneumonia," *Journal of the American Medical Association* 311, no. 21 (June 2014): 2199–208.
3. Sameer Arora et al., "Twenty Year Trends and Sex Differences in Young Adults Hospitalized with Acute Myocardial Infarction: The ARIC Community Surveillance Study," *Circulation* 139, no. 8 (February 2019): 1047–56.
4. Julinda Mehilli and Patrizia Presbitero, "Coronary Artery Disease and Acute Coronary Syndrome in Women," *Heart* 106, no. 7 (April 2020): 487–92.

NOTES

5. Alzheimer's Association, "2020 Alzheimer's Disease Facts and Figures Special Report, On the Front Lines: Primary Care Physicians and Alzheimer's Care in America," https://www.alz.org/media/Documents/alzheimers-facts-and-figures_1.pdf.

6. European Society of Cardiology, "Heart Disease Deaths Rising in Young Women" (February 2021), https://www.escardio.org/The-ESC/Press-Office/Press-releases/Heart-disease-deaths-rising-in-young-women.

7. Oras A. Alabas et al., "Sex Differences in Treatments, Relative Survival, and Excess Mortality Following Acute Myocardial Infarction: National Cohort Study Using Swedeheart Registry," *Journal of the American Heart Association* 6, no. 12 (December 2017): e007123.

8. J. Hector Pope et al., "Missed Diagnoses of Acute Cardiac Ischemia in the Emergency Department," *New England Journal of Medicine* 342, no. 16 (April 2000): 1163–70.

9. Michael G. Nanna et al., "Sex Differences in the Use of Statins in Community Practice," *Circulation: Cardiovascular Quality and Outcomes* 12, no. 8 (August 2019): e005562

10. "Cardiology's Problem Women," *The Lancet* 393, no. 10175 (March 2019): 959.

11. Ibid.

12. O. A. Iakoubova et al.,"Polymorphism in KIF6 Gene and Benefit from Statins after Acute Coronary Syndromes: Results from the PROVE IT-TIMI 22 Study," *Journal of the American College of Cardiology* 51, no. 4 (January 2008): 449–55.

13. Kwang Kon Koh et al., "Atorvastatin Causes Insulin Resistance and Increases Ambient Glycemia in Hypercholesterolemic Patients," *Journal of the American College of Cardiology* 55, no. 12 (March 2010): 1209–16.

14. Peter S. Sever et al., "Prevention of Coronary and Stroke Events with Atorvastatin in Hypertensive Patients Who Have Average or Lower-Than-Average Cholesterol Concentrations, in the Anglo-Scandinavian Cardiac Outcomes Trial—Lipid Lowering Arm (ASCOT-LLA): A Multicentre Randomised Controlled Trial," *The Lancet* 361, no. 9364 (April 2003): 1149–58.

15. Bairey Merz et al., "Knowledge, Attitudes, and Beliefs Regarding Cardiovascular Disease in Women: The Women's Heart Alliance," *Journal of the American College of Cardiology* 70, no. 2 (July 2017): 123–32.

16. American Heart Association, "Common Myths about Heart Disease," https://www.goredforwomen.org/en/about-heart-disease-in-women/facts/common-myths-about-heart-disease.

17. Nanette K. Wenger, "Prevention of Cardiovascular Disease in Women: Highlights for the Clinician of the 2011 American Heart Association Guidelines," *Advances in Chronic Kidney Disease* 20, no. 5 (September 2013): 419–22.

18. Scott M. Grundy et al., "AHA/ACC/AACVPR/AAPA/ABC/ACPM/ADA/AGS/APhA/ASPC/NLA/PCNA Guideline on the Management of

Blood Cholesterol: A Report of the American College of Cardiology/ American Heart Association Task Force on Clinical Practice Guidelines," *Journal of the American College of Cardiologists* 73, no. 24 (June 2019): e285–350.

19. W. P. Castelli, "Cholesterol and Lipids in the Risk of Coronary Artery Disease—The Framingham Heart Study," *The Canadian Journal of Cardiology* 4, Supplement A (July 1988): 5A–10A.

20. John G. Canto et al., "Association of Age and Sex with Myocardial Infarction Symptom Presentation and In-Hospital Mortality," *Journal of the American Medical Association* 307, no. 8 (February 2012): 813–22.

21. Garima Arora and Vera Bittner, "Chest Pain Characteristics and Gender in the Early Diagnosis of Acute Myocardial Infarction," *Current Cardiology Reports* 17, no. 2 (February 2015): 5.

22. Brendan M. Everett et al., "High Sensitivity Cardiac Troponin I and B-Type Natriuretic Peptide as Predictors of Vascular Events in Primary Prevention: Impact of Statin Therapy," *Circulation* 131, no. 21 (May 2015): 1851–60.

23. Ronit Calderon-Margalit et al., "Prospective Association of PCOS with Coronary Artery Calcification and Carotid-Intima-Media Thickness: The Coronary Artery Risk Development in Young Adults Women's Study," *Arterioschlerosis, Thrombosis, and Vascular Biology* 34, no. 12 (December 2014): 2688–94.

24. Bulent Yilmaz et al., "Metabolic Syndrome, Hypertension, and Hyperlipidemia in Mothers, Fathers, Sisters, and Brothers of Women with Polycystic Ovary Syndrome: A Systematic Review and Meta-Analysis," *Fertility and Sterility* 109, no. 2 (February 2018): 356–64.

25. Marise M. Wagner et al., "Association between Miscarriage and Cardio-vascular Disease in a Scottish Cohort," *Heart* 101, no. 24 (December 2015): 1954–60.

26. Leanne Bellamy et al., "Type 2 Diabetes Mellitus after Gestational Diabetes: A Systematic Review and Meta-Analysis," *The Lancet* 373 (May 2009): 1773–79; Caroline K. Kramer, Sara Campbell, and Ravi Retnakaran, "Gestational Diabetes and the Risk of Cardiovascular Disease in Women: A Systematic Review and Meta-Analysis," *Diabetologia* 62, no. 6 (March 2019): 905–14.

27. Pensée Wu et al., "Preeclampsia and Future Cardiovascular Health: A Systematic Review and Meta-Analysis," *Circulation Cardiovascular Quality Outcomes* 10, no. 2 (July 2017): e003497.

28. Ibid.

29. Jacques E. Rossouw et al., "Risks and Benefits of Estrogen Plus Progestin in Healthy Postmenopausal Women: Principal Results from the Women's Health Initiative Randomized Controlled Trial," *Journal of the American Medical Association* 288, no. 3 (July 2002): 321–33.

30. H. G. Burger et al., "Evidence-Based Assessment of the Impact of the WHI on Women's Health," *Climacteric* 15, no. 3 (June 2012): 281–87.

31. Xiolin Xu, Mark Jones, and Gita D. Mishra, "Age at Natural Menopause and Development of Chronic Conditions and Multimorbidity: Results from an Australian Prospective Cohort," *Human Reproduction* 35, no. 1 (January 2020): 203–11; Samar R. El Khoudary et al., "Menopause Transition and Cardiovascular Disease Risk: Implications for Timing of Early Prevention," *Circulation* 142, no. 25 (December 2020): e506–e532.

32. Matthew Nudy, Vernon M. Chinchilli, and Andrew J. Foy, "A Systematic Review and Meta-Regression Analysis to Examine the 'Timing Hypothesis' of Hormone Replacement Therapy on Mortality, Coronary Heart Disease, and Stroke," *International Journal of Cardiology Heart and Vasculature* 22 (January 2019): 123–31.

33. Candyce H. Kroenke et al., "Effects of a Dietary Intervention and Weight Change on Vasomotor Symptoms on the Women's Health Initiative," *Menopause* 19, no. 9 (September 2012): 980–88.

34. Debra J. Anderson et al., "Obesity, Smoking, and Risk of Vasomotor Menopausal Symptoms: A Pooled Analysis of Eight Cohort Studies," *American Journal of Obstetrics and Gynecology* 222, no. 5 (May 2020): 478.

35. American Heart Association, "The Facts about Women and Heart Disease," https://www.goredforwomen.org/en/about-heart-disease-in -women/facts.

36. Bernhard Haring et al., "Cardiovascular Disease and Cognitive Decline in Postmenopausal Women: Results from the Women's Health Initiative Memory Study," *Journal of the American Heart Association* 2, no. 6 (November 2013): e000369.

37. American Heart Association, "American Heart Association Recommen-dations for Physical Activity for Adults and Kids," Updated April 12, 2018, https://www.heart.org/en/healthy-living/fitness/fitness-basics/aha -recs-for-physical-activity-in-adults.

38. T. S. Han et al., "Waist Circumference Reduction and Cardiovascular Benefits during Weight Loss in Women," *International Journal of Obesity and Related Metabolic Disorders* 21, no. 2 (February 1997): 1127–34.

39. James F. Burke and Leslie E. Skorlarus, "Are More Young People Having Strokes? A Simple Question with an Uncertain Answer," *JAMA Neurology* 74, no. 6 (June 2017): 639–41.

40. James J. DiNicolantonio, Sean C. Lucan, and James H. O'Keefe, "The Evidence for Saturated Fat and for Sugar Related to Coronary Heart Disease," *Progress in Cardiovascular Diseases* 58, no. 5 (March–April 2016): 464–72.

41. Richard F. Hamman et al., "Effect of Weight Loss with Lifestyle Intervention on Risk of Diabetes," *Diabetes Care* 29, no. 9 (September 2006): 21027.

42. O. Akinseye, N. Ojike, and S. K. Williams et al., "Increased risk of stroke among hypertensive patients with abnormally short sleep duration: Analysis of the National Health Interview Survey." *Journal of the American Society of Hypertension* 9, no. 4 (June 2015).

43. Centers for Disease Control and Prevention, "Tobacco Related Mortality," Updated April 28, 2020, https://www.cdc.gov/tobacco/data _statistics/fact_sheets/health_effects/tobacco_related_mortality/in dex.htm.

44. James A. Palmer et al., "Differential Risk of ST-Segment Elevation of Myocardial Infarction in Male and Female Smokers," *Journal of the American College of Cardiology* 73, no. 25 (July 2019): 3259–66.

45. Allan Hacksaw et al., "Low Cigarette Consumption and Risk of Coronary Heart Disease and Stroke: Meta-Analysis of 141 Cohort Studies in 55 Study Reports," *British Medical Journal* 369 (January 2018): j5855; National Cancer Institute, "No Safe Level of Smoking: Even Low-Intensity Smokers Are at Increased Risk of Earlier Death," December 5, 2016, https://www.cancer.gov/news-events/press-releases/2016/low -intensity-smoking-risk.

46. Centers for Disease Control and Prevention, "Tobacco Related Mortality," April 28, 2020, https://www.cdc.gov/tobacco/data_statistics/fact_sheets /health_effects/tobacco_related_mortality/index.htm.

47. Centers for Disease Control and Prevention, High Blood Pressure, "Facts about Hypertension," September 8, 2020, https://www.cdc.gov/blood pressure/facts.htm.

48. Blood Pressure Lowering Treatment Trialists' Collaboration "Pharma-cological Blood Pressure Lowering for Primary and Secondary Prevention of Cardiovascular Disease Across Different Levels of Blood Pressure: An Individual Participant-Level Data Meta-Analysis," *Lancet* 397, no. 10285 (2021): 1625–36.

49. Oluwaseun Akinseye et al., "Increased Risk of Stroke among Hypertensive Patients with Abnormally Short Sleep Duration: Analysis of the National Health Interview Survey," *Journal of the American Society of Hypertension* 9, no. 4 (June 2015: e3.

50. Eric Suni, "How Sleep Deprivation Affects Your Heart," December 4, 2020, https://www.sleepfoundation.org/sleep-deprivation/how-sleep -deprivation-affects-your-hear.

Chapter 6: Lifesaving Lessons We've Learned From Looking at More Than Ten Thousand Arteries

1. Salim S. Virani et al., "Heart Disease and Stroke Statistics—2020 Update: A Report from the American Heart Association," *Circulation* 141, no. 9 (January 2020): e139–596.

2. Mary G. George, Xin Tong, and Barbara A. Bowman, "Prevalence of Cardiovascular Risk Factors and Strokes in Younger Adults," *Neurology* 74, no. 6 (June 2017): 695–70.

3. Michelle Leppert et al., "Young Women Had More Strokes than Young Men in a Large, United States Claims Sample," *Stroke* 51, no. 11 (September 2020): 3352–55.

4. Merel S. Ekker et al., "Stroke Incidence in Young Adults According to Age, Subtype, Sex, and Time Trends," *Neurology* 92, no.21 (May 2019): e2444–54.

5. Jukka Putaala et al., "Demographic and Geographic Vascular Risk Factor Differences in European Young Adults with Ischemic Stroke: The 15 Cities Young Stroke Study," *Stroke* 43, no. 10 (October 2012): 2624–30.

6. Eric Greb, "Incidence of Stroke, but Not MI, Increasing in Young People," https://www.medscape.com/viewarticle/941674.

7. Michael O'Riordan, "The 'fiction' of primary prevention: Role of IVUS in identifying early atherosclerosis," *Medscape*, April 23, 2004, https://www.medscape.com/viewarticle/784686.

8. Tarun Girotra et al., "A Contemporary and Comprehensive Analysis of the Costs of Stroke in the United States," *Journal of the Neurological Sciences* 410, no. 116643 (March 2020), 15;410:116643. doi: 10.1016/j.jns.2019 .116643. Epub 2019 Dec 24. PMID: 31927342.

9. Ibid.; Valery L. Feigin et al., "Burden of Neurological Disorders Across the US from 1990–2017," *Neurology* 78, no. 2 (February 2021): 165–87.

10. Girotra et al., "A Contemporary and Comprehensive Analysis of the Costs of Stroke in the United States"; Feigin et al., "Burden of Neurological Disorders Across the US from 1990–2017."

11. Erling Falk, Prediman Shah, and Valentin Fuster, "Coronary Plaque Disruption," *Circulation* 92, no. 3 (August 1995): 657–71; Marcio S. Bittencourt et al., "Prognostic Value of Non-Obstructive and Obstructive Coronary Artery Disease Detected by Coronary Computed Tomography Angiography To Identify Cardiovascular Events," *Circulation: Cardiovascular Imaging* 7, no. 2 (March 2014): 282–91; Thomas M. Maddox et al., "Nonobstructive Coronary Artery Disease and Risk of Myocardial Infarction," *Journal of the American Medical Association* 312, no. 17 (November 2014): 1754–63; Zorin Makarović et al., "Nonobstructive Coronary Artery Disease—Clinical Relevance, Diagnosis, Management and Proposal of New Pathophysiological Classification," *Acta Clinica Croatica* 57, no. 3 (September 2018): 528–41.

12. Olli Patrakka et al., "Oral Bacterial Signatures in Cerebral Thrombi in Patients with Acute Ischemic Stroke Treated with Thrombectomy," *Journal of the American Heart Association* 8, no. 11 (May 2019): e012330.

13. Anne Langsted, Børge G. Nordestgaard, and Pia R. Kamstrup, "Elevated Lipoprotein and Risk of Ischemic Stroke," *Journal of the American College of Cardiology* 74, no.1 (July 2019): 54–66.

14. Kåre Berg, "A New Serum Type System in Man—the LP System," *Acta Pathologica et Microbiologica Scandinavica* 59, no.3 (November 1963): 369–82.

15. P. M. Ridker, C. H. Hennekens, and M. J. Stampfer, "A Prospective Study of Lipoprotein(a) and the Risk of Myocardial Infarction," *Journal of the American Medical Association* 270, no. 18 (November 1993): 2195–99;

Robert Clarke et al., "Genetic Variants Associated with Lp(a) Lipoprotein Level and Coronary Disease," *New England Journal of Medicine* 361, no. 26 (December 2009): 2518–28.

16. Lotte C. A. Stiekema et al., "Persistent Arterial Wall Inflammation in Patients with Elevated Lipoprotein(a) Despite Strong Low-Density Lipoprotein Cholesterol Reduction by Proprotein Convertase Subtilisin/ Kexin Type 9 Antibody Treatment," *European Heart Journal* 40, no. 33 (September 2019): 2775–81.

17. Allison W. Peng et al., "Very High Coronary Artery Calcium (≥1000) and Association with Cardiovascular Disease Events, Non-Cardiovascular Outcomes, and Mortality: Results from MESA," *Circulation* 143, no. 16 (April 2021): 1571–83; Akira Fujiyoshi et al., "Coronary Artery Calcium and Risk of Dementia in MESA (Multi-Ethnic Study of Atherosclerosis)," *Circulation Cardiovascular Imaging* 10, no. 5 (May 2017): e005349.

18. Mohammadhassan Mirbolouk et al., "The Association of Coronary Artery Calcium Score and Mortality Risk among Smokers: The Coronary Artery Calcium Consortium," *Atherosclerosis* 294 (February 2020): 33–40.

19. Naveen R. Parva et al., "Prevalence of Vitamin D Deficiency and Associated Risk Factors in the US Population (2011–2012)," *Cureus* 10, no. 6 (June 2018). doi:10.7759/cureus.2741.

20. Laurie Margolies et al., "Digital Mammography and Screening for Coronary Artery Disease," *Journal of the American College of Cardiology* 9, no. 4 (April 2016): 350–60.

21. Michelle A. Rotter et al., "Breast Arterial Calcifications (BACs) Found on Screening Mammography and Their Association with Cardiovascular Disease," *Menopause* 15, no. 2 (March 2008): 276–81.

22. Kiran R. Nandalur et al., "Carotid Artery Calcification on CT May Independently Predict Stroke Risk," *American Journal of Roentgenology* 186, no. 2 (February 2006): 547–52.

23. Stanley N. Cohen et al., "Carotid Calcification on Panoramic Radiographs: An Important Marker for Vascular Risk," *Oral and Maxillofacial Radiology* 94, no. 4 (October 2002): 510–14; Mohammed M. Chowdhury et al., "Lower Limb Arterial Calcification (LLAC) Scores in Patients with Symptomatic Peripheral Arterial Disease Are Associated with Increased Cardiac Mortality and Morbidity," *PLoS ONE* 12, no. 9 (September 2017): e0182952; Jean-Marc Bugnicourt et al., "Presence of Intracranial Artery Calcification Is Associated with Mortality and Vascular Events in Patients with Ischemic Stroke after Hospital Discharge: A Cohort Study," *Stroke* 42, no. 12 (December 2011): 3447–53; Michael H. Criqui et al., "Abdominal Aortic Calcium, Coronary Artery Calcium, and Cardiovascular Morbidity and Mortality in the Multi-Ethnic Study of Atherosclerosis," *Arteriosclerosis, Thrombosis, and Vascular Biology* 34, no. 7 (July 2014): 1574–79.

Chapter 7: Tests That Could Save Your Life

1. Lai Lai Fan, Bai Hui Chen, and Zhi Juan Dai, "The Relation between Gallstone Disease and Cardiovascular Disease," *Scientific Reports* 7, no. 15104 (November 2017).
2. Wei-Hung Chen, "Hashimoto's Thyroiditis, Risk of Coronary Heart Disease, and L-Thyroxine Treatment: A Nationwide Cohort Study," *The Journal of Clinical Endocrinology and Metabolism* 100, no. 1 (January 2015): 109–14.
3. Jiahua Fan et al., "Small dense LDL Cholesterol Is Associated with Metabolic Syndrome Traits Independently of Obesity and Inflammation," *Nutrition & Metabolism* 16, no. 7 (January 2019).
4. Amy Berrington de Gonzalez et al., "Projected Cancer Risks from Computed Tomography Scans Performed in the United States in 2007," *Archives of Internal Medicine* 169, no. 22 (December 2009): 2071–77.
5. E. Stephen Amis Jr. et al., "American College of Radiology White Paper on Radiation Dose in Medicine," *Journal of the American College of Radiology* 4, no. 5 (May 2007): 272–84.
6. Peter Willeit et al., "Carotid Intima-Media Thickness Progression as Surrogate Marker for Cardiovascular Risk," *Circulation* 142, no. 7 (June 2020): 621–42.
7. Mamoud Zureik et al., "Echogenic Carotid Plaques Are Associated with Aortic Arterial Stiffness in Subjects with Subclinical Carotid Atherosclerosis," *Hypertension* 41, no. 3 (March 2003): 519–27.
8. Society of Atherosclerosis Imaging and Prevention Developed in Collaboration with the International Atherosclerosis Society, "Appropriate Use Criteria for Carotid Intima Media Thickness Testing," *Atherosclerosis* 214, no. 1 (January 2011): 43–46.
9. Hannah Gardener et al., "Ultrasound Markers of Carotid Atherosclerosis and Cognition: The Northern Manhattan Study," *Stroke* 48, no. 7 (July 2017): 1855–61.
10. Amy L. Doneen and Bradley F. Bale, "Carotid Intima-Media Thickness Testing as an Asymptomatic Cardiovascular Disease Identifier and Method for Making Therapeutic Decisions," *Postgraduate Medicine* 125, no. 2 (March 2013): 108–23.
11. Henry G. Cheng et al., "Effect of Comprehensive Cardiovascular Disease Risk Management on Longitudinal Changes in Carotid Artery Intima-Media Thickness in a Community-Based Prevention Clinic," *Archives of Medical Science* 12, no. 4 (August 2016): 728–35.
12. K. Craig Kent et al., "Analysis of Risk Factors for Abdominal Aortic Aneurysm in a Cohort of More Than 3 Million Individuals," *Journal of Vascular Surgery* 52, no. 3 (September 2010): 539–48.
13. Atul Mathur et al., "Aortic Aneurysm," *Journal of Translational Internal Medicine* 4, no. 1 (April 2016): 35–41.

14. Centers for Disease Control and Prevention, "Underlying Cause of Death 1999–2019," http://wonder.cdc.gov/ucd-icd10.html.

15. Derek Klarin et al., "Genetic Architecture of Abdominal Aortic Aneurysm in the Million Veteran Program," *Circulation* 142, no. 17 (October 2020): 1633–46.

16. Michael H. Criqui et al., "Abdominal Aortic Calcium, Coronary Artery Calcium, and Cardiovascular Morbidity and Mortality in the Multi-Ethnic Study of Atherosclerosis," *Arteriosclerosis, Thrombosis, and Vascular Biology* 34, no. 7 (July 2014): 1574–79.

17. Anna Helgadottir et al., "The Same Sequence Variant on 9p21 Associates with Myocardial Infarction, Abdominal Aortic Aneurysm and Intracranial Aneurysm," *Nature Genetics* 40, no. 2 (February 2008): 217–24.

18. Pavel Poredos and Borut Jug, "The Prevalence of Peripheral Arterial Disease in High Risk Subjects and Coronary or Cerebrovascular Patients," *Angiology* 58, no. 3 (June 2007): 309–15.

19. Jeffrey T. Lu and Mark A. Creager, "The Relationship of Cigarette Smoking to Peripheral Arterial Disease," *Reviews in Cardiovascular Medicine* 5, no. 4 (Fall 2004): 189–93.

20. Vascular Disease Foundation, "Life Saving Tips about…Smoking and PAD," http://vasculardisease.org/flyers/lifesaving-tips-on-smoking-and -pad-flyer.pdf.

21. Centers for Disease Control and Prevention, "Peripheral Arterial Disease (PAD) Fact Sheet," https://www.cdc.gov/dhdsp/data_statistics/fact_sheets /fs_pad.htm.

22. Nico Mihatov and Eric A. Secemsky, "Peripheral Matters/Peripheral and Coronary Artery Disease: Two Sides of the Same Coin," *Cardiology Magazine* 48 no. 9 (September 20, 2019): 38, https://www.acc.org /latest-in-cardiology/articles/2019/09/14/24/42/peripheral-and -coronary-artery-disease-two-sides-of-the-same-coin; Emile R. Mohler III, "Peripheral Arterial Disease: Identification and Implications," *Archives of Internal Medicine* 163, no. 19 (October 2003): 2306–14.

23. Mohler III, "Peripheral Arterial Disease: Identification and Implications."

24. Benjamin T. Fitzgerald, William M. Scalia, and Gregory M. Scalia, "Female False Positive Exercise Stress ECG Testing—Fact Versus Fiction," *Heart Lung & Circulation* 28, no. 5 (May 2019): 735–41.

25. Erling Falk, Prediman K. Shah, and Valentin Fuster, "Coronary Plaque Disruption," *Circulation* 92, no. 3 (August 1995): 657–71.

26. "Final Recommendation Statement: Cardiovascular Disease Risk: Screening with Electrocardiography," June 12, 2018, https://www .uspreventiveservicestaskforce.org/uspstf/document/Recommendation StatementFinal/cardiovascular-disease-risk-screening-with -electrocardiography; Roger Chou, "Cardiac Screening with Electrocardiography, Stress Echocardiography, or Myocardial Perfusion Imaging: Advice for High-Value Care from the American College of Physicians," *Annals of Internal Medicine* 162, no. 6 (March 2015): 438–47;

Lionel S. Lim et al., "Atherosclerotic Cardiovascular Disease Screening in Adults: American College of Preventive Medicine Position Statement on Preventive Practice," *American Journal of Preventive Medicine* 40, no. 3 (March 2011): e1–10; American Academy of Family Physicians, "Cardiovascular Disease Risk: Clinical Preventive Service Recommendation," https://www.aafp.org/family-physician/patient-care/clinical-recommendations/all-clinical-recommendations/coronary-heart-disease.htm;

27. Daniel S. Berman et al., "Relationship between Stress-Induced Myocardial Ischemia and Atherosclerosis Measured by Coronary Calcium Tomography," *Journal of the American College of Cardiology* 44, no. 4 (August 2004): 923–30.

28. Jose Milei et al., "Perinatal and Infant Early Atherosclerotic Coronary Lesions," *The Canadian Journal of Cardiology* 24, no. 2 (February 2008): 137–41; Claudio Napoli et al., "Fatty Streak Formation Occurs in Human Fetal Aortas and Is Greatly Enhanced by Maternal Hypercholesterolemia Intimal Accumulation of Low Density Lipoprotein and Its Oxidation Precede Monocyte Recruitment into Early Atherosclerotic Lesions," *Journal of Clinical Investigation* 100, no. 11 (December 1997): 2680–90.

29. Young Mi Hong, "Atherosclerotic Cardiovascular Disease Beginning in Childhood," *Korean Circulation Journal* 40, no. 1 (January 2010): 1–9.

30. Rishi Puri et al., "Impact of Statins on Serial Coronary Calcification During Atheroma Progression and Regression," *Journal of the American College of Cardiology* 65, no. 13 (April 2015): 1273–82; Brian G. Kral et al., "Noncalcified Coronary Plaque Volumes in Healthy People with a Family History of Early Onset Coronary Artery Disease," *Circulation: Cardiovascular Imaging* 7, no. 3 (May 2014): 446–53; Ryan D. Madderet et al., "Large Lipid-Rich Coronary Plaques Detected by Near-Infrared Spectroscopy at Non-Stented Sites in the Target Artery Identify Patients Likely to Experience Future Major Adverse Cardiovascular Events," *European Heart Journal Cardiovascular Imaging* 17, no. 4 (April 2016): 393–99; Jie Sun et al., "Carotid Plaque Lipid Content and Fibrous Cap Status Predict Systemic CV Outcomes: The MRI Substudy in AIM-HIGH," *Journal of the American College of Cardiology Cardiovascular Imaging* 10, no. 3 (March 2017): 241–49; Lei Xing et al., "Clinical Significance of Lipid-Rich Plaque Detected by Optical Coherence Tomography: A 4-Year Follow-Up Study," *Journal of the American College of Cardiology* 69, no. 20 (May 2017): 2502–13.

31. Catherine E. Handy et al., "The Association of Coronary Artery Calcium with Noncardiovascular Disease: The Multi-Ethnic Study of Atherosclerosis," *Journal of the American College of Cardiology Cardiovascular Imaging* 9, no. 5 (May 2016): 568–76.

32. Akira Fujiyoshi et al., "Coronary Artery Calcium and Risk of Dementia in MESA (Multi-Ethnic Study of Atherosclerosis)," *Circulation: Cardiovascular Imaging* 10, no. 5 (May 2017): e005349; Handy et al., "The Association of Coronary Artery Calcium with Noncardiovascular Disease."

33. John Jeffrey Carr et al., "Association of Coronary Artery Calcium in Adults Aged 32 to 46 Years with Incident Coronary Heart Disease and Death," *Cardiology* 2, no. 4 (April 2017): 391–99.
34. Morteza Naghavi et al., "From Vulnerable Plaque to Vulnerable Patient— Part III: Executive Summary of the Screening for Heart Attack Prevention and Education (SHAPE) Task Force Report," *American Journal of Cardiology* 98, no. 2A (July 2006): 2H–15H.
35. John A. Rumberger et al., "Coronary Artery Calcium Area by Electron- Beam Computed Tomography and Coronary Atherosclerotic Plaque Area A Histopathologic Correlative Study," *Circulation* 92, no. 8 (October 1995): 2157–62.
36. L.P. Casalino et al., "Frequency of Failure to Inform Patients of Clinically Significant Outpatient Test Results," *Archives of Internal Medicine* 169, no. 12 (2009): 1123–29.

Chapter 8: Are Your Arteries on Fire?

1. Paul M. Ridker et al., "Comparison of C-reactive Protein and Low-Density Lipoprotein Cholesterol Levels in the Prediction of First Cardiovascular Events," *New England Journal of Medicine* 347, no. 20 (November 2002): 1557–65; Paul M. Ridker et al., "C-reactive Protein and Other Markers of Inflammation in the Prediction of Cardiovascular Disease in Women," *New England Journal of Medicine* 342, no. 12 (March 2000): 836–43.
2. Eung Ju Kim et al., "Metabolic Activity of the Spleen and Bone Marrow in Patients with Acute Myocardial Infarction Evaluated by 18F- Fluorodeoxyglucose Positron Emission Tomograpic Imaging," *Circulation: Cardiovascular Imaging* 7, no. 3 (May 2014): 454–60; Konstantinos Toutouzas et al., "Incremental Predictive Value of Carotid Inflammation in Acute Ischemic Stroke," *Stroke* 46, no. 1 (November 2014): 272–74; Tae Nyun Kim et al., "Vascular Inflammation in Patients with Impaired Glucose Tolerance and Type 2 Diabetes: Analysis with 18F-Fluorodeoxyglucose Positron Emission Tomography," *Circulation: Cardiovascular Imaging* 3, no. 2 (January 2010): 142–48; Amit Shah et al., "Sex and Age Differences in the Association of Depression with Obstructive Coronary Artery Disease and Adverse Cardiovascular Events," *Journal of American Heart Association* 3, no. 3 (June 2014); Alejandro R. Chade, "Small Vessels, Big Role: Renal Microcirculation and Progression of Renal Injury," *Hypertension*, 69, no. 4 (April 2017): 551– 63; Rocco J. Cannistraro et al., "CNS Small Vessel Disease: A Clinical Review," *Neurology* 92, no. 24 (June 2019): 1146–56; Antoine M. Hakim, "Small Vessel Disease," *Frontiers in Neurology* 10 (September 2019): 1020; Martin Reriani et al., "Microvascular Endothelial Dysfunction Predicts the Development of Erectile Dysfunction in Men with Coronary Atherosclerosis with Critical Stenoses," *Coronary Artery Disease* 25, no. 7 (November 2014): 552–57; Kenneth Cusi et al., "Long-Term Pioglitazone Treatment for Patients with Nonalcoholic Steatohepatitis and Prediabetes or Type 2

Diabetes Mellitus: A Randomized, Controlled Trial Long-Term Pioglitazone for Patients with NASH and Prediabetes or T2DM," *Annals of
Internal Medicine* 165, no. 5 (September 2016): 305–15;

    Una L. Kelly et al., "High Density Lipoproteins Are a Potential
Therapeutic Target for Age-Related Macular Degeneration," *Journal of
Biological Chemistry* 295, no. 39 (September 2020): 13601–16; Evi Paouri
and Spiros Georgopoulos, "Systemic and CNS Inflammation Crosstalk:
Implications for Alzheimer's Disease," *Current Alzheimer Research* 16, no. 6
(July 2019): 559–74; Nisha Nigil Haroon et al., "Patients with Ankylosing
Spondylitis Have Increased Cardiovascular and Cerebrovascular Mortality:
A Population-Based Study," *Annals of Internal Medicine* 163, no. 6 (September
2015): 409–16; David Furman et al., "Chronic Inflammation in the
Etiology of Disease Across the Life Span," *Nature Medicine* 25, no. 12
(December 2019): 1822–132.

3. Furman et al., "Chronic Inflammation in the Etiology of Disease Across
the Life Span."

4. G. Lyman Duff and Gardner C. MacMillan, "Pathology of Atherosclerosis,"
American Journal of Medicine 11, no. 1 (July 1951): 92–108.

5. Eugene Braunwald, "Shattuck Lecture Cardiovascular Medicine at the
Turn of the Millennium: Triumphs, Concerns, and Opportunities," *New
England Journal of Medicine* 337 (November 1997): 1360–69; Amit
Sachdeva et al., "Lipid Levels in Patients Hospitalized with Coronary
Artery Disease: An Analysis of 136,905 Hospitalizations in Get with The
Guidelines," *American Heart Journal* 157, no. 1 (January 2009): 111–17.

6. Harvard Health Publishing, "Inflammation: A Unifying Theory of
Disease," May 2020, https://www.health.harvard.edu/staying-healthy
/inflammation-a-unifying-theory-of-disease.

7. Per Fogelstrand and Jan Borén, "Retention of Atherogenic Lipoproteins
in the Artery Wall and Its Role in Atherogenesis," *Nutrition, Metabolism
and Cardiovascular Disease* 22, no. 1 (January 2012): 1–7.

8. Martin Flajnik and Masanori Kasahara, "Origin and Evolution of the
Adaptive Immune System: Genetic Events and Selective Pressures,"
Nature Reviews Genetics 11, no. 1 (January 2010): 47–59.

9. "The Interleukin-6 Receptor as a Target for Prevention of Coronary
Heart Disease: A Mendelian Radomisation Analysis," *The Lancet* 379, no.
9822 (March 2012): 1214–24.

10. Paul M. Ridker, "Antiinflammatory Therapy with Canakinumab for
Atherosclerotic Disease," *New England Journal of Medicine* 377, no. 12
(September 2017): 1119–31.

11. "A First: Drug Lowers Heart Risks by Curbing Inflammation," https://www
.cnbc.com/2017/08/27/a-first-drug-lowers-heart-risks-by-curbing
-inflammation.html; Laura Donnelly, "New Wonder Drug Hailed as Biggest
Breakthrough in Fight against Heart Attacks and Cancer, *The Telegraph*,
August 27, 2017, https://www.telegraph.co.uk/science/2017/08/27/new
-wonder-drug-hailed-biggest-breakthrough-fight-against-heart.

12. Brendan M. Everett et al., "Inhibition of Interleukin-1β and Reduction in Atherothrombotic Cardiovascular Events in the CANTOS Trial," *Journal of the American College of Cardiology* 76, no. 14 (October 2020): 1660–70.

13. "A First: Drug Lowers Heart Risks by Curbing Inflammation."

14. Aaron R. Folsom et al., "American Heart Association's Life's Simple 7: Avoiding Heart Failure and Preserving Cardiac Structure and Function," *American Journal of Medicine* 128, no. 9 (September 2015): 970–76; Amanda M. Fretts et al., "Life's Simple 7 and Incidence of Diabetes among American Indians: The Strong Heart Family Study," *Diabetes Care* 37, no. 8 (August 2014): 2240–45; Paul Muntner et al., "Cardiovascular Risk Factors in CKD Associate with Both ESRD and Mortality," *Journal of the American Society of Nephrology* 24, no. 7 (June 2013): 1159–65; Evan L. Thacker et al., "The American Heart Association Life's Simple 7 and Incident Cognitive Impairment: The REasons for Geographic And Racial Differences in Stroke (REGARDS) Study," *Journal of the American Heart Association* 3, no. 3 (June 2014): e000635;

Agneta Akesson et al., "Low-Risk Diet and Lifestyle Habits in the Primary Prevention of Myocardial Infarction in Men: A Population-Based Prospective Cohort Study," *Journal of the American College of Cardiology* 64, no. 13 (September 2014): 1299–1306.

Andrea K. Chomistek et al., "Healthy Lifestyle in the Primordial Prevention of Cardiovascular Disease among Young Women," *Journal of the American College of Cardiology* 65, no. 1 (January 2015): 43–51.

15. Xiao-Ni Yan et al., "Lipoprotein(a) Is Associated with the Presence and Severity of New-Onset Coronary Artery Disease in Postmenopausal Women," *Journal of Women's Health* 29, no. 4 (April 2020): 503–10

16. Paul M. Ridker et al., "Rosuvastatin to Prevent Vascular Events in Men and Women with Elevated C-Reactive Protein," *New England Journal of Medicine* 359, no. 21 (November 2008): 2195–207.

17. Ermanno Rossi et al., "Increased Plasma Levels of Platelet-Derived Growth Factor (PDGF-BB + PDGF-AB) in Patients with Never-Treated Mild Essential Hypertension," *American Journal of Hypertension* 11, no. 10 (October 1998): 1239–43; Gary K. Owens, Meena S. Kumar, and Brian R. Wamhoff, "Molecular Regulation of Vascular Smooth Muscle Cell Differentiation in Development and Disease," *Physiological Reviews* 84, no. 3 (July 2004): 767–801.

18. Clémence Cheignon et al., "Oxidative Stress and the Amyloid Beta Peptide in Alzheimer's Disease," *Redox Biology* 14 (April 2018): 450–64; Ferdinando Giacco and Michael Brownlee, "Oxidative Stress and Diabetic Complications," *Circulation Research* 107, no. 9 (October 2010): 1058–70; Simone Reuter et al., "Oxidative Stress, Inflammation, and Cancer: How Are They Linked?," *Free Radical Biology and Medicine* 49, no. 11 (December 2010): 1603–16; Mengxue Wang et al., "Systematic Understanding of Pathophysiological Mechanisms of Oxidative Stress-Related Conditions—Diabetes Mellitus, Cardiovascular Diseases, and

Ischemia–Reperfusion Injury" *Frontiers in Cardiovascular Medicine* 8, no. 649785 (April 2021); Joanna Kruk, Katarzyna Kubasik-Kladna, and Hassan Y. Aboul-Enein, "The Role Oxidative Stress in the Pathogenesis of Eye Diseases: Current Status and a Dual Role of Physical Activity," *Mini Reviews in Medicinal Chemistry* 16, no. 3 (2015): 241–57; Eveliina Pollari et al., "The Role of Oxidative Stress in Degeneration of the Neuromuscular Junction in Amyotrophic Lateral Sclerosis," *Frontiers in Cellular Neuroscience* 8, no. 131 (May 2014): 1–8.

19. Mehdi H. Shishehbor et al., "Systemic Elevations of Free Radical Oxidation Products of Arachidonic Acid Are Associated with Angiographic Evidence of Coronary Artery Disease," *Free Radical Biology and Medicine* 41, no. 11 (December 2006): 1678–83.

20. James H. O'Keefe et al., "Potential Adverse Cardiovascular Effects from Excessive Endurance Exercise," *Mayo Clinic Proceedings* 87, no. 6 (June 2012): 587–95.

21. Fibrinogen Studies Collaboration, "Plasma Fibrinogen Level and the Risk of Major Cardiovascular Diseases and Nonvascular Mortality: An Individual Participant Meta-Analysis," *Journal of the American Medical Association* 294, no. 14 (October 2005): 1799–1809.

22. Michiel L. Bots et al., "Level of Fibrinogen and Risk of Fatal and Non-Fatal Stroke EUROSTROKE: A Collaborative Study among Research Centres in Europe," *Journal of Epidemiology and Community Health* 56, Supplement 1 (February 2002): i14–8.

23. Fibrinogen Studies Collaboration, "Plasma Fibrinogen Level and the Risk of Major Cardiovascular Diseases and Nonvascular Mortality: An Individual Participant Meta-Analysis," *Journal of the American Medical Association* 294, no. 14 (October 2005): 1799–1809.

24. The Emerging Risk Factors Collaboration, "C-Reactive Protein, Fibrinogen, and Cardiovascular Disease Prediction," *New England Journal of Medicine* 367, no. 14 (October 2012): 1310–20.

25. Paul M. Ridker, Robert J. Glynn, and Charles H. Hennekens, "C-reactive Protein Adds to the Predictive Value of Total and HDL Cholesterol in Determining Risk of First Myocardial Infarction," *Circulation* 97, no. 20 (May 1998): 2007–11.

26. Ridker et al., "C-reactive Protein and Other Markers of Inflammation in the Prediction of Cardiovascular Disease in Women."

27. Thomas J. Wang et al., "Multiple Biomarkers for the Prediction of First Major Cardiovascular Events and Death," *New England Journal of Medicine* 355, no. 25 (December 2006): 2631–39.

28. Johan Ärnlöv et al., "Low-Grade Albuminuria and Incidence of Cardiovascular Disease Events in Nonhypertensive and Nondiabetic Individuals: The Framingham Heart Study," *Circulation* 112, no. 7 (August 2005): 969–75.

29. Jose Maria Pascual et al., "Prognostic Value of Microalbuminuria During Antihypertensive Treatment in Essential Hypertension," *Hypertension* 64, no. 6 (December 2014): 1228–34.

30. Carolina A. Garza et al., "Association between Lipoprotein-Associated Phospholipase A2 and Cardiovascular Disease: A Systematic Review," *Mayo Clinic Proceedings* 82, no. 2 (February 2007): 159–65; Alexander Thompson et al., "Lipoprotein-Associated Phospholipase A(2) and Risk of Coronary Disease, Stroke, and Mortality: Collaborative Analysis of 32 Prospective Studies," *The Lancet* 375, no. 9725 (May 2010): 1536–44.

31. Heidi Mochari, John T. Grbic, and Lori Mosca, "Usefulness of Self-Reported Periodontal Disease to Identify Individuals with Elevated Inflammatory Markers at Risk of Cardiovascular Disease," *American Journal of Cardiology* 102, no. 11 (December 2008): 1509–13.

32. Wolfgang Lösche et al., "Lipoprotein-Associated Phospholipase A2 and Plasma Lipids in Patients with Destructive Periodontal Disease," *Journal of Clinical Periodontology* 32, no. 6 (April 2005): 640–44.

33. Jane F. Ferguson et al., "Translational Studies of Lipoprotein-Associated Phospholipase A2 in Inflammation and Atherosclerosis," *Journal of American College of Cardiology* 59, no. 8 (February 2012): 764–72; Michael H. Davidson et al., "Consensus Panel Recommendation for Incorporating Lipoprotein-Associated Phospholipase A2 Testing into Cardiovascular Disease Risk Assessment Guidelines," *American Journal of Cardiology* 101, no. 12A (June 2008): 51F–57F.

34. Mónica Acevedo et al., "Comparison of Lipoprotein-Associated Phospholipase A2 and High Sensitive C-Reactive Protein as Determinants of Metabolic Syndrome in Subjects without Coronary Heart Disease: In Search of the Best Predictor," *International Journal of Endocrinology* (May 2015): 934681.

35. Eric H. Yang et al., "Lipoprotein Associated Phospholipase A_2 Is an Independent Marker for Coronary Endothelial Dysfunction in Humans," *Arteriosclerosis, Thrombosis, and Vascular Biology* 26, no. 1 (January 2006): 106–11.

36. Wolfgang Koenig et al., "Lipoproteinassociated Phospholipase A2 Predicts Future Cardiovascular Events in Patients with Coronary Heart Disease Independently of Traditional Risk Factors, Markers of Inflammation, Renal Function, and Hemodynamic Stress," *Atherosclerosis, Thrombosis, and Vascular Biology* 26, no. 7 (July 2006): 1586–93.

37. Marijn C. Meuwese et al., "Serum Myeloperoxidase Levels Are Associated with the Future Risk of Coronary Artery Disease in Apparently Healthy Individuals: The EPIC-Norfolk Prospective Population Study," *Journal American College of Cardiology* 50, no. 2 (July 2007): 159–65.

38. Ramon A. Partida et al., "Plaque Erosion: A New in Vivo Diagnosis and a Potential Major Shift in the Management of Patients with Acute Coronary Syndromes," *European Heart Journal* 39, no. 22 (June 2018): 2070–76.

39. Claire L. Heslop, Jiri J. Forhlich, and John S. Hill, "Myeloperoxidase and C-reactive Protein Have Combined Utility for Long-Term Prediction of Cardiovascular Mortality after Coronary Angiography," *Journal of the American College of Cardiology* 55, no. 11 (March 2010): 11029.

40. Marie-Louise Brennan et al., "Prognostic Value of Myeloperoxidase in Patients with Chest Pain," *New England Journal of Medicine* 349, no. 17 (October 2003): 1595–1604.

41. Ahmed Tawakol et al., "Relation between Resting Amygdalar Activity and Cardiovascular Events: A Longitudinal and Cohort Study," *The Lancet* 389, no. 10071 (January 2017): 834–45.

42. Samia Mora et al., "Physical Activity and Reduced Risk of Cardiovascular Events: Potential Mediating Mechanisms," *Circulation* 116, no. 19 (November 2007): 2110–18.

43. Yikyung Park et al., "Dietary Fiber Intake and Mortality in the NIH-AARP Diet and Health Study," *Archives of Internal Medicine* 171, no. 12 (June 2011): 1061–68.

44. Vasanti S. Malik and Frank B. Hu, "Fructose and Cardiometabolic Health: What the Evidence from Sugar-Sweetened Beverages Tells Us," *Journal of the American College of Cardiology* 66, no. 14 (October 2015): 1615–24.

Chapter 9: The Deadly Pandemic You've Never Heard Of

1. Paul W. F. Wilson et al., "Metabolic Syndrome as a Precursor of Cardiovascular Disease and Type 2 Diabetes Mellitus," *Circulation* 112, no. 20 (November 2005): 3066–72.

2. Sandra J. Lewis et al., "Self-Reported Prevalence and Awareness of Metabolic Syndrome: Findings from SHIELD," *International Journal of Clinical Practice* 62, no. 8 (August 2008): 1168–76.

3. Mohammad G. Saklayen, "The Global Epidemic of the Metabolic Syndrome," *Current Hypertension Reports* 20, no. 2 (February 2018): 12.

4. Grishma Hirode and Robert J. Wong, "Trends in the Prevalence of Metabolic Syndrome in the United States, 2011–2016," *Journal of the American Medical Association* 323, no. 24 (June 2020): 2526–28.

5. "More Young Americans Developing Unhealthy Predictors of Heart Disease," June 2020, https://consumer.healthday.com/diabetes-information-10/metabolic-syndrome-news-761/more-young-americans-developing-unhealthy-predictors-of-heart-disease-758871.html.

6. Katherine Esposito et al., "Metabolic Syndrome and Risk of Cancer: A Systematic Review and Meta-Analysis," *Diabetes Care* 35, no. 11 (November 2012): 2402–11; Yeo Jin Kim et al., "Associations between Metabolic Syndrome and Type of Dementia: Analysis Based on the National Health Insurance Service Database of Gangwon Province in South Korea," *Diabetology & Metabolic Syndrome* 13, no. 4 (January 2021); Scott M. Grundy et al., "Diagnosis and Management of the Metabolic Syndrome: An American Heart Association/National Heart, Lung, and Blood Institute Scientific Statement," *Circulation* 112, no. 17 (October 2005): 2735–52; Gang Hu et al., "Prevalence of the Metabolic Syndrome and Its Relation to All-Cause and Cardiovascular Mortality in Nondiabetic European Men and Women," *Archives of Internal Medicine* 164, no. 10 (May 2004): 1066–76.

NOTES

7. Paul L. Hess et al., "The Metabolic Syndrome and Risk of Sudden Cardiac Death: The Atherosclerosis Risk in Communities Study," *Journal of the American Heart Association* 6, no. 8 (August 2017): e006103; Ting Huai Shi, BinhuanWang, and Sundar Natarajan, "The Influence of Metabolic Syndrome in Predicting Mortality Risk among US Adults: Importance of Metabolic Syndrome Even in Adults with Normal Weight," *Preventing Chronic Disease* 17, no. E36 (May 2020): 1–10.

8. Sara Ghoneim et al., "The Incidence of COVID-19 in Patients with Metabolic Syndrome and Non-Alcoholic Steatohepatitis: A Population-Based Study," *Metabolism Open* 8 (December 2020): 100057.

9. Joana Araújo, Jianwen Cai, and June Stevens, "Prevalence of Optimal Metabolic Health in American Adults: National Health and Nutrition Examination Survey 2009–2016," *Metabolic Syndrome and Related Disorders* 17, no. 1 (February 2019): 46–52.

10. "Non-Alcoholic Fatty Liver Disease," October 21, 2020, https://www.mayoclinic.org/diseases-conditions/nonalcoholic-fatty-liver-disease/symptoms-causes/syc-20354567.

11. Ki-Chul Sung and Sun H. Kim, "Interrelationship between Fatty Liver and Insulin Resistance in the Development of Type 2 Diabetes," *The Journal of Clinical Endocrinology & Metabolism* 96, no. 4 (April 2011): 1093–97.

12. Ifigenia Kostoglou-Athanassiou and P. Athanassiou, "Metabolic Syndrome and Sleep Apnea" *Hippokratia* 12, no. 2 (May 2008): 81–6.

13. Steven R. Coughlin et al., "Obstructive Sleep Apnoea Is Independently Associated with an Increased Prevalence of Metabolic Syndrome," *European Heart Journal* 25, no. 9 (May 2004): 735–41.

14. Felipe Lobelo et al., "Routine Assessment and Promotion of Physical Activity in Healthcare Settings: A Scientific Statement from the American Heart Association," *Circulation* 137, no. 18 (May 2018): e495–522.

15. Chi Pang Wen and Xifeng Wu, "Stressing Harms of Physical Inactivity to Promote Exercise," *The Lancet* 380, no. 9838 (July 2012): 192–93.

16. "Metabolic Syndrome: Other Names," National Heart, Lung, and Blood Institute, http://www.nhlbi.nih.gov/health/dci/Diseases/ms/ms_othernames.html.

17. Cuilin Zhang et al., "Abdominal Obesity and the Risk of All-Cause, Cardiovascular, and Cancer Mortality: Sixteen Years of Follow-Up in US Women," *Circulation* 117, no. 13 (April 2008): 1658–67.

18. Geum Joon Cho et al., "Association between Waist Circumference and Dementia in Older Persons: A Nationwide Population-Based Study," *Obesity (Silver Spring)* 27, no. 11 (November 2019): 1883–91.

19. The InterAct Consortium, "Long-Term Risk of Incident Type 2 Diabetes and Measures of Overall and Regional Obesity: The Epic-InterAct Case-Cohort Study," *Plos Medicine* 9, no. 6 (June 2012): e10011230; Silke Feller, Heiner Boeing, and Tobias Pischon, "Body Mass Index, Waist Circumference and the Risk of Type 2 Diabetes Mellitus," *Deutsches Ärzetblatt International* 107, no. 26 (July 2010): 470–76.

20. American Psychological Association, "Fat Shaming in the Doctor's Office Can Be Mentally and Physically Harmful," August 3, 2017, https://www.apa.org/news/press/releases/2017/08/fat-shaming.

21. Ilze Mentoor, Maritza Kruger, and Theo Nell, "Metabolic Syndrome and Body Shape Predict Differences in Health Parameters in Farm Working Women," *BMC Public Health* 18, no. 1 (April 2018): 453.

22. "An International Atherosclerosis Society Position Paper: Global Recommendations for the Management of Dyslipidemia—Full Report," *Journal of Clinical Lipidology* 8, no. 1 (January 2014): 29–60.

23. Gary R. Hunter et al., "Exercise Training Prevents Regain of Visceral Fat for 1 Year Following Weight Loss," *Obesity (Silver Spring)* 18, no. 4 (April 2010): 690–95.

24. Vasanti S. Malik et al., "Sugar-Sweetened Beverages and Risk of Metabolic Syndrome and Type 2 Diabetes," *Diabetes Care* 33, no. 11 (November 2010): 2477–83; Zhila Semnani-Azad et al., "Association of Major Food Sources of Fructose-Containing Sugars with Incident Metabolic Syndrome: A Systematic Review and Meta-Analysis," *JAMA Network Open* 3, no. 7 (July 2020): e209993.

25. John M. Flack and Bemi Adekola, "Blood Pressure and the New ACC/AHA Hypertension Guidelines," *Trends in Cardiovascular Medicine* 30, no. 3 (May 2019): 160–64.

26. Centers for Disease Control and Prevention, "Hypertension Cascade: Hypertension Prevalence, Treatment and Control Estimates among US Adults Aged 18 Years and Older Applying the Criteria from the American College of Cardiology and American Heart Association's 2017 Hypertension Guideline—NHANES 2013–2016," https://millionhearts.hhs.gov/data-reports/hypertension-prevalence.html.

27. Ibid.

28. Zinat Nadia Hatmi, Nasrin Jalilian, and Ali Pakravan, "The Relationship between Premature Myocardial Infarction with TC/HDL-C Ratio Subgroups in a Multiple Risk Factor Model," *Advanced Journal of Emergency Medicine* 12, no. 3 (May 2019): e24.

29. G. L. Vega et al., "Triglyceride-to-High-Density-Lipoprotein-Cholesterol Ratio Is an Index of Heart Disease Mortality and of Incidence Of Type 2 Diabetes Mellitus in Men," *Journal of Investigative Medicine* 62, no. 2 (February 2014): 345-49; M. Prasad et al., "Triglyceride and Triglyceride/ HDL (High Density Lipoprotein) Ratio Predict Major Adverse Cardiovascular Outcomes in Women with Non-Obstructive Coronary Artery Disease," *J Am Heart Assoc* 8, no. 9 (May 2019): e009442.

30. Lucas Schwingshackl and Georg Hoffmann, "Monounsaturated Fatty Acids, Olive Oil and Health Status: A Systematic Review and Meta-Analysis of Cohort Studies," *Lipids in Health and Disease* 13, no. 154 (October 2014); María-Isabel Covas et al., "The Effect of Polyphenols in Olive Oil on Heart Disease Risk Factors: A Randomized Trial," *Annals of Internal Medicine* 145, no. 5 (September 2006): 333–41; María-Jesús Oliveras-López et al., "Extra Virgin Olive Oil (EVOO) Consumption and

Antioxidant Status in Healthy Institutionalized Elderly Humans," *Archives of Gerontology and Geriatrics* 57, no. 2 (September–October 2013): 234–42.

31. Dan Li et al., "Purified Anthocyanin Supplementation Reduces Dyslipidemia, Enhances Antioxidant Capacity, and Prevents Insulin Resistance in Diabetic Patients," *The Journal of Nutrition* 145, no. 4 (April 2015): 742–48; Yu Qin et al., "Anthocyanin Supplementation Improves Serum LDL- and HDL-Cholesterol Concentrations Associated with the Inhibition of Cholesteryl Ester Transfer Protein in Dyslipidemic Subjects," *American Journal of Clinical Nutrition* 90, no. 3 (September 2009): 485–92.

32. J. Michael Gaziano et al., "Fasting Triglycerides, High-Density Lipoprotein, and Risk of Myocardial Infarction," *Circulation* 96, no. 8 (October 1997): 2520–25.

33. Tracey McLaughlin et al., "Is There a Simple Way to Identify Insulin-Resistant Individuals at Increased Risk of Cardiovascular Disease?" *American Journal of Cardiolology* 96, no. 3 (August 2005): 399–404; Chaoyang Li et al., "Does the Association of the Triglyceride to High-Density Lipoprotein Cholesterol Ratio with Fasting Serum Insulin Differ by Race/Ethnicity?" *Cardiovascular Diabetology* 7, no. 1 (February 2008): 1–9.

34. Michael Miller et al., "Triglycerides and Cardiovascular Disease: A Scientific Statement from the American Heart Association," *Circulation* 123, no. 20 (May 2011): 2292–333.

35. Charles J. Glueck et al., "Associations between Serum 25-Hydroxyvitamin D and Lipids, Lipoprotein Cholesterols, and Homocysteine," *North American Journal of Medical Sciences* 8, no. 7 (July 2016): 284–90; Xiongjing Jiang et al., "Vitamin D Deficiency Is Associated with Dyslipidemia: A Cross-Sectional Study in 3788 Subjects," *Current Medical Research and Opinion* 3, no. 6 (June 2019): 1059–63; Richard C. Strange, Kate E. Shipman, and Sudarshan Ramachandran, "Metabolic Syndrome: A Review of the Role of Vitamin D in Mediating Susceptibility and Outcome," *World Journal of Diabetes* 6, no. 7 (July 2015): 896–911.

36. Susan P. Helmrich et al., "Physical Activity and Reduced Occurrence of Non-Insulin-Dependent Diabetes Mellitus," *New England Journal of Medicine* 325, no. 3 (July 1991): 147–52; Susumu Sawada et al., "Long-Term Trends in Cardiorespiratory Fitness and the Incidence of Type 2 Diabetes," *Diabetes Care* 33, no. 6 (June 2010): 1353–57.

37. Sheri R. Colberg et al., "Physical Activity/Exercise and Diabetes: A Position Statement of the American Diabetes Association," *Diabetes Care* 39, no. 11 (November 2016): 2065–79.

38. William C. Knowler et al., "Diabetes Prevention Program Research Group Reduction in the Incidence of Type 2 Diabetes with Lifestyle Intervention or Metformin," *New England Journal of Medicine* 346, no. 6 (February 2002): 393–403.

39. "Glucose Tolerance and Mortality: Comparison of WHO and American Diabetes Association Diagnostic Criteria. The DECODE Study Group.

European Diabetes Epidemiology Group. Diabetes Epidemiology: Collaborative Analysis of Diagnostic Criteria in Europe," *Lancet* 1354, no. 9179 (1999): 617–21.

40. B. J. Neth and S. Craft, "Insulin Resistance and Alzheimer's Disease: Bioenergetic Linkages," *Frontiers of Aging Neuroscience* 9 (2017): 345.
41. E. Onyebuchi et al., "Can Admission and Fasting Glucose Reliably Identify Undiagnosed Diabetes in Patients with Acute Coronary Syndrome?," *Diabetes Care* 31, no. 10 (October 2008): 1955–59.
42. "National Diabetes Statistics Report 2020: Estimates of Diabetes and Its Burden on the United States," Centers for Disease Control and Prevention, https://www.cdc.gov/diabetes/pdfs/data/statistics/national -diabetes-statistics-report.pdf.
43. Centers for Disease Control and Prevention, "Diabetes Basics: Prediabetes," June 11, 2020, https://www.cdc.gov/diabetes/basics/prediabetes.html.
44. Muhammad A. Abdul-Ghani et al., "Minimal Contribution of Fasting Hyperglycemia to the Incidence of Type 2 Diabetes in Subjects with Normal 2-h Plasma Glucose," *Diabetes Care* 33, no. 3 (March 2010): 557–61.
45. R. Loh et al., "Effects of Interrupting Prolonged Sitting with Physical Activity Breaks on Blood Glucose, Insulin and Triacylglycerol Measures: A Systematic Review and Meta-Analysis," *Sports Medicine* 50 (2020): 295–330.

Chapter 10: Healthy Gums and Teeth Help You Live Longer

1. Paul I. Eke et al., "Prevalence of Periodontitis in Adults in the United States: 2009 and 2010," *Journal of Dental Research* 91, no. 10 (August 2012): 914–20.
2. Quan Shi et al., "Association between Myocardial Infarction and Peri-odontitis: A Meta-Analysis of Case-Control Studies," *Frontiers in Physiology* 7, no. 519 (November 2016).
3. Jae-Hong Lee et al., "Association of Lifestyle-Related Comorbidities with Periodontitis: A Nationwide Cohort Study in Korea," *Medicine* 94, no. 37 (September 2015): e1567.
4. Philip M. Preshaw et al., "Periodontitis and Diabetes: A Two-Way Relationship," *Diabetologia* 55, no. 1 (January 2012): 21–31.
5. Ibid.
6. Dominique S. Michaud et al., "Periodontal Disease Assessed Using Clinical Dental Measurements and Cancer Risk in the ARIC Study," *Journal of the National Cancer Institute* 110, no. 8 (August 2018): 843–54.
7. Jo L. Freudenheim et al., "Periodontal Disease and Breast Cancer: Prospective Cohort Study of Postmenopausal Women," *Cancer Epidemiology, Biomarkers & Prevention* 25, no. 1 (January 2016): 43–50.
8. Qianting Wang et al., "The Association between Chronic Periodontitis and Vasculogenic Erectile Dysfunction: A Systematic Review and Meta-Analysis," *Journal of Clinical Periodontology* 43, no. 3 (March 2016): 206–15.

NOTES

9. Abubekir Eltas et al., "The Effect of Periodontal Treatment in Improving Erectile Dysfunction: A Randomized Controlled Trial," *Journal of Clinical Periodontology* 40, no. 2 (February 2013): 148–54; Vijendra P. Singh et al., "Oral Health and Erectile Dysfunction," *Journal of Human Reproductive Sciences* 10, no. 3 (October 2017): 162–66.

10. Sheena E. Ramsay et al., "Influence of Poor Oral Health on Physical Frailty: A Population-Based Cohort Study of Older British Men," *Journal of the American Geriatrics Society* 66, no. 3 (March 2018): 473–79.

11. Sushil Kaur, Saralouise White, and P. Mark Bartold, "Periodontal Disease and Rheumatoid Arthritis: A Systematic Review," *Journal of Dental Research* 92, no. 5 (May 2013): 399–408.

12. P. Ortiz et al., "Periodontal Therapy Reduces the Severity of Active Rheumatoid Arthritis in Patients Treated with or with Tumor Necrosis Factor Inhibitors," *Journal of Periodontology* 80, no. 4 (April 2009): 535–40.

13. Chang-Kai Chen, Yung-Tsan Wu, and Yu-Chao Chang, "Association between Chronic Periodontitis and the Risk of Alzheimer's Disease: A Retrospective, Population-Based, Matched-Cohort Study," *Alzheimer's Research & Therapy* 9, no. 1 (August 2017).

14. Priya Nimish Deo and Revati Deshmukh, "Oral Microbiome: Unveiling the Fundamentals," *Journal of Oral and Maxillofacial Pathology* 23, no. 1 (January–April 2019): 122–28.

15. Guodong Jia et al., "The Oral Microbiota—A Mechanistic Role for Systemic Diseases," *British Dental Journal* 224, no. 6 (March 2018): 447–55.

16. Herbert M. Cobe, "Transitory Bacteremia," *Oral Surgery, Oral Medicine and Oral Pathology* 7, no. 6 (June 1954): 609–15.

17. Ingar Olsen, "Update on Bacteraemia Related to Dental Procedures," *Transfusion and Apheresis Science* 39, no. 2 (October 2008): 173–78.

18. Peter B. Lockhart et al., "Periodontal Disease and Atherosclerotic Vascular Disease: Does the Evidence Support an Independent Association?: A Scientific Statement from the American Heart Association," *Circulation* 125, no. 20 (May 2012): 2520–44.

19. Bradley F. Bale, Amy L. Doneen, and David J. Vigerust, "High-Risk Periodontal Pathogens Contribute to the Pathogenesis of Atherosclerosis," *Postgrad Medical Journal* 93, no. 1098 (April 2017): 215–20.

20. Per Fogelstrand and Jan Borén, "Retention of Atherogenic Lipoproteins in the Artery Wall and Its Role in Atherogenesis," *Nutrition, Metabolism and Cardiovascular Diseases* 22, no. 1 (January 2012): 1–7.

21. Tanja Pessi et al., "Bacterial Signatures in Thrombus Aspirates of Patients with Myocardial Infarction," *Circulation* 127, no. 11 (March 2013): 1219–28.

22. Damir Vakhitov et al., "Bacterial Signatures in Thrombus Aspirates of Patients with Lower Limb Arterial and Venous Thrombosis," *Journal of Vascular Surgery* 67, no. 6 (June 2018): 19027.

23. Kamile Leonardi Dutra et al., "Diagnostic Accuracy of Cone-Beam Computed Tomography and Conventional Radiography on Apical Periodontitis: A Systematic Review and Meta-Analysis," *Journal of Endodontics* 42, no. 3 (March 2016): 356–64.

24. Sonja Sälzer et al., "Efficacy of Inter-Dental Mechanical Plaque Control in Managing Gingivitis—A Meta-Review," *Journal of Clinical Periodontology* 42, Suppl 16 (April 2015): S92–105.

25. Annlia Paganini-Hill, Stuart C. White, and Kathryn A. Atchison, "Dental Health Behaviors, Dentition, and Mortality in the Elderly: The Leisure World Cohort Study," *Journal of Aging Research* 2011 (June 2011): 156061.

Chapter 11: Mining Your DNA for Actionable Health Insights

1. Jelena Kornej et al., "Epidemiology of Atrial Fibrillation in the 21st Century: Novel Methods and New Insights," *Circulation Research* 127, no. 1 (June 2020): 4–20.

2. Lisa Gannett ,"The Human Genome Project," in *The Stanford Encyclopedia of Philosophy,* ed. Edward N. Zalta (2019), https://plato.stanford.edu /archives/win2019/entries/human-genome/.

3. Stephen R. Houser, "The American Heart Association's New Institute for Precision Cardiovascular Medicine," *Circulation* 134, no. 24 (December 2016): 1913–14.

4. Bradley F. Bale, Amy L. Doneen, and David J. Vigerust, "Precision Healthcare of Type 2 Diabetic Patients through Implementation of Haptoglobin Genotyping," *Frontiers in Cardiovascular Medicine* 5, no. 141 (October 2018).

5. Jane Kaye, "The Regulation of Direct-to-Consumer Genetic Tests," *Human Molecular Genetics* 17, no. R2 (October 2008): R180–83.

6. "Home Genetic Testing: A Nationally Representative Multi-Mode Survey," *Consumer Reports,* October 2020, https://article.images.consumerreports .org/prod/content/dam/surveys/Consumer%20Reports%20 Home%20Genetic%20Testing%20October%202020.

7. J. Scott Roberts et al., "Direct-to-Consumer Genetic Testing: User Motivations, Decision Making, and Perceived Utility of Results," *Public Health Genomics* 20, no. 1 (January 2017): 36–45.

8. Kathryn A. Phillips et al., "Genetic Test Availability and Spending: Where Are We Now? Where Are We Going?" *Health Affairs (Project Hope)* 37, no. 5 (May 2018): 710–16.

9. Melissa A. Austin et al., "Genetic Causes of Monogenic Heterozygous Familial Hypercholesterolemia: A HuGE Prevalence Review," *American Journal of Epidemiology* 160, no. 5 (September 2004): 407–20.

10. Euan A. Ashley et al., "Genetics and Cardiovascular Disease: A Policy Statement from the American Heart Association," *Circulation* 126, no. 1 (May 2012): 142–57; Seema Mital et al., "Enhancing Literacy in

Cardiovascular Genetics: A Scientific Statement from the American Heart Association," *Circulation Cardiovascular Genetics* 9, no. 5 (October 2016): 448–67.

11. Glenn E. Palomaki, Stephanie Melillo, and Linda A. Bradley, "Association between 9p21 Genomic Markers and Heart Disease: A Meta-Analysis," *Journal of the American Medical Association* 303, no. 7 (February 2010): 648–56.

12. Anna Helgadottir et al., "A Common Variant on Chromosome 9p21 Affects the Risk of Myocardial Infarction," *Science* 316, no. 5830 (June 2007): 1491–93; Anna Helgadottir et al., "The Same Sequence Variant on 9p21 Associates with Myocardial Infarction, Abdominal Aortic Aneurysm and Intercranial Aneurysm," *Nature Genetics* 40, no. 2 (February 2008): 217–24.

13. Ibid.

14. Ibid.

15. Weili Zhang et al., "Variants on Chromosome 9p21.3 Correlated with ANRIL Expression Contribute to Stroke Risk and Recurrence in a Large Prospective Stroke Population," *Stroke* 43, no. 1 (January 2012): 14–21.

16. Ibid.

17. Anna Helgadottir et al., "The Same Sequence Variant on 9p21 Associates with Myocardial Infarction, Abdominal Aortic Aneurysm and Intercranial Aneurysm," *Nature Genetics* 40, no. 2 (February 2008): 217–24.

18. Alessandro Doria et al., " Interaction between Poor Glycemic Control and 9p21 Locus on Risk of Coronary Artery Disease in Type 2 Diabetes," *Journal of the American Medical Association* 300, no. 20 (November 2008): 2389–97.

19. Emma Tikkanen, Stefan Gustafsson, Erik Ingelsson, "Associations of Fitness, Physical Activity, Strength, and Genetic Risk with Cardiovascular Disease: Longitudinal Analyses in the UK Biobank Study," *Circulation* 137, no. 24 (June 2018): 2583–91.

20. Doria et al., " Interaction between Poor Glycemic Control and 9p21 Locus on Risk of Coronary Artery Disease in Type 2 Diabetes."

21. Jay S. Skyler et al., "American Diabetes Association; American College of Cardiology Foundation, American Heart Association, Intensive Glycemic Control and the Prevention of Cardiovascular Events: Implications of the ACCORD, ADVANCE, and VA Diabetes Trials: A Position Statement of the American Diabetes Association and a Scientific Statement of the American College of Cardiology Foundation and the American Heart Association," *Diabetes Care* 32, no. 7 (July 2009): 187–92.

22. "Glycemic Targets: Standards of Medical Care in Diabetes—2021, American Diabetes Association," *Diabetes Care* 44, Suppl 1 (January 2021): S73–84.

23. Centers for Disease Control and Prevention, "National Center for Health Statistics, Underlying Cause of Death 1999–2018," http://wonder.cdc .gov/ucd-icd10.html.

24. I-Min Lee et al., "Effect of Physical Inactivity on Major Non-Communicable Diseases Worldwide: An Analysis of Burden of Disease and Life Expectancy," *The Lancet* 380, no. 9838 (July 2012): 219–29.

25. Jacob Raber, Yadong Huang, and J. Wesson Ashford, "ApoE Genotype Accounts for the Vast Majority of AD Risk and AD Pathology," *Neurobiology of Aging* 25, no. 5 (May–June 2004): 641–50.

26. Peter S. Sever et al., "Prevention of Coronary and Stroke Events with Atorvastatin in Hypertensive Patients Who Have Average or Lower-Than-Average Cholesterol Concentrations, in the Anglo-Scandinavian Cardiac Outcome Trial—Lipid Lowering Arm (ASCOT–LLA): A Multicentre Randomised Controlled Trial," *The Lancet* 361, no. 9364 (April 2003): 1149–58.

27. Centers for Disease Control and Prevention, "Atrial Fibrillation," https://www.cdc.gov/heartdisease/atrial_fibrillation.htm.

28. Laila Staerk et al., "Lifetime Risk of Atrial Fibrillation According to Optimal, Borderline, or Elevated Levels of Risk Factors: Cohort Study Based on Longitudinal Data from the Framingham Heart Study," *British Medical Journal* 361 (April 2018): k1453.

29. Peter M. Okin et al., "Effect of Lower On-Treatment Systolic Blood Pressure on the Risk of Atrial Fibrillation in Hypertensive Patients," *Hypertension* 66, no. 2 (July 2015): 368–73.

30. Miguel Á. Martínez-González et al., "Extravirgin Olive Oil Consumption Reduces Risk of Atrial Fibrillation: The PREDIMED (Prevención con Dieta Mediterránea) Trial," *Circulation* 130, no. 1 (July 2014): 18–26.

31. James H. O'Keefe et al., "Effects of Habitual Coffee Consumption on Cardiometabolic Disease, Cardiovascular Health, and All-Cause Mortality," Journal of the American College of Cardiology 62, no 12 (September 2013): 1043-1051; Amatul S. Hasan et al., "Coffee, Caffeine, and Risk of Hospitalization for Arrhythmias," poster presented at the EPIINPAM 2010 Annual Conference, San Francisco, CA, March 2010 Abstract P461, https://www.bsu.edu/Academics/CollegesandDepartments/CEPP/Research/CEPPProgramResearch/-/media/WWW/DepartmentalContent/CEPP/PDFs/4Abstract.ashx.

32. Bradley F. Bale et al., "Precision Healthcare of Type 2 Diabetic Patients through Implementation of Haptoglobin Genotyping," *Frontiers in Cardiovascular Medicine* 5, no. 141 (October 2018).

33. Andrew P. Levy et al., "Haptoglobin Phenotype Is an Independent Risk Factor for Cardiovascular Disease in Individuals with Diabetes: The Strong Heart Study," *Journal of the American College of Cardiology* 40, no. 11 (December 2002): 1984–90.

34. Michel R. Langlois and Joris R. Delanghe, "Biological and Clinical Significance of Haptoglobin Polymorphism in Humans, *Clinical Chemistry* 42, no. 10 (October 1996): 1589–1600.

35. Amit Tripathi et al., "Identification of Human Zonulin, A Physiological Modulator of Tight Junctions, as Prehaptoglobin-2," *Proceedings of the*

National Academy Sciences of the United States of America 106, no. 39 (September 2009): 16799–804.

36. Alessio Fasano, "Zonulin and Its Regulation of Intestinal Barrier Function: The Biological Door to Inflammation, Autoimmunity, and Cancer," *Physiology Review* 91, no. 1 (January 2011): 151–75.

37. "Familial Hypercholesterolemia (FH)," Centers for Disease Control and Prevention, Updated March 20, 2020, https://www.cdc.gov/genomics /disease/fh/FH.htm.

38. Ibid

39. "Familial Hypercholesterolemia (FH)," American Heart Association, Updated November 9, 2020, https://www.heart.org/en/health-topics /cholesterol/causes-of-high-cholesterol/familial-hyper cholesterolemia-fh.

Chapter 12: Three Smart Strategies to Protect Your Memory

1. Alzheimer's Disease International. (2020) "Dementia Statistics," https:// www.alzint.org/about/dementia-facts-figures/dementia-statistics/.

2. R. Brookmeyer et al., "National estimates of the prevalence of Alzheimer's disease in the United States." *Alzheimer's & Dementia: The Journal of the Alzheimer's Association* 7, no. 1 (2011): 61–73; C. Ballard et al., "Alzheimer's disease," *The The Lancet* 377, no. 9770 (2011): 1019–31.

3. Alzheimer's Association, "2020 Alzheimer's Disease Facts and Figures," *Alzheimers Dement* 16, no. 3 (2020): 391.

4. Ibid.

5. Ibid.

6. Ibid.

7. Ibid

8. Ibid

9. G. Livingston et al., "Dementia Prevention, Intervention, and Care: 2020 Report of the Lancet Commission," *The Lancet* 396, no. 10248 (2020): 413–46. doi: 10.1016/S0140-6736(20)30367-6. Epub 2020 Jul 30.

10. World Health Organization, "Risk Reduction of Cognitive Decline and Dementia: WHO Guidelines" (2019), https://apps.who.int/iris/bitstream /handle/10665/312180/9789241550543-eng.pdf.

11. G. Livingston et al., "Dementia Prevention, Intervention, and Care," *The Lancet* 396, no. 10248 (2020): 413–46. doi: 10.1016/S0140-6736(20)30367-6. Epub 2020 Jul 30.

12. K. Dhana et al., "Healthy Lifestyle and the Risk of Alzheimer Dementia: Findings from 2 Longitudinal Studies," *Neurology* 95 no. 4 (2020): e374–e383.

13. Alzheimer's Association, "Your Brain," https://www.alz.org/espanol /about/brain/02.asp.

14. M. Rusanen et al., "Heavy Smoking in Midlife and Long-Term Risk of Alzheimer Disease and Vascular Dementia," *Arch Intern Med* 171, no. 4 (2011): 333–39.

15. G. Paroni, P. Bisceglia, and D. Seripa, "Understanding the Amyloid Hypothesis in Alzheimer's Disease," *J Alzheimers Dis* 68, no. 2 (2019): 493–510, doi:10.3233/JAD-180802. PMID: 30883346.

16. G. Livingston et al., " Dementia Prevention, Intervention, and Care," *The Lancet* 396, no. 10248 (2020): 413–46. doi: 10.1016/S0140-6736(20)30367-6. Epub 2020 Jul 30.

17. E. Y. Cornwell and L. J. Waite, "Measuring Social Isolation among Older Adults Using Multiple Indicators from the NSHAP Study," *J Gerontol B Psychol Sci Soc Sci* 64, Suppl 1 (2009): i38–46. Epub 2009 Jun 9.

18. G. Livingston et al., "Dementia prevention, intervention, and care: 2020 report of the Lancet Commission," Lancet 396, 10248 (2020): 413–446, doi: 10.1016/S0140-6736(20)30367-6.

19. C. Valls-Pedret et al., "Mediterranean Diet and Age-Related Cognitive Decline: A Randomized Clinical Trial," *JAMA Intern Med* 175, no. 7 (2015): 1094–103. Erratum in *JAMA Intern Med* 178, no. 12 (2018): 1731–32.

20. Time Gard et al., "The Potential Effects of Meditation on Age-Related Cognitive Decline: A Systematic Review," *Annals of the New York Academy of Sciences* 1307 (2014): 89–103.

21. R. Wilson et al., "Participation in cognitively stimulating activities and risk of incident Alzheimer disease," *Journal of the American Medical Association* 267, no. 16 (2002): 742–48, doi: 10.1001/jama.287.6.742. PMID: 11851541; F. Craik et al., "Delaying the onset of Alzheimer disease: bilingualism as a form of cognitive reserve," *Neurology* 75, no. 19 (2010): 1726–29, doi: 10.1212/WNL.0b013e3181fc2a1c; N. Scarmeas et al., "Physical activity, diet, and risk of Alzheimer disease," *Journal of the American Medical Association* 302, no. 6 (2009): 627–37, doi: 10.1001/jama.2009.1144; K. Ertel et al., "Effects of social integration on preserving memory function in a nationally representative US elderly population," *Am J Public Health* (2008): 1215–20, doi: 10.2105/AJPH.2007.113654: P. S. Pressman et al., "Observing conversational laughter in frontotemporal dementia," *J Neurol Neurosurg Psychiatry* 88, no. 5 (2017), 418–24, doi: 10.1136/jnnp-2016-314931.

22. E. Shokri-Kojori et al., "β-Amyloid Accumulation in the Human Brain after One Night of Sleep Deprivation," *Proceedings of the National Academy of Sciences of the United States of America* 115, no. 17 (2018): 4483–88, doi: 10.1073/pnas.1721694115.

23. M. S. Tsai et al., "Risk of Alzheimer's Disease in Obstructive Sleep Apnea Patients With or Without Treatment: Real-World Evidence," *Laryngoscope* 130, no. 9 (September 2020): 2292-22.

24. Thomas J. Littlejohns et al., "Vitamin D and the Risk of Dementia and Alzheimer Disease," *Neurology* 83, no. 10 (September 2014): 920–28.

25. M. Beydoun et al., "Clinical and Bacterial Markers of Periodontitis and Their Association with Incident All-Cause and Alzheimer's Disease Dementia in a Large National Survey," *Journal of Alzheimer's Disease* 75, no. 1 (2020): 157–72.

26. S. Dominy et al., "Porphyromonas gingivalis in Alzheimer's disease brains: Evidence for disease causation and treatment with small-molecule inhibitors," J Science Advances 5, no. 1 (2019).

27. A. Solomon et al., "Midlife Serum Cholesterol and Increased Risk of Alzheimer's and Vascular Dementia Three Decades Later," *Dement Geriatr Cogn Disord* 28, no. 1 (2009): 75–80; K. J. Anstey et al., "Updating the Evidence on the Association between Serum Cholesterol and Risk of Late-Life Dementia: Review and Meta-Analysis." *Journal of Alzheimer's Disease* 56, no. 1 (2017): 215–28.

28. Anstey et al., "Updating the Evidence on the Association between Serum Cholesterol and Risk of Late-Life Dementia."

29. S. J. Taler, "Initial Treatment of Hypertension," *New England Journal of Medicine* 2018, no. 378 (2018): 636–44, doi: 10.1056/NEJMcp1613481. PMID: 29443671.

30. C. A. Emdin, "Blood Pressure and Risk of Vascular Dementia: Evidence from Primary Care Registry and a Cohort Study of Transient Ischemic Attack and Stroke," *Stroke* 47, no. 6 (2016): 1429–35.

31. C. Lane et al., 2019. "Associations between Blood Pressure across Adulthood and Late-Life Brain Structure and Pathology in the Neuroscience Substudy of the 1946 British Birth Cohort: An Epidemiological Study," *Lancet Neurology;* 18, no. 210 (2019:942–52.

32. K. Kowalski & A. Mulak, "Brain-Gut-Microbiota Axis in Alzheimer's Disease," *Journal of Neurogastroenterology and Motility* 25, no. 1 (2019): 48–60.

33. F. Zhu, C. Li, F. Chu, X Tian, and J. Zhu, "Target Dysbiosis of Gut Microbes as a Future Therapeutic Manipulation in Alzheimer's Disease," *Front Aging Neurosci* 12 (2020): 544235.

34. B. J. Neth and S. Craft (2017). "Insulin Resistance and Alzheimer's Disease: Bioenergetic Linkages." *Front Aging Neurosci* 9 (2017).

35. S. T. Ferreira and W. L. Klein, "The Abeta Oligomer Hypothesis for Synapse Failure and Memory Loss in Alzheimer's Disease," *Neurobiol Learn Mem* 96, no. 4 (2011): 529–43.

36. Ibid.

37. J. Verghese et al., "Leisure Activities and the Risk of Dementia in the Elderly," *New England Journal of Medicine* 348, no. 25 (2003): 2508–16.

38. "Why Do We Like to Dance—And Move to the Beat?" *Scientific American* (2008), https://www.scientificamerican.com/article/experts-dance/.

39. "Dancing and the Brain," Harvard Medical School (2015), https://hms.harvard.edu/news-events/publications-archive/brain/dancing-brain.

Chapter 13: Lifestyle: the Ultimate Miracle Cure

1. Felipe Lobelo et al., "Routine Assessment and Promotion of Physical Activity in Healthcare Settings: A Scientific Statement from the American Heart Association," *Circulation* 137, no. 18 (May 2018): e495-522.

NOTES

2. Lorenzo Galluzzi and Guido Kroemer, "Autophagy Mediates the Metabolic Benefits of Endurance Training," *Circulation Research* 110, no. 1 (May 2012): 1276–78; Congcong He et al., "Exercise-Induced BCL–2-Regulated Autophagy Is Required for Muscle Glucose Homeostasis," *Nature* 481, no. 7382 (January 2012): 511–15.

3. Klodian Dhana et al., "Healthy Lifestyle and the Risk of Alzheimer's Dementia: Findings from Two Longitudinal Studies," *Neurology* 95, no. 4 (July 2020): e374–83; Andrea Chomistek et al., "Healthy Lifestyle in the Primordial Prevention of Cardiovascular Disease among Young Women," *Journal of the American College of Cardiology* 65, no. 1 (January 2015): 43–51.

4. Nisa M. Maruthur et al., "Early Response to Preventive Strategies in the Diabetes Prevention Program," *Journal of General Internal Medicine* 28, no. 12 (December 2013): 1629–36.

5. William E Kraus et al., "2 Years of Calorie Restriction and Cardiometabolic Risk (CALERIE): Exploratory Outcomes of a Multicentre, Phase 2, Randomised Controlled Trial," *The Lancet Diabetes & Endocrinology* 7, no. 9 (September 2019): 673–83.

6. Dena Bravata et al., "Using Pedometers to Increase Physical Activity and Improve Health: A Systematic Review," *Journal of the American Medical Association* 298, no. 19 (November 2007): 2296–304; Stanford Medicine News Center, "Pedometers Help People Stay Active, Stanford Study Finds," November 20, 2007, https://med.stanford.edu/news/all-news /2007/11/pedometers-help-people-stay-active-stanford-study-finds .html.

7. Liliana Laranjo et al., "Do Smartphone Applications and Activity Trackers Increase Physical Activity in Adults? Systematic Review, Meta-Analysis and Metaregression," *British Journal of Sports Medicine* 55, no. 8 (April 2021): 422–32.

8. Clara K. Chow et al., "Association of Diet, Exercise, and Smoking Modification with Risk of Early Cardiovascular Events after Acute Coronary Syndromes," *Circulation* 121, no. 6 (February 2010): 750–58.

9. American Heart Association, "Life's Simple 7" (2021), https://www .heart.org/en/professional/workplace-health/lifes-simple-7.

10. Donald M. Lloyd-Jones et al., "Defining and Setting National Goals for Cardiovascular Health Promotion and Disease Reduction: The American Heart Association's Strategic Impact Goal through 2020 and Beyond," *Circulation* 121, no. 4 (February 2010): 586–613; Liyuan Han et al., "National Trends in American Heart Association Revised Life's Simple 7 Metrics Associated with Risk of Mortality among US Adults," *Journal of the American Medical Association Network Open* 2, no. 10 (October 2019): e1913131; Laura D. Ellingson et al., "Active and Sedentary Behaviors Influence Feelings of Energy and Fatigue in Women," *Medicine and Science in Sports and Exercise* 46, no. 1 (January 2014): 192–200; Stephen R. Bird and John A. Hawley, "Update on the Effects of Physical Activity on

Insulin Sensitivity in Humans," *BMJ Open Sport & Exercise Medicine* 2, no. 1 (March 2017): e000143; Matthew A. Nystoriak and Aruni Bhatnagar, "Cardiovascular Effects and Benefits of Exercise," *Frontiers in Cardiovascular Medicine* 5, no. 135 (September 2018), Neve J. Kirk-Sanchez and Ellen L. McGough, "Physical Exercise and Cognitive Performance in the Elderly: Current Perspectives," *Clinical Interventions in Aging* 2014, no. 9 (December 2013): 51–62; Pei-YuYang et al., "Exercise Training Improves Sleep Quality in Middle-Aged and Older Adults with Sleep Problems: A Systematic Review," *Journal of Physiotherapy* 58, no. 3 (September 2012): 157–63; Amelia M. Stanton, Ariel B. Handy, and Cindy M. Meston, "The Effects of Exercise on Sexual Function in Women," *Sexual Medicine Reviews* 6, no. 4 (October 2018): 548–57; Kirkpatrick B. Fergus et al., "Exercise Improves Self-Reported Sexual Function among Physically Active Adults," *Journal of Sexual Medicine* 16, no. 8 (August 2019): 1236–45.

11. Ytaka Nakashima, Thomas N. Wight, and Katsuo Sueishi, "Early Atherosclerosis in Humans: Role of Diffuse Intimal Thickening and Extracellular Matrix Proteoglycans," *Cardiovascular Research* 79, no. 1 (July 2008): 14–23; Per Fogelstrand and Jan Borén, "Retention of Atherogenic Lipoproteins in the Artery Wall and Its Role in Atherogenesis," *Nutrition, Metabolism and Cardiovascular Diseases* 22, no. 1 (January 2012): 1–7.

12. Achmad Rudijanto, "The Role of Vascular Smooth Muscle Cells on the Pathogenesis of Atherosclerosis," *Acta Medica Indonesiana* 39, no. 2 (April–June 2007): 86–93; Amanda C. Doran, Nahum Meller, and Coleen A. McNamara, "Role of Smooth Muscle Cells in the Initiation and Early Progression of Atherosclerosis," *Arteriosclerosis, Thrombosis, and Vascular Biology* 28, no. 5 (May 2008): 812–19.

13. Ytaka Nakashima, Thomas N. Wight, and Katsuo Sueishi, "Early Atherosclerosis in Humans: Role of Diffuse Intimal Thickening and Extracellular Matrix Proteoglycans," *Cardiovascular Research* 79, no. 1 (July 2008): 14–23.

14. Brian R. Kupchak et al., "Beneficial Effects of Habitual Resistance Exercise Training on Coagulation and Fibrinolytic Responses," *Thrombosis Research* 131, no. 6 (June 2013): e227–34.

15. Mi-Na Gim and Jung-Hyun Choi, "The Effects of Weekly Exercise Time on VO2max and Resting Metabolic Rate in Normal Adults," *Journal of Physical Therapy Science* 28, no. 4 (April 2016): 1359–63; Jonathan Myers, Peter Kokkinos, and Eric Nyelin, "Physical Activity, Cardiorespiratory Fitness, and the Metabolic Syndrome," *Nutrients* 11, no. 7 (July 2019): 1652; Julia C. Basso and Wendy A Suzuki, "The Effects of Acute Exercise on Mood, Cognition, Neurophysiology, and Neurochemical Pathways: A Review," *Brain Plasticity* 2, no. 2 (March 2017): 127–52.

16. Dick H. J. Thijssen, "Association of Exercise Preconditioning with Immediate Cardioprotection: A Review," *JAMA Cardiology* 3, no. 2 (February 2018): 169–76.

NOTES

17. Mark A. Tully et al., "Randomised Controlled Trial of Home-Based Walking Programmes at and Below Current Recommended Levels of Exercise in Sedentary Adults," *Journal of Epidemiology and Community Health* 61, no. 9 (September 2007): 778–83.

18. Steven C. Moore et al., "Association of Leisure-Time Physical Activity with Risk of 26 Types of Cancer in 1.44 Million Adults," *JAMA Internal Medicine* 176, no. 6 (June 2016): 816–25; Rajesh Shigdel et al., "Cardiorespiratory Fitness and the Risk of First Acute Myocardial Infarction: The HUNT Study," *Journal of the American Heart Association* 8, no. 9 (May 2019): e010293; Susumu Sawada et al., "Long-Term Trends in Cardiorespiratory Fitness and the Incidence of Type 2 Diabetes," *Diabetes Care* 33, no. 6 (June 2010): 1353–57.

19. Alpa V. Patel et al., "Walking Reduces Mortality in a Large Prospective Cohort of Older U.S. Adults," *American Journal of Preventive Medicine* 54, no. 1 (January 2018): 10–19.

20. James H. O'Keefe et al., "Potential Adverse Cardiovascular Effects Excessive Endurance Exercise," *Mayo Clinic Proceedings* 87, no. 6 (June 2012): 587–95.

21. Aron S. Buchman et al., "Physical Activity, Common Brain Pathologies, and Cognition in Community-Dwelling Older Adults," *Neurology* 92, no. 8 (February 2019): e811–22.

22. Orjan Ekblom et al., "Increased Physical Activity Post Myocardial Infarction Is Related to Reduced Mortality: Results from the SWEDEHEART Registry," *Journal of the American Heart Association* 7, no. 24 (December 2018): e010108.

23. Elena Salmoirago-Blotcher et al., "Tai Chi Is a Promising Exercise Option for Patients with Coronary Heart Disease Declining Cardiac Rehab," *Journal of the American Heart Association* 6, no. 10 (October 2017): e00663.

24. Arnt E. Tjønna et al., "Aerobic Interval Training Versus Continuous Moderate Exercise as a Treatment for the Metabolic Syndrome: A Pilot Study," *Circulation* 118, no. 4 (July 2008): 346–54.

25. Rania Mekary et al., "Weight Training, Aerobic Physical Activities, and Long-Term Waist Circumference Change in Men," *Obesity (Silver Spring)* 23, no. 2 (February 2015): 461–67.

26. Gary R. Hunter et al., "Exercise Training Prevents Regain of Visceral Fat for 1 Year Following Weight Loss," *Obesity (Silver Spring)* 18, no. 4 (April 2010): 690–95.

27. Cynthia M. Kroeger et al., "Improvement in Coronary Heart Disease Risk Factors during an Intermittent Fasting/Calorie Restriction Regimen: Relationship to Adipokine Modulations," *Nutrition & Metabolism* 9, no. 1 (October 2012): 98.

28. Rafael deCabo and Mark P. Mattison, "Effects of Intermittent Fasting on Health, Aging, and Disease," *New England Journal of Medicine* 381, no. 26 (December 2019): 2541–51; Bradley F. Bale and Amy L. Doneen,

"Autophagy, Senescence, and Arterial Inflammation: Relationship to Arterial Health and Longevity," *Alternative Therapies in Health & Medicine* 19, no. 4 (July–August 2013): 8–10.

29. Salim Jusuf et al., "Effect of Potentially Modifiable Risk Factors Associated with Myocardial Infarction in 52 Countries (The INTERHEART Study): Case-Control Study," *The Lancet* 364, no. 9438 (September 2004): 937–52.

30. Ahmed Tawakol et al., "Relation between Resting Amygdalar Activity and Cardiovascular Events: A Longitudinal and Cohort Study," *The Lancet* 389, no. 10071 (February 2017): 834–45.

31. Soudabeh Sadeghimoghaddam et al., "The Effect of Two Methods of Relaxation and Prayer Therapy on Anxiety and Hope in Patients with Coronary Artery Disease: A Quasi–Experimental Study," *Iranian Journal of Nursing and Midwifery Research* 24, no. 2 (March–April 2019): 102–7.

32. Tim Gard, Britta K. Hölzel, and Sara W. Lazar, "The Potential Effects of Meditation on Age-Related Cognitive Decline: A Systematic Review," *Annals of the New York Academy of Sciences* 1307 (May 2014): 89–103.

33. J. David Creswell et al., "Alterations in Resting-State Functional Connectivity Link Mindfulness Meditation with Reduced Interleukin-6: A Randomized Controlled Trial," *Biological Psychiatry* 80, no. 1 (July 2016): 53–61.

34. Manoj K. Bhasin et al., "Specific Transcriptome Changes Associated with Blood Pressure Reduction in Hypertensive Patients after Relaxation Response Training," *Journal of Alternative and Complementary Medicine* 24, no. 5 (May 2018): 486–504.

35. Samuel Y. S. Wong et al., "Treating Subthreshold Depression in Primary Care: A Randomized Controlled Trial of Behavioral Activation with Mindfulness," *Annals of Family Medicine* 16, no. 2 (March 2018): 111–19.

36. Steven Bell et al., "Association between Clinically Recorded Alcohol Consumption and Initial Presentation of 12 Cardiovascular Diseases: Population Based Cohort Study Using Linked Health Records," *British Medical Journal* 356 (March 2017): j909.

37. Michaël Schwarzinger et al., "Contribution of Alcohol Use Disorders to the Burden of Dementia in France 2008–13: A Nationwide Retrospective Cohort Study," *The Lancet Public Health* 3, no. 3 (March 2018): e124–32.

38. Justin S. Sadhu et al., "Association of Alcohol Consumption after Development of Heart Failure with Survival among Older Adults in the Cardiovascular Health Study," *JAMA Network Open* 1, no. 8 (December 2018): e186383.

39. "Dietary Guidelines for Americans, 2020–2025," U.S. Department of Agriculture and U.S. Department of Health and Human Services, December 2020, https://www.dietaryguidelines.gov/resources/2020-2025 -dietary-guidelines-online-materials.

40. S. Jane Henley et al., "Alcohol Control Efforts in Comprehensive Cancer Control Plans and Alcohol Use among Adults in the United States,"

Alcohol and Alcoholism: International Journal of the Medical Council on Alcoholism 49, no. 6 (November 2014): 661–67.

41. Gemma Chiva-Blanch and Lina Badimon, "Benefits and Risks of Moderate Alcohol Consumption on Cardiovascular Disease: Current Findings and Controversies," *Nutrients* 12, no. 1 (January 2020): 108.

42. Tanya Chikritzhs, Kaye Fillmore, and Tim Stockwell, "A Healthy Dose of Skepticism: Four Good Reasons to Think Again about Protective Effects of Alcohol on Coronary Heart Disease," *Drug Alcohol Review* 28, no. 4 (July 2009): 441–44.

43. Craig S. Knott et al., "All Cause Mortality and the Case for Age Specific Alcohol Consumption Guidelines: Pooled Analyses of Up to 10 Population Based Cohorts," *British Medical Journal* 350 (February 2015): h384.

44. Marie K. Dam et al., "Five Year Change in Alcohol Intake and Risk of Breast Cancer and Coronary Heart Disease among Postmenopausal Women: Prospective Cohort Study," *British Medical Journal* 353 (May 2016): 12314.

45. Aleksandr Voskoboinik et al., "Moderate Alcohol Consumption Is Associated with Atrial Electrical and Structural Changes: Insights from High-Density Left Atrial Electroanatomic Mapping," *Heart Rhythm* 16, no. 2 (February 2019): 251–59.

46. Ibid.

47. Renata Micha et al., "Association between Dietary Factors and Mortality from Heart Disease, Stroke, and Type 2 Diabetes in the United States," *Journal of the American Medical Association* 317, no. 9 (March 2017): 912–24.

48. Marta Guasch-Ferré et al., "Nut Consumption and Risk of Cardiovascular Disease," *Journal of the American College of Cardiology* 70, no. 20 (November 2017): 2519–32.

49. "Nuts for Nuts? Daily Serving May Help Control Weight and Benefit Health," *ScienceDaily*, November 5, 2018, https://www.sciencedaily.com/releases/2018/11/181105081742.htm.\

50. Rajiv Chowdhury et al., "Association between Fish Consumption, Long Chain Omega 3 Fatty Acids, and Risk of Cerebrovascular Disease: Systematic Review and Meta-Analysis," *British Medical Journal* 345 (October 2012): e6698.

51. American Society for Nutrition, "Millions of Cardiovascular Deaths Attributed to Not Eating Enough Fruits and Vegetables," June 8, 2019, https://nutrition.org/millions-of-cardiovascular-deaths-attributed-to-not-eating-enough-fruits-and-vegetables/.

52. Huaidong Du et al., "Fresh Fruit Consumption and Major Cardiovascular Disease in China," *New England Journal of Medicine* 374, no. 14 (April 2016): 1332–43.

53. Huaidong Du et al., "Fresh Fruit Consumption in Relation to Incident Diabetes and Diabetic Vascular Complications: A 7-y Prospective Study of 0.5 Million Chinese Adults," *PLoS Medicine* 14, no. 4 (April 2017): e1002279.

54. Yikyung Park et al., "Dietary Fiber Intake and Mortality in the NIH-AARP Diet and Health Study," *Archives of Internal Medicine* 171, no. 12 (June 2011): 1061–68.

55. Andrew Reynolds et al., " Carbohydrate Quality and Human Health: A Series of Systematic Reviews and Meta-Analyses," *The Lancet* 393, no. 10170 (February 2019): 434–45.

56. Brian Buijsse et al., "Chocolate Consumption in Relation to Blood Pressure and Risk of Cardiovascular Disease in German Adults," *European Heart Journal* 31, no. 13 (2010): 1616–23. doi: 10.1093/eurheartj/ehq068.

57. Victor Zhong et al., "Associations of Processed Meat, Unprocessed Red Meat, Poultry, or Fish Intake with Incident Cardiovascular Disease and All-Cause Mortality," *JAMA Internal Medicine* 180, no. 4 (April 2020): 503–12.

58. Kathryn E. Bradbury, Neil Murphy, and Timothy J. Key, "Diet and Colorectal Cancer in UK Biobank: A Prospective Study," *International Journal of Epidemiology* 49, no. 1 (February 2020): 246–58.

59. Vasanti S. Malik and Frank B. Hu, "Fructose and Cardiometabolic Health: What the Evidence from Sugar-Sweetened Beverages Tells Us," *Journal of the American College of Cardiology* 66, no. 14 (October 2015): 1615–24.

60. Anthony Crimarco et al., "A Randomized Crossover Trial on the Effect of Plant-Based Compared with Animal-Based Meat on Trimethylamine-N-Oxide and Cardiovascular Disease Risk Factors in Generally Healthy Adults: Study with Appetizing Plantfood—Meat Eating Alternative Trial (SWAP-ME)," *The American Journal of Clinical Nutrition* 112, no. 5 (November 2020): 1188–99.

61. US Food & Drug Administration, "Quitting Smoking: Closer with Every Attempt," May 1, 2020, https://www.fda.gov/tobacco-products/health -information/quitting-smoking-closer-every-attempt#references.

62. U.S. Department of Health and Human Services, "The Health Consequences of Smoking—50 Years of Progress: A Report of the Surgeon General" (2014).

63. U.S. Department of Health and Human Services, "Surgeon General Releases First Report Focused on Smoking Cessation in 30 Years," January 23, 2020, https://www.hhs.gov/about/news/2020/01/23/surgeon -general-releases-first-report-focused-on-smoking-cessation-in-30-years .html.

64. Nicola Lindson-Hawley et al., "Gradual versus Abrupt Smoking Cessation: A Randomized, Controlled Noninferiority Trial," *Annals of Internal Medicine*, 164, no. 9 (May 2016): 585–92.

65. James A. K. Erskine, George J. Georgiou, and Lia Kvavilashvili, "I Suppress, Therefore I Smoke: Effects of Thought Suppression on Smoking Behavior," *Psychological Science* 21, no. 9 (September 2010): 1225–30.

66. Jamie Hartmann-Boyce et al., "Behavioural Interventions for Smoking Cessation: An Overview and Network Meta-Analysis," *Cochrane Database of Systematic Reviews* 1 (January 2021): CD013229.

67. Glenn N. Levine et al., "Sexual Activity and Cardiovascular Disease: A Scientific Statement from the American Heart Association," *Circulation* 125, no. 8 (February 2012): 1058–72.

68. Gali Cohen et al., "Resuming Sexual Activity after Acute Myocardial Infarction Enhances Long Term Survival," *European Journal of Preventive Cardiology* (September 2020).

69. Huang-Kuang Chen et al., "A Prospective Cohort Study on the Effect of Sexual Activity, Libido and Widowhood on Mortality among the Elderly People: 14-Year Follow-Up of 2453 Elderly Taiwanese," *International Journal of Epidemiology* 36, no. 5 (October 2007): 1136–42.

70. Cohen et al., "Resuming Sexual Activity after Acute Myocardial Infarction Enhances Long Term Survival."

71. Jennifer R. Rider et al., "Ejaculation Frequency and Risk of Prostate Cancer: Updated Results with an Additional Decade of Follow-up," *European Urology* 70, no. 6 (December 2016): 974–82.

72. Lia M. Jiannine, "An Investigation of the Relationship between Physical Fitness, Self-Concept, and Sexual Functioning," *Journal of Education and Health Promotion* 7, no. 57 (May 2018); Amelia M. Stanton, Ariel B. Handy, and Cindy M. Meston, "The Effects of Exercise on Sexual Function in Women," *Sexual Medicine Reviews* 6, no. 4 (October 2018): 548–57; Helle Gerbild et al., "Physical Activity to Improve Erectile Function: A Systematic Review of Intervention Studies," *Sexual Medicine* 6, no. 2 (June 2018): 75–89; Kilpatrick B. Fergus et al., "Exercise Improves Self-Reported Sexual Function among Physically Active Adults," *Journal of Sexual Medicine* 16, no. 8 (August 2019): 1236–45.

73. Kaori Sakurada et al., "Associations of Frequency of Laughter with Risk of All-Cause Mortality and Cardiovascular Disease Incidence in a General Population: Findings from the Yamagata Study," *Journal of Epidemiology* 30, no. 4 (April 2020): 188–93.

74. Seung Hee Lee-Kwan et al., "Disparities in State-Specific Adult Fruit and Vegetable Consumption—United States," *Morbidity and Mortality Weekly Report* 66, no. 45 (November 2017): 1241–47.

75. Sari Voutilainen et al., "Carotenoids and Cardiovascular Health," *American Journal of Clinical Nutrition* 83, no. 6 (June 2006): 1265–71; Paola Palozza et al., "Effect of Lycopene and Tomato Products on Cholesterol Metabolism," *Annals of Nutrition and Metabolism* 61, no. 2 (2012): 126–34; Ingrid Delbone Figueiredo et al., "Lycopene Improves the Metformin Effects on Glycemic Control and Decreases Biomarkers of Glycoxidative Stress in Diabetic Rats," *Diabetes, Metabolic Syndrome and Obesity: Targets and Therapy* 13 (September 2020): 3117–35.

76. Jouni Karppi et al., "Serum Lycopene Decreases the Risk of Stroke in Men: A Population-Based Follow-Up Study," *Neurology* 79, no. 15 (October 2012): 1540–47.

77. Elizabeth E. Devore et al., "Dietary Intakes of Berries and Flavonoids in Relation to Cognitive Decline," *Annals of Neurology* 72, no. 1 (July 2012): 135–43.

78. Huaidong Du et al., "Fresh Fruit Consumption and Major Cardiovascular Disease in China," *New England Journal of Medicine* 374, no. 14 (April 2016): 1332–43.
79. Dong D. Wang et al., "Fruit and Vegetable Intake and Mortality: Results from 2 Prospective Cohort Studies of US Men and Women and a Meta-Analysis of 26 Cohort Studies," *Circulation* 143, no. 17 (April 2021): 1642–54.
80. Hsin-Chia Hung et al., "Fruit and Vegetable Intake and Risk of Major Chronic Disease," *Journal of the National Cancer Institute* 96, no. 21 (November 2004): 1577–84.
81. Tomoyo Yamada et al., "Frequency of Citrus Fruit Intake Is Associated with the Incidence of Cardiovascular Disease: The Jichi Medical School Cohort Study," *Journal of Epidemiology* 21, no. 3 (March 2011): 169–75; Hsin-Chia Hung et al., "Fruit and Vegetable Intake and Risk of Major Chronic Disease," *Journal of the National Cancer Institute* 96, no. 21 (November 2004): 1577–84.
82. Edward G. Miller et al., "Further Studies on the Anticancer Activity of Citrus Limonoids," *Journal of Agricultural and Food Chemistry* 52, no. 15 (July 2004): 4908–12.
83. Satya P. Sharma et al., "Paradoxical Effects of Fruit on Obesity," *Nutrients* 8, no. 10 (October 2016), 633.

Chapter 14: Are You Getting the Right Medications and Supplements, at the Right Dose?

1. Agneta Akesson et al., "Low-Risk Diet and Lifestyle Habits in the Primary Prevention of Myocardial Infarction in Men: A Population-Based Prospective Cohort Study," *Journal of the American College of Cardiology* 64, no. 13 (September 2014): 1299–1306; Dariush Mozaffarian, "The Promise of Lifestyle for Cardiovascular Health: Time for Implementation," *Journal of the American College of Cardiology* 64, no. 13 (September 2014): 1307–9.
2. Centers for Disease Control and Prevention, "Prediabetes: Your Chance to Prevent Type 2 Diabetes," June 11, 2020, https://www.cdc.gov/diabetes/basics/prediabetes.html.
3. Ibid.
4. Stephen D. Fihn, "ACCF/AHA/ACP/AATS/PCNA/SCAI/STS Guideline for the Diagnosis and Management of Patients with Stable Ischemic Heart Disease: Executive Summary: A Report of the American College of Cardiology Foundation/American Heart Association Task Force on Practice Guidelines, and the American College of Physicians, American Association for Thoracic Surgery, Preventive Cardiovascular Nurses Association, Society for Cardiovascular Angiography and Interventions, and Society of Thoracic Surgeons," *Circulation* 126, no. 25 (December 2012): 3097–137.

5. William E. Boden and Bernard J. Gersh, "Defining the Proper SYNTAX for Long-Term Benefit of Myocardial Revascularization with Optimal Medical Therapy," *Journal of the American College of Cardiology* 78, no. 1 (July 2021): 39–41.

6. Hideyuki Kawashima et al., "Impact of Optimal Medical Therapy on 10-Year Mortality after Coronary Revascularization," *Journal of the American College of Cardiology* 78, no. 1 (July 2021): 27–38.

7. Akesson et al., "Low-Risk Diet and Lifestyle Habits in the Primary Prevention of Myocardial Infarction in Men"; Mozaffarian, "The Promise of Lifestyle for Cardiovascular Health"; Paula Chu et al., "Comparative Effectiveness of Personalized Lifestyle Management Strategies for Cardiovascular Disease Risk Reduction," *Journal of the American Heart Association* 5, no. 3 (March 2016): e002737.

8. Olivier Milleron et al., "Benefits of Obstructive Sleep Apnoea Treatment in Coronary Artery Disease: A Long-Term Follow-Up Study," *European Heart Journal* 25, no. 9 (May 2004): 728–34.

9. Emmi Tikkanen, Stefan Gustafsson, and Erik Ingelsson, "Associations of Fitness, Physical Activity, Strength, and Genetic Risk with Cardiovascular Disease: Longitudinal Analyses in the UK Biobank Study, *Circulation* 137, no. 24 (June 2018): 2583–91; Jose M. Marin et al., "Long-Term Cardiovascular Outcomes in Men with Obstructive Sleep Apnoea-Hypopnoea with or without Treatment with Continuous Positive Airway Pressure: An Observational Study," *Lancet* 365, no. 9464 (March 2005): 1046–53.

10. Hanmin Wang et al., "Vitamin D and Chronic Diseases," *Aging and Disease* 8, no. 3 (May 2017): 346–53; Erika Rimondi et al., "Role of Vitamin D in the Pathogenesis of Atheromatosis," *Nutrition, Metabolism & Cardiovascular Diseases* 31, no. 1 (January 2021): 344–353.

11. Carl J. Lavie et al., "Vitamin D and Cardiovascular Disease? Will It Live Up to Its Hype?" *Journal of American College of Cardiology* 58, no. 15 (October 2011): 1547–56; Michael F. Holic, "Vitamin D Deficiency," *New England Journal of Medicine* 357, no. 3 (July 2007): 266–81; Tara Dall and Joan Anderson, "Vitamin D: Merging Research into a Clinical Lipid Practice," *The Lipid Spin* 6, no. 3 (2008): 4–8.

12. Muhammad Amer and Rehan Qayyum, "Relation between Serum-25 Hydroxyvitamin D and C-Reactive Protein in Asymptomatic Adults (from the Continuous National Health and Nutrition Examination Survey 2001 to 2006)," *American Journal of Cardiology* 109, no. 2 (January 2012): 226–30, doi: 10.1016/j.amjcard.2011.08.032;

Epub P. Barton Duell and William E. Connor, "Vitamin D Deficiency Is Associated with Myalgias in Hyperlipidemic Subjects Taking Statins," Presentation 3701, American Heart Association Scientific Sessions, November 12, 2008; Waqas Ahmed et al., "Low Serum 25 (OH) Vitamin D Levels (<32ng/mL) Are Associated with Reversible Myositis-Myalgia in Statin-Treated Patients," *Translational Research: The Journal of Laboratory and Clinical Medicine* 153, no. 1 (January 2009): 11-6; Thomas J.

Littlejohns et al., "Vitamin D and the Risk of Dementia and Alzheimer Disease," *Neurology* 83, no. 10 (September 2014): 920–28; Mahtab Niroomand et al., "Does High-Dose Vitamin D Supplementation Impact Insulin Resistance and Risk of Development of Diabetes in Patients with Pre-Diabetes? A Double-Blind Randomized Clinical Trial," *Diabetes Research Clinical Practice* 148 (February 2019): 1–9.

13. Niroomand et al., "Does High-Dose Vitamin D Supplementation Impact Insulin Resistance and Risk of Development of Diabetes in Patients with Pre-Diabetes?"

14. Ammar W. Ashor et al., "Limited Evidence for a Beneficial Effect of Vitamin C Supplementation on Biomarkers of Cardiovascular Diseases: An Umbrella Review of Systematic Reviews and Meta-Analysis," *Nutrition Research* 61 (January 2019): 1–12.

15. Zhi-Hao Li et al., "Associations of Habitual Fish Oil Supplementation with Cardiovascular Outcomes and All Cause Mortality: Evidence from a Large Population Based Cohort Study," *British Medical Journal* 368 (March 2020): m456.

16. Aldo A. Bernasconi et al., "Effect of Omega 3 Dosage on Cardiovascular Outcomes: An Updated Meta-Analysis," *Mayo Clinic Proceedings* 96, no. 2 (February 2021): 304–13.

17. Hua Qu et al., "Effects of Coenzyme Q-10 on Statin-Induced Myopathy: An Updated Meta-Analysis of Randomized Controlled Trials," *Journal of the American Heart Association* 7, no. 19 (October 2018): e009835.

18. Hong-Mei Yan et al., "Efficacy of Berberine in Patients with Non-Alcoholic Fatty Liver Disease," *PLoS ONE* 10, no. 8 (August 2015): e0134172.

19. Robert W. Allen et al., "Cinnamon Use in Type 2 Diabetes: An Updated Systematic Review and Meta-Analysis," *Annals of Family Medicine* 11, no. 5 (September–October 2013): 452–59.

20. Giulio R. Romeo et al., "Influence of Cinnamon on Glycemic Control in Subjects with Prediabetes: A Randomized Controlled Trial," *Journal of the Endocrine Society* 4, no. 11 (July 2020).

21. Dawn Connelly, "A History of Aspirin," *The Pharmaceutical Journal*, September 26, 2014, https://pharmaceutical-journal.com/article/infographics/a-history-of-aspirin.

22. Jolanta M. Siller-Matula, "Hemorrhagic Complications Associated with Aspirin: An Underestimated Hazard in Clinical Practice," *Journal of the American Medical Association* 307, no. 21 (June 2012): 2318–20.

23. Philip B. Gorelick and Steven M. Weisman, "Risk of Hemorrhagic Stroke with Aspirin Use: An Update," *Stroke* 36, no. 8 (August 2005): 18017; Antithrombotic Trialists' (ATT) Collaboration, "Aspirin in the Primary and Secondary Prevention of Vascular Disease: Collaborative Meta-Analysis of Individual Participant Data from Randomized Trials," *The Lancet* 373, no. 9678 (May 2009): 1849–60.

24. Paola Patrignani and Carlo Patrono, "Aspirin and Cancer," *Journal of the American College of Cardiology* 68, no. 9 (August 2016): 967–76.

25. Silke Kern et al., "Does Low-Dose Acetylsalicylic Acid Prevent Cognitive Decline in Women with High Cardiovascular Risk? A 5-year Follow-Up of a Non-Demented Population-Based Cohort of Swedish Elderly Women," *BMJ Open* 2, no. 5 (October 2012): e001288; Hui Li et al., "Aspirin Use on Incident Dementia and Mild Cognitive Decline: A Systemic Review and Meta-Analysis," *Frontiers in Aging Neuroscience* 12 (February 2021): 578071.

26. Jillian T. Henderson et al., "Low Dose Aspirin for Prevention of Morbidity and Mortality from Preeclampsia: A Systematic Evidence Review from the U.S. Preventive Services Task Force," *Annals of Internal Medicine* 160, no. 10 (May 2014): 695–703.

27. U.S. Preventive Services Task Force, "Final Recommendation Statement: Aspirin Use to Prevent Cardiovascular Disease and Colorectal Cancer: Preventive Medication," April 11, 2016, https://www.uspreventiveservices taskforce.org/uspstf/document/RecommendationStatementFinal/aspirin -to-prevent-cardiovascular-disease-and-cancer.

28. Dylan R. Collins et al., "Global Cardiovascular Risk Assessment in the Primary Prevention of Cardiovascular Disease in Adults: Systematic Review of Systematic Reviews," *BMJ Open* 7, no. 3 (March 2017): e013650.

29. Rachel S. Eidelman et al., "An Update on Aspirin in the Primary Prevention of Cardiovascular Disease," *Archives of Internal Medicine* 163, no. 17 (September 2003): 2006–10.

30. John J. McNeil et al., "Effect of Aspirin on Cardiovascular Events and Bleeding in the Healthy Elderly," *New England Journal of Medicine* 379, no. 16 (September 2018): 1509–18.

31. Armen Yuri Gasparyan, Timothy Watson, and Gregory Y. H. Lip, "The Role of Aspirin in Cardiovascular Prevention: Implications of Aspirin Resistance," *Journal of the American College of Cardiology* 51, no. 19 (May 2008): 1829–43.

32. George Krasopoulos et al., "Aspirin "Resistance and Risk of Cardiovascular Morbidity: A Systematic Review and Meta-Analysis," *British Medical Journal* 336, no. 7637 (January 2008): 195–98.

33. Nicholas J. Leeper et al., "Statin Use in Patients with Extremely Low Low-Density Lipoprotein Levels Is Associated with Improved Survival," *Circulation* 116, no. 6 (August 2007): 613–18.

34. Paul M. Ridker et al., "Rosuvastatin to Prevent Vascular Events in Men and Women with Elevated C-Reactive Protein," *New England Journal of Medicine* 359, no. 21 (November 2008): 2195–207.

35. M. R. Law, N. J. Wald, and A. R. Rudnicka, "Quantifying Effect of Statins on Low Density Lipoprotein Cholesterol, Ischaemic Heart Disease, and Stroke: Systematic Review and Meta-Analysis," *British Medical Journal* 326, no. 7404 (June 2003): 1423.

36. Harvey D. White et al., "Changes in Lipoprotein-Associated Phospholipase A2 Activity Predict Coronary Events and Partly Account for the Treatment Effect of Pravastatin: Results from the Long-Term Intervention with Pravastatin in Ischemic Disease Study," *Journal of the American Heart Association* 2, no. 5 (October 2013): e000360; Parmanand Singh et al.,

"Coronary Plaque Morphology and the Anti-Inflammatory Impact of Atorvastatin: A Multicenter 18F-Fluorodeoxyglucose Positron Emission Tomographic/Computed Tomographic Study," *Circulation Cardiovascular Imaging* 9, no. 12 (December 2016): e004195.

37. Caroline A. Garza et al., "Association between Lipoprotein-Associated Phospholipase A2 and Cardiovascular Disease: A Systematic Review," *Mayo Clinic Proceedings* 82, no. 2 (February 2007): 159–65; Alexander Thompson et al., "Lipoprotein-Associated Phospholipase A(2) and Risk of Coronary Disease, Stroke, and Mortality: Collaborative Analysis of 32 Prospective Studies," *The Lancet* 375, no. 9725 (May 2010): 1536–44.

38. Harvey D. White et al., "Changes in Lipoprotein-Associated Phospholipase A2 Activity Predict Coronary Events and Partly Account for the Treatment Effect of Pravastatin: Results from the Long-Term Intervention with Pravastatin in Ischemic Disease Study," *Journal of the American Heart Association* 2, no. 5 (September 2013): e000360.

39. Pasquale Pignatelli et al., "Immediate Antioxidant and Antiplatelet Effect of Atorvastatin via Inhibition of Nox2," *Circulation* 126, no. 1 (July 2012): 92–103.

40. R. S. Rosenson and C. C. Tangney, "Antiatherothrombotic Properties of Statins: Implications of Cardiovascular Event Reduction," *Journal of the American Medical Association* 279, no. 20 (May 1998): 1643–50; Antonio M. Gotto Jr. and John A. Farmer, "Pleiotropic Effects of Statins: Do They Matter?" *Current Opinion in Lipidology* 12, no. 4 (August 2001): 391–94; David J. Maron, Sergio Fazio, and MacRae F. Linton, "Current Perspectives on Statins," *Circulation* 101, no. 2 (January 2000): 207–21; C. Michael White, "Pharmacological Effects of HMG CoA Inhibitors Other Than Lipoprotein Modulation," *Journal of Clinical Pharmacology* 39, no. 2 (February 1999): 111–18.

41. Sharath Subramanian et al., "High-Dose Atorvastatin Reduces Periodontal Inflammation: A Novel Pleiotropic Effect of Statins," *Journal of the American College of Cardiology* 62, no. 25 (December 2013): 2382–91.

42. Peter Meisel et al., "Statins and Tooth Loss," *Journal of Periodontology* 85, no. 6 (June 2014): e160–68.

43. C. Cramer et al., "Use of Statins and Incidence of Dementia and Cognitive Impairment without Dementia in a Cohort Study," *Neurology* 71, no. 5 (July 2008): 344–50.

44. Julie M. Zissimopoulos et al., "Sex and Race Differences in the Association between Statin Use and the Incidence of Alzheimer Disease," *JAMA Neurology* 74, no. 2 (February 2017): 225–32.

45. Kwang Kon Koh et al., "Atorvastatin Causes Insulin Resistance and Increases Ambient Glycemia in Hypercholesterolemic Patients," *Journal of the American College of Cardiology* 55, no. 12 (March 2010): 1209–16.

46. Peter S. Sever et al., "Prevention of Coronary and Stroke Events Atorvastatin in Hypertensive Patients Who Have Average or Lower-Than-Average Cholesterol Concentration in the Anglo-Scandanavian

Cardiac Outcomes Trial—Lipid Lowering Arm (ASCOT-LLA): A Multicentre Randomised Controlled Trial," *The Lancet* 361, no. 934 (April 2003): 1149–58

47. Samia Mora et al., "Statins for the Primary Prevention of Cardiovascular Events in Women with Elevated High-Sensitivity C-Reactive Protein or Dyslipidemia: Results from the Justification for the Use of Statins in Prevention: An Intervention Trial Evaluating Rosuvastatin (JUPITER) and Meta-Analysis of Women from Primary Prevention Trials," *Circulation* 121, no. 9 (March 2010): 1069–77.

48. Olga Iakoubova et al., "Association of the Trp719Arg Polymorphism in Kinesin-Like Protein 6 with Myocardial Infarction and Coronary Heart Disease in 2 Prospective Trials: The CARE and WOSCOPS Trials," *Journal of the American College of Cardiology* 51, no. 4 (January 2008): 435–43; Dov Shiffman et al., "Effect of Pravastatin Therapy on Coronary Events in Carriers of the KIF6 719Arg Allele from the Cholesterol and Recurrent Events Trial," *American Journal of Cardiology* 105, no. 9 (May 2010): 1300–1305.

49. Donna K. Arnett et al., "ACC/AHA Guideline on the Primary Prevention of Cardiovascular Disease: A Report of the American College of Cardiology/American Heart Association Task Force on Clinical Practice Guidelines," *Circulation* 140, no. 11 (September 2019): e596–646;

50. Peter W. F. Wilson et al., "Systematic review for the 2018 AHA/ACC/ AACVPR/AAPA/ABC/ACPM/ADA/AGS/APhA/ASPC/NLA/PCNA Guideline on the Management of Blood Cholesterol: A Report of the American College of Cardiology/American Heart Association Task Force on Clinical Practice Guidelines," *Journal of the American College of Cardiology* 73, no. 24 (June 2019): 3210–27.

51. Connie B. Newman et al., "Statin Safety and Associated Adverse Events: A Scientific Statement from the American Heart Association," *Arteriosclerosis Thrombosis and Vascular Biology* 39, no. 2 (February 2019): e38–81.

52. NIA Press Team, "Could Taking Statins Prevent Dementia, Disability?" National Institute on Aging, October 23, 2019, https://www.nia.nih.gov /news/could-taking-statins-prevent-dementia-disability.

53. Sasa Vukelic and Kathy K. Griendling, "Angiotensin II, from Vaso-constrictor to Growth Factor: A Paradigm Shift," *Circulation Research* 114, no. 5 (February 2014): 754–57.

54. Vincenza Snow et al., "Primary Care Management of Chronic Stable Angina or Asymptomatic or Known Coronary Artery Disease: A Clinical Practice Guideline from the American College of Physicians," *Annals of Internal Medicine* 141, no. 7 (October 2004): 562–67.

55. The SPRINT Research Group, "A Randomized Trial of Intensive versus Standardized Blood-Pressure Control," *New England Journal of Medicine* 373 (November 2015): 2103–16.

56. Louise Pilote et al., "Mortality Rates in Elderly Patients Who Take Dif-ferent Angiotensin-Converting Enzyme Inhibitors after Acute Myocardial

Infarction: A Class Effect? *Annals of Internal Medicine* 141, no. 2 (July 2004): 102–12.

57. Jackie Bosch et al., "Long-Term Effects of Ramipril on Cardiovascular Events and on Diabetes: Results of the HOPE Study Extension," *Circulation* 112, no. 9 (August 2005): 1339–46.

58. Jun Cheng et al., "Effect of Angiotensin-Converting Enzyme Inhibitors and Angiotensin II Receptor Blockers on All-Cause Mortality, Cardiovascular Death, and Cardiovascular Events in Patients with Diabetes Mellitus: A Meta-Analysis," *JAMA Internal Medicine* 174, no. 5 (May 2014): 773–85.

59. Fabrizio deOliveira et al., "Pharmacogenetics of Angiotensin-Converting Enzyme Inhibitors in Patients with Alzheimer's Disease Dementia," *Current Alzheimer Research* 15, no. 4 (February 2018): 386–98.

60. Sripal Bangalore et al., "Angiotensin Receptor Blockers and Risk of Myocardial Infarction: Meta-Analyses and Trial Sequential Analyses of 147 020 Patients from Randomized Trials," *British Medical Journal* 342 (April 2011): d2234.

61. John J. V. McMurray, "Systolic Heart Failure," *New England Journal of Medicine* 362 (January 2010): 228–38.

62. Jun Cheng et al., "Effect of Angiotensin-Converting Enzyme Inhibtors and Angiotensin II Receptor Blockers on All-Cause Mortality, Cardiovascular Death, and Cardiovascular Events in Patients with Diabetes Mellitus: A Meta-Analysis," *JAMA Internal Medicine* 174, no. 5 (May 2014): 773–85.

63. Tony Antoniou et al., "Trimethoprim-Sulfamethoxazole-Induced Hyperkalemia in Patients Receiving Inhibitors of the Renin-Angiotensin System: A Population-Based Study," *Archives of Internal Medicine* 170, no. 12 (June 2010): 1045–49.

64. Hui Wen Sim et al., "Beta-Blockers and Renin-Angiotensin System Inhibitors in Acute Myocardial Infarction Managed with Inhospital Coronary Revascularization," *Scientific Reports* 10, no. 1 (September 2020): 15184.

65. Yuesong Pan et al., "Outcomes Associated with Clopidogrel-Aspirin Use in Minor Stroke or Transient Ischemic Attack: A Pooled Analysis of Clopidogrel in High-Risk Patients with Acute Non-Disabling Cerebrovascular Events (CHANCE) and Platelet-Oriented Inhibition in New TIA and Minor Ischemic Stroke (POINT) Trials," *JAMA Neurology* 76, no. 12 (December 2019): 1466–73.

66. Islam Osman and Laksham Segar, "Pioglitazone, a PPARγ Agonist, Attenuates PDGF-Induced Vascular Smooth Muscle Cell Proliferation through AMPK-Dependent and AMPK-Independent Inhibition of mTOR/p70S6K and ERK Signaling," *Biochemical Pharmacology* 101 (February 2016): 54–70; Santiago Redondo et al., "Pioglitazone Induces Vascular Smooth Muscle Cell Apoptosis through a Peroxisome Proliferator-Activated Receptor-γ, Transforming Growth Factor-β1, and a Smad2-Dependent Mechanism," *Diabetes* 54, no. 3 (March 2005): 811–17; Paul M. Vanhoutte, "Endothelial Dysfunction: The First Step toward Coronary Arteriosclerosis," *Circulation Journal* 73, no. 4 (April 2009): 595–601; Akisuki Morikawa et al., "Pioglitazone Reduces Urinary Albumin Excretion in Renin-Angiotensin

System Inhibitor-Treated Type 2 Diabetic Patients with Hypertension and Microalbuminuria: The APRIME Study," *Clinical and Experimental Nephrology* 15, no. 6 (December 2011): 848–53; Mandy Bloch et al., "High-Mobility Group A1 Protein: A New Coregulator of Peroxisome Proliferator-Activated Receptor-Gamma-Mediated Transrepression in the Vasculature," *Circulation Research* 110 no. 3 (February 2012): 394–405; Markolf Hanefeld, "The Role of Pioglitazone in Modifying the Atherogenic Lipoprotein Profile," *Diabetes, Obesity and Metabolism* 11, no. 8 (June 2009): 742–56; Theodore Mazzone et al., "Effect of Pioglitazone Compared with Glimepiride on Carotid Intima-Media Thickness in Type 2 Diabetes: A Randomized Trial," *Journal of the American Medical Association* 296, no. 21 (December 2006): 2572–81; Peter D. Reaven et al., "Pioglitazone Reduces Long-Term Progression of Carotid Atherosclerosis in IGT," Presentation, American Diabetes Association 2009 Scientific Sessions, June 7, 2009, New Orleans, LA.

67. Steven E. Nissen et al., "Comparison of Pioglitazone vs Glimepiride on Progression of Coronary Atherosclerosis in Patients with Type 2 Diabetes: The Periscope Randomized Controlled Trial," *Journal of the American Medical Association* 299, no. 13 (April 2008): 1561–73.

68. Helen Strongman et al., "Pioglitazone and Cause-Specific Risk of Mortality in Patients with Type 2 Diabetes: Extended Analysis from a European Multidatabase Cohort Study," *BMJ Open Diabetes Research & Care* 5, no. 1 (May 2017): e000364.

69. Lawrence H. Young et al., "Cardiac Outcomes after Ischemic Stroke or TIA: Effects of Pioglitazone in Patients with Insulin Resistance with Diabetes," *Circulation* 135, no. 20 (May 2017): 1882–93.

Chapter 15: Achieving Optimal Arterial Wellness

1. Centers for Disease Control and Prevention, "Underlying Cause of Death, 1999–2018," CDC Wonder online database, http://wonder.cdc.gov/ucd-icd10.html.

2. H. C. Kung and J. Q. Xu, "Hypertension-Related Mortality in the United States, 2000–2013," NCHS Data Brief, No. 193 (Hyattsville, MD: National Center for Health Statistics, 2015).

3. P. K. Whelton et al., "ACC/AHA/AAPA/ABC/ACPM/AGS/APhA/ASH/ASPC/NMA/PCNA Guideline for the Prevention, Detection, Evaluation, and Management of High Blood Pressure in Adults: Executive Summary: A Report of the American College of Cardiology/American Heart Association Task Force on Clinical Practice Guidelines," *Hypertension* 71, no. 6 (2018): 1269–1324.

4. S. J. Taler, "Initial Treatment of Hypertension," *N Engl J Med* 2018, no. 378 (2018): 636–44.

5. Centers for Disease Control and Prevention (CDC), *Hypertension Cascade: Hypertension Prevalence, Treatment and Control Estimates among US Adults Aged 18 Years and Older Applying the Criteria from the American College of*

*Cardiology and American Heart Association's 2017 Hypertension Guideline —
NHANES 2013–2016* (Atlanta, GA: US Department of Health and
Human Services, 2019).

6. C. Lane et al., "Associations Between Blood Pressure Across Adulthood
    and Late-Life Brain Structure and Pathology in the Neuroscience
    Substudy of the 1946 British Birth Cohort: An Epidemiological Study,"
    The Lancet Neurology 19 (August 2019) Oct;18(10):942-952. doi: 10.1016/
    S1474-4422(19)30228-5. Epub 2019 Aug 20. Erratum in: Lancet Neurol.
    2020 Jul;19(7):e6. PMID: 31444142; PMCID: PMC6744368.

7. B. Bale, "Optimizing Hypertension Management in Underserved Rural
    Populations," *J Natl Med Assoc* 102, no. 1 (January 2010): 102(1):10-7. doi:
    10.1016/s0027-9684(15)30470-3. PMID: 20158131.

8. Centers for Disease Control and Prevention, "Prediabetes: Your Chance
    to Prevent Type 2 Diabetes," June 11, 2020, https://www.cdc.gov
    /diabetes/basics/prediabetes.html.

9. J. Benjamin Emelia et al., American Heart Association Council on
    Epidemiology and Prevention Statistics Committee and Stroke Statistics
    Subcommittee. Heart Disease and Stroke Statistics-2019 Update: A
    Report From the American Heart Association. Circulation. 2019 Mar
    5;139(10):e56-e528. doi: 10.1161/CIR.0000000000000659. Erratum in:
    Circulation. 2020 Jan 14;141(2):e33. PMID: 30700139.

10. American Heart Association, "Heart-Health Screenings," https://www
    .heart.org/en/health-topics/consumer-healthcare/what-is
    -cardiovascular-disease/heart-health-screenings.

11. K. Kario et al., "Morning Home Blood Pressure Is a Strong Predictor of
    Coronary Artery Disease: The HONEST Study," *J Am Coll Cardiol, 67,* no.
    13 (2016), 1519–27.

12. E. Casiglia et al., "Poor Reliability of Wrist Blood Pressure Self-
    Measurement at Home: A Population-Based Study," *Hypertension* 68, no.
    4 (2016): 896–903.

13. A. Tsimploulis et al., "Systolic BP and Outcomes in Patients with HFpEF,"
    JAMA Cardiology, February 14, 2018, http://207.231.204.201/internal
    medicine/clinical-edge/summary/cardiology/systolic-bp-and
    -outcomes-patients-hfpef?group_type=week.

14. I Betti et al., "The PROBE-HF Study," *J Cardiac Fail* 15 (June 2009):
    377–84.

15. O. Melander et al., "Novel and conventional biomarkers for prediction of
    incident cardiovascular events in the community.," *Journal of the American
    Medical Association,* 302, no. 1, 2009 Jul 1;302(1):49-57. doi: 10.1001/
    jama.2009.943. PMID: 19567439; PMCID: PMC3090639.

16. M. Ostovanch et al., "Change in NT-ProBNP Level and Risk of Dementia
    in Multi-Ethnic Study of Atherosclerosis (MESA)," *Hypertension* 75
    (2020): 316–23

17. Betti et al., "The PROBE-HF Study."

INDEX